Medicine & Society
In America

Medicine & Society
In America

Advisory Editor

Charles E. Rosenberg
Professor of History
University of Pennsylvania

A

HISTORY

OF THE

MASSACHUSETTS

GENERAL HOSPITAL

[To August 5, 1851.]

By N. I. BOWDITCH

ARNO PRESS & THE NEW YORK TIMES
New York   1972

Reprint Edition 1972 by Arno Press Inc.

Reprinted from a copy in
The Library of The College of
Physicians of Philadelphia

LC# 74-180558
ISBN 0-405-03938-7

Medicine and Society in America
ISBN for complete set: 0-405-03930-1
See last pages of this volume for titles.

Manufactured in the United States of America

HISTORY

OF THE

MASSACHUSETTS GENERAL HOSPITAL.

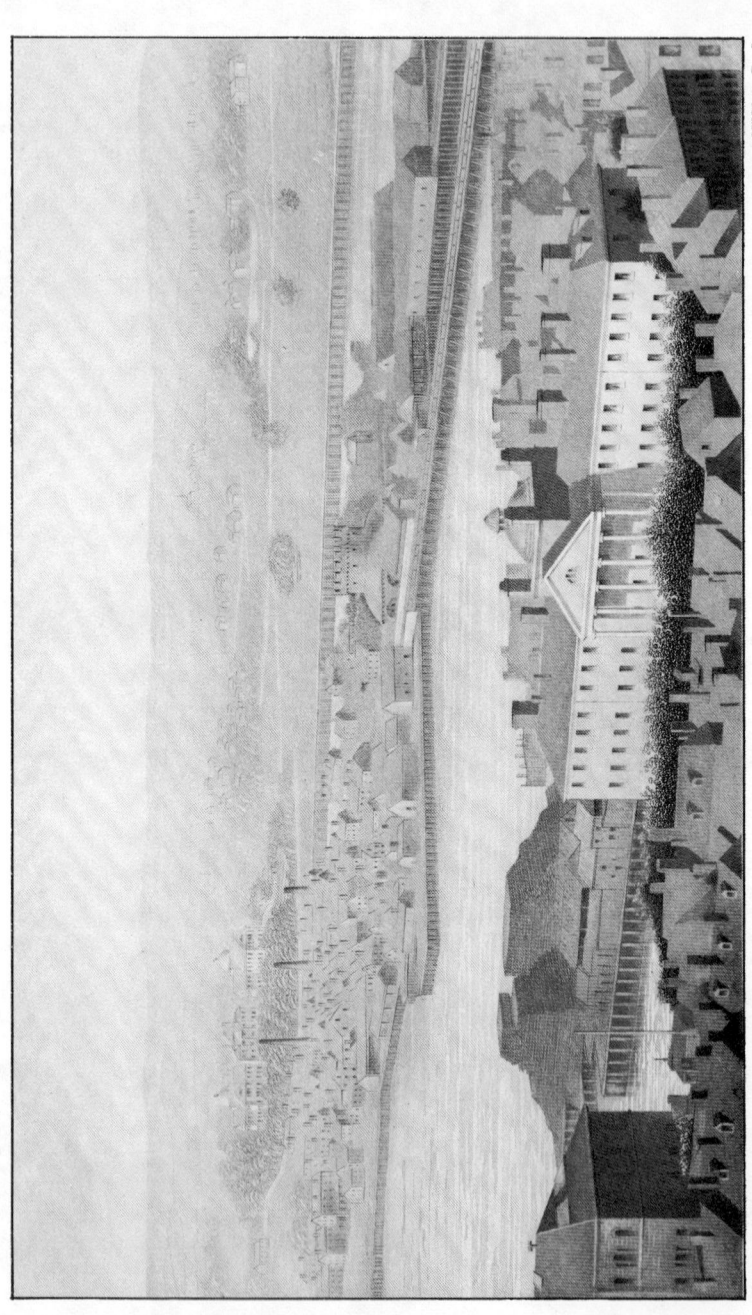

Dagᵗ of Southworth. J.W. Watts Engʳ.

The Massachusetts General Hospital.

A

HISTORY

OF THE

MASSACHUSETTS

GENERAL HOSPITAL.

[To August 5, 1851.]

By N. I. BOWDITCH.

"Drink . weary . pilgrim . drink . and . pray .
For . the . kind . soul . of . Sybil . Grey .
Who . built . this . cross . and . well . "
SCOTT'S MARMION.

[Privately Printed in 1851.]

Second Edition, with a Continuation to 1872.

Prepared by Request, in a Vote of the Trustees, chiefly from the Records and Annual Reports.

BOSTON:
PRINTED BY THE TRUSTEES FROM THE BOWDITCH FUND.
1872.

Entered according to Act of Congress, in the year 1872, by
THE MASSACHUSETTS GENERAL HOSPITAL,
In the Office of the Librarian of Congress, at Washington.

CAMBRIDGE:
PRESS OF JOHN WILSON AND SON.

PREFATORY NOTE TO THIS EDITION,

BY THE EDITOR.

THE following is an extract from the will of the late NATHANIEL I. BOWDITCH : —

"In 1851 I published for private distribution, at the cost of eleven hundred dollars, a History of the Massachusetts General Hospital. I now give to that Corporation the copyright of said work and the plates prepared for it in the frontispiece and the likeness of Dr. James Jackson. Also, the sum of two thousand dollars, to be put at interest till another edition shall be deemed desirable by the Trustees, when said sum, with its accumulations, or such part thereof as may be needed, shall be appropriated to that object. A volume of the proof-sheets of this work is in my possession, containing various manuscript additions and corrections made by me, which I should wish to have incorporated in any new edition.

"It would gratify me to have my friend and classmate, Edward Wigglesworth, superintend the printing of any such new edition."

Mr. BOWDITCH's History was highly valued by the friends and institutions on whom he bestowed copies, and it had an especial interest for professional men and for those engaged in the care and administration of Hospitals. It had become difficult for many who much desired it to obtain possession of the work. The Trustees were therefore concerned to procure its reproduction. Mr. EDWARD WIGGLESWORTH declined to undertake its editorship.

PREFATORY NOTE.

At a meeting of the Trustees of the Hospital, on Nov. 17, 1871, the following vote was passed: —

"*Voted*, That our associate, Dr. George E. Ellis, be appointed Editor of the proposed new edition of Mr. Bowditch's History of the Hospital, with a continuation by himself to this time; with full power to make such additions as he deems advisable, while conforming to the terms of Mr. Bowditch's will, and to contract for the printing of the same."

In executing the trust thus committed to him, the Editor has had in his hands Mr. BOWDITCH's private copy of his book, with all the changes in text and margin which he desired to be introduced in a new edition. These have been made with an attempt at strict carefulness in the following pages. In all other respects the volume is an exact and literal reproduction of Mr. BOWDITCH's work.

Under the proper date in the Continuation of the History, requested by his associates in the government of the Hospital, the Editor has sought to pay an appropriate tribute to the Author, his own much esteemed friend.

The aim has been to construct that Continuation after the plan of the original work. There are some entries on the Hospital records, which, being of a strictly private or personal nature, are not set forth in print. When next after a like interval of years a third edition of this History may be produced, it may be considered desirable to arrange its contents in two volumes. The present Editor thought it preferable to include the contents thus far within a single pair of covers, though the book may be a bulky one.

The Treasurer in his last report credits the Bowditch History Fund, with its accretions, at $5,561.91.

G. E. E.

BOSTON, July, 1872.

PREFACE,

[By Mr. Bowditch.]

The Massachusetts General Hospital — with its two departments, the Hospital for the sick in Allen Street and the Asylum for the Insane in Somerville — is one of the largest and most important of the charitable institutions of this Commonwealth. Superintended by officers faithful to their trust, it has ever, in a high degree, enjoyed the confidence of the community, and been the object of public and private munificence. A brief history of this Institution, — of its small beginnings, its early difficulties, and its ultimate success, — an account of what has been done for it, and of what it has itself done in return, — will perhaps, to its friends and benefactors at least, prove not wholly devoid of interest. I have been personally connected with it, in the offices of Secretary and Trustee, for twenty-five years; and my father-in-law, Ebenezer Francis, Esq., was one of its earliest and most active Managers. Our joint recollection extends back through the whole period of its existence. The materials for such a history were thus, to a considerable extent, either already possessed by me or placed easily within my reach. Their selection and arrangement have been " a labor of love."

The frontispiece* is an engraving on steel, representing a section of the panorama of Boston and its vicinity, taken by means of a daguerreotype from the top of the State House. In the foreground appears the Hospital; at the left corner is part

---

* [This frontispiece is retained, though the erection of new buildings, the filling up of flats, the extension of the Hospital grounds, and many changes in the landscape, give the view an historical interest, rather than present it as a representation of what now is.]

of the Medical College, the scene of a late fearful tragedy; and, in the background beyond the river, the hill is crowned by the Asylum, a peaceful retreat, standing forth from amid the foliage and shrubbery by which it is sheltered and secluded. I have been permitted by the Trustees to use a separate engraving of the Asylum, which has for several years belonged to the Corporation. The likeness of Dr. JAMES JACKSON was also executed for this publication from a daguerreotype, of which it is a very accurate copy, though the happiest expression has not been secured. The engraving of Dr. WARREN is from an existing plate, which he kindly placed at my disposal. After the volume was in the press, I learned, for the first time, that my friend and co-trustee, GEORGE M. DEXTER, Esq., had already prepared, at great labor and expense, large and elegant engravings of the interior and exterior of the Hospital, which, at a future day, he intended to publish, with some description of the establishment, historical as well as architectural. Of all these engravings, he, with great liberality, offered me the free use. This courtesy, however, I felt that I ought not to accept. His intended publication he will, as is hoped, yet complete. Its design is truly magnificent, and will not be superseded by the present compilation. If, indeed, that shall be regarded as letter-press worthy of accompanying his architectural illustrations, I may well be satisfied.

The chapter on the Ether-discovery is very much longer than I desired or expected. It contains nothing new, except perhaps the award of the French academy, and also a note showing the extent to which ether is used in the Hospital. Readers of the present generation will probably omit it entirely; but the extracts from various pamphlets which it contains, familiar as these now are, may hereafter be of some interest and value, when time shall have rendered the originals difficult of access. The short letter of Dr. HENRY J. BIGELOW, in page 344, presents, as I conceive, in almost the condensed form of an algebraic equation, a clear, striking, and conclusive view of the merits of the whole controversy. The Academy, as will be seen, accords to

Dr. MORTON the idea, thought, or purpose (*pensée*) of making this discovery, and to Dr. C. T. JACKSON the fact (*le fait observé*) of the safety of the agent used; and attributes the final result equally to them both, regarding the mental pre-occupation or engrossment (*préoccupation*) of the one, and the observations of the other, alike indispensable. This award is obviously an entire triumph of Dr. MORTON over the *exclusive* claims of his opponent, and must be to him the more gratifying, inasmuch as it has been gained from a tribunal, most if not all of whose members, though strangers to himself, are the scientific correspondents or personal friends of Dr. JACKSON.

It is due to the Institution to say, that this is in no sense an official publication, but merely a private and humble contribution in its behalf, — a slight and inadequate expression of the interest felt in its welfare by one who has ever regarded as among his happiest hours those which he has been privileged to pass in its service.

BOSTON, October, 1851.

CONTENTS.

CHAPTER I.

PAGE

Urgent Need of Hospital. Bequest of William Phillips, 1804. Circular Letter, 1810. Charter, 1811. Subsequent Acts to 1851. Rights under Life-Insurance Charters. Grant of Province House. Lease of Same for One Hundred Years, &c. 1

CHAPTER II.

1813–1817.

Organization. Trustees elected, 1813. Liberal Subscriptions. Purchases of Two Estates. Deed of Asylum Estate, on Condition. Defect of Title in Hospital Estate, but Claim favorably compromised. Its greatly increased Value. Choice of Dr. James Jackson and Dr. John C. Warren as Physician and Surgeon of Hospital. Lieutenant-Governor William Phillips increases his Father's Gift of Five Thousand to Twenty Thousand Dollars. Common Seal 15

CHAPTER III.

1818–1822.

Thomas H. Perkins, Chairman. Dr. Rufus Wyman chosen Physician of Asylum. Corner-stone of Hospital laid, July 4, 1818. Addresses on the Occasion. Tax on Licenses asked for. Colonel May, Chairman. Address by Richard Sullivan, 1819. Capuchin Chapel. Death of James Prince, Treasurer. Election and Death of William Cochran. Election of N. P. Russell. Death of James Perkins, Vice-President. Tolls on Canal Bridge.

CONTENTS.

Nathaniel Fletcher, Superintendent of Hospital. First Patient, Sept. 3, 1821. Bequests of Thomas Oliver, Samuel Eliot, Beza Tucker, &c. Donations of Horace Gray, &c. Address to Public, 1822. State of Finances, &c. 36

CHAPTER IV.

JANUARY, 1823, TO JUNE, 1827.

Mummy from Thebes. Fifty Thousand Dollars invested in Massachusetts Hospital Life Insurance Company. West Wing of Hospital finished. Debt created. Bequest of John M'Lean, over One Hundred Thousand Dollars. Legacies of Abraham Touro, Eleanor Davis, &c. Death of Mr. Fletcher. Nathan Gurney elected Superintendent. Gift of a Sow. Lafayette. Annual Free Beds. Portraits of Benefactors. Colonel May resigns. Joseph Head, Chairman. Erysipelas at Hospital. Patients removed. Measures in Honor of John M'Lean. Value of his Bequest as compared with Life Insurance Charters . . . 61

CHAPTER V.

JUNE, 1827, THROUGH 1832.

Bequest of William Phillips. Varioloid at Hospital. Domestic Coffee. Donation Book. New Building at Asylum. Fire at Hospital. Auditor of Accounts. Silver Spoons. Ebenezer Francis, Chairman. Mr. Joy's Brick-kiln. Death of Mrs. Gurney. Wedding at Hospital. Death of General Cobb. Dr. George Hayward chosen Junior Surgeon. Colored Patient. Plank Sidewalk. Bequest of Jeremiah Belknap. Donation of Joseph Lee. Lying-in Hospital. Edward Tuckerman, Chairman. Donations of John P. Cushing and John C. Gray. Bequest of Isaiah Thomas. Cholera Patients. Dr. Wyman's Illness and Two Resignations. Dr. Walker's Services. Munificent Bequest of Miss Mary Belknap, One Hundred Thousand Dollars. Services of Joseph Head. Portrait of Mr. Belknap: how painted. Bequest of Miss Margaret Tucker. A Painted Letter. Belknap Ward. Prosperous Condition of the Institution 80

CONTENTS. xi

CHAPTER VI.

1833–1837.

PAGE

Death of Gardiner Greene, President. Resignation of Mr. Gurney. Choice of Gamaliel Bradford. Final Resignation of Dr. Wyman, and Choice of Dr. Thomas G. Lee. Columbus Tyler elected Steward of Asylum. Services of Mrs. Tyler. Bequest of Jonathan Moseley. Portrait of Thomas Oliver. Resignation of Joseph Head, President. George Bond, Chairman. Diet at Hospital. Free Beds for Life. Bequest of Miss Susan Richardson. Piano-forte and Billiard Table at Asylum. Trustees' Meeting: Nobody Present. Death of Dr. Lee, and Votes of Trustees. Dr. Luther V. Bell elected his Successor. Colored Patient. Interesting Report of S. A. Eliot on occasion of Non-observance of Rules and Regulations. Resignation of Dr. James Jackson: his Character and Services. Resignation of Mr. Russell, the Treasurer, and Choice of Henry Andrews. Summary. Great Changes of the Officers. Donations only a Thousand Dollars for the Five Years 113

CHAPTER VII.

1838–1842

Death of Dr. Bradford. Charles Sumner elected Superintendent. His Resignation. John M. Goodwin chosen his Successor. Index to Medical and Surgical Records. Railroads at the Asylum. Pitiful Land Damages. A Water Bed. Miss Brimmer's Bequest. John M'Lean's Portrait. Warren Fund. Small Pox at Hospital. Death of George Bond, Chairman of Trustees: his Character and Services. Robert Hooper, jun., Chairman. Bust of Dr. James Jackson 146

CHAPTER VIII.

1843–1847.

Donation Book completed by Mr. Rogers. Varioloid again in Hospital. Mr. Appleton's Donation, Ten Thousand Dollars.

CONTENTS.

PAGE

Israel Munson's Bequest, Twenty Thousand Dollars. Sears Free Beds. Lands in Somerville taxed. Two Wings added to Hospital: Subscription of Sixty-two Thousand Five Hundred and Fifty Dollars. Services of Mr. Rogers. Miss Taylor's Illness. Dr. Bell's Visit to Europe at Request of Butler Hospital, of Rhode Island. Bequest of John Parker, Ten Thousand Dollars. Statue of Apollo. Lying-in Department discussed. Daniel Waldo's Bequest, Forty Thousand Dollars. Death of Mr. Goodwin. Anecdote of him. Richard Girdler elected. Tomb of Thomas Oliver. New Kitchen at Hospital. Enlarged Medical and Surgical Staff. Medical College. John Redman's Bequest, One Hundred Thousand Dollars. William Oliver's, Fifty Thousand Dollars. Out-door Patients. Hospital Fence. Monument to Jeremiah and Mary Belknap. Addition to Dwelling-house at Asylum. Bequest of Sarah Clough, a Domestic. Ether Discovery. Sickness at Asylum. Death of Several Patients, and of Two Children of Dr. Bell 169

CHAPTER IX.

1847–1849.

The Ether Discovery, and Controversy between Drs. Morton and Jackson. List of more than two dozen Pamphlets. Extracts from a few of them. Hospital Report. Vindication of Same. Dr. Smilie's Address. Congress Report. The Casket and Ribbon. Award of the French Academy. Extent to which Ether is used at the Hospital 215

CHAPTER X.

1848–1851.

Wedding at Hospital. Gift of Trustees. Cost of the Two New Wings, &c. Death of Dr. Enoch Hale. All further Ether Controversy declined. Gas. Devise of John D. Williams of Store worth Seventeen Thousand Dollars. Free Beds placed at Disposal of his Executors. Bequest of B. R. Nichols, Six Thousand Dollars. Bequests of John Bromfield, in all Forty

CONTENTS. xiii

PAGE

Thousand Dollars. Mr. Hooper resigns as Chairman, and is elected Vice-President. Bequest of Henry Todd, Five Thousand Dollars. Death of Dr. John D. Fisher. Addition to Lodge at the Asylum. Post-mortem Examinations. Death of Signor Sarti. New Donation of William Appleton, Twenty Thousand Dollars. Night Watch at Asylum. Resignation of Dr. Hayward: his long and valuable Services. Votes of Trustees. Varioloid at Hospital. Votes of Trustees. Legacy of Dr. Charles W. Wilder, Twenty Thousand. Dollars. Lee Donations of 1830. Dix Ward at Asylum named in honor of Miss Dix 349

CHAPTER XI.

Visits of Trustees: their great Regularity. Incidents and Anecdotes of Life in the Asylum and in the Hospital. Death of a Little Italian Boy and of a Female Attendant 383

CHAPTER XII.

The Members of the Corporation. List of Trustees. Remarks and Anecdotes. List of Officers. List of Subscriptions. Summary of the same to 1843. Enlargement of Hospital in 1844. Free-bed Subscription List. Legacies, Donations, and Devises. Receipts from Life Office, &c. Grand Summary of all these Donations. Tables of Admissions and Discharges at the Asylum and at the Hospital. Concluding Remarks 410

CONTINUATION.

CHAPTER XIII.

FROM AUGUST 5, 1851, TO MARCH 16, 1856.

Mr. Bowditch's History: Its Value. Thanks of the Committee of Trustees. Claim of the Corporation on a Life Insurance Company. Pipes for the Cochituate Water. Visitors to the Railroad Jubilee. Charges for Out-of-town Patients. Dr. Warren's Gift of Surgical Instruments. Indexes to Hospital Records. Contract for Water. Office of Chemist and Microscopist. Dr. J. Bacon, jun., elected thereto. Case of Alleged Abuse at Asylum Investigated. Bequest from Mrs. Salisbury. Report for 1851. Improvements at the Asylum. Organization for 1852. Tribute to Mr. Rogers. A Question of Prerogative. Legacy from J. Ingersoll. Sad Occurrence at the Hospital. Resignation of Dr. J. C. Warren. Annual Meeting. Organization for 1853. Report for 1852. Resignation of Mr. Goodhue. New Supervisors at the Asylum. Another Offering from Mr. Bowditch. Tribute to Hon. S. Appleton. Hospital Index. Additional Physician at Asylum. Annual Meeting. Organization for 1854. Report for 1853. Bequest of Judah Touro. Death of Dr. Shattuck. Building of a Foul Ward. Dr. J. Homans elected a Consulting Physician. Dr. M. Ranney, Assistant-Physician at Asylum. Pathological Museum. Gift from S. Appleton's Estate. Gift of J. B. Bradlee. Dr. C. Ellis, Curator of the Pathological Cabinet. Death of Dr. S. Parkman. Dr. G. H. Gay elected a Visiting Surgeon. Annual Meeting, 1855. Organization. Report for 1854. Tribute to J. P. Bigelow. Microscopist at the Hospital. Resignation of Dr. J. Bigelow. Additional Rooms at Hospital. Bequest of Miss E. Pratt. New Fence at Hospital. Annual Meeting. Organization for 1856. Report for 1855. Resignation of Dr. Bell: his Farewell. 459

CHAPTER XIV.

March 16, 1856, to February 5, 1862.

Routine Business at the Meetings of the Trustees. New Fence at the Hospital. Dr. C. Booth elected Superintendent of the Asylum, and Dr. J. C. Smith an Assistant Physician. Resignation of Dr. Perry. Notice of the death of Dr. J. C. Warren. Proposal for a Sea-Wall on the Hospital Bounds. Bequest of William Read. Important Votes concerning the Asylum. Annual Meeting. Organization for 1857. Report for 1856. Illness of Dr. Booth. Contribution to Dr. Morton. Dr. L. M. Sargent, jun., chosen Artist of the Hospital. Gift from Dr. J. M. Warren. Death of

CONTENTS. XV

PAGE

Dr. Booth. Temporary Service of Dr. Bell. Annual Meeting. Organization for 1858. Report for 1857. Bequests of M. P. Sawyer and W. Pickman. Dr. J. E. Tyler, Superintendent of the Asylum. Bequest of Dr. J. G. Treadwell. Office of Resident Physician at the Hospital. Resignation of Superintendent Girdler, and of the Secretary. Malignant Fever at the Hospital. Donation from Executors of Thomas Dowse. T. B. Hall chosen Secretary. Dr. B. S. Shaw chosen Resident Physician, and Dr. S. L. Abbot, Physician to Out-Patients, at the Hospital. Application of a Female Student. Mr. and Mrs. Gallison chosen Steward and Matron of the Hospital. Thanks to Capt. Girdler. Tribute to Dr. Storer. Dr. F. Minot chosen a Visiting Physician. Bequest of Mrs. A. Austin. Establishment of the Treadwell Library. Estate of M. P. Sawyer. Filling of Flats. Annual Meeting. Organization for 1859. Report for 1858. Resignation of the Treasurer, and Election of Mr. Stevenson. More Land at the Asylum. Bequests of George Hills and of Mrs. S. B. Thompson. Annual Meeting. Organization for 1860. Report for 1859. Dr. Tyler's Report. Important Votes. Bequest of Jonathan Phillips. Reduction of Expenses. Annual Meeting. Organization for 1861. Report for 1860. New Cottage at the Asylum. Death of Mr. Bowditch. Sketch of his Life and Character. His Work on Suffolk Surnames. The Civil War. Preparations to receive Diseased and Wounded Soldiers. A New Form of Bond for Patients at the Asylum. Absence of the Chairman. Bounds of the Hospital Grounds. Donation by Mr. W. Appleton 510

CHAPTER XV.

FEB. 5, 1862, TO FEB. 22, 1867.

Annual Meeting and Organization for 1862. Report for 1861. Death of the President, Mr. Appleton, and Tribute to him. Invalid Soldiers at the Hospital. Bequest from Miss Townsend. United States Sanitary Commission ask the Services of Dr. Shaw and Dr. Tyler. Resignation of the Steward and Matron of the Asylum. Services of Dr. Morrill Wyman. Legislation on Asylums. Annual Meeting. Organization for 1863. Report for 1862. Resignation of Dr. Townsend. Dr. Tyler's Tribute to Dr. Bell. Sketch of him. New Cottage for Males at the Asylum. Resignation of Dr. Bacon as Chemist. House Pupils to board at the Hospital. Dr. J. C. White elected Chemist. Bequest of John Pickens. Death of Dr. Hayward. Dr. Townsend elected Consulting Physician. Additional Surgical House Pupils. Litigation concerning Bequest of Miss Loring. Bequest of Dr. B. D. Greene. Hours for the Visits of Surgeons and Physicians. A Surgeon to Out-Patients. Annual Meeting. Organization for 1864. Report for 1863. Historical Pamphlets presented by Dr. Shaw. Legacy of William Oliver. Resignation of Secretary Hall. Election of Mr. W. S. Dexter. Resignation of Dr. Bowditch, and choice of Dr. C. Ellis as a Visiting Physician. Other Changes among the Officers. Tribute to Dr. J. B. S. Jackson. Bequest of Miss Sever. Annual Meeting. Organization for 1865. Report for 1864. Death of J. Amory Davis. Resignation and Appointments at the Asylum. Other Resignations. Annual Meeting. Organization for 1866. Report for 1865. Important Report on the Finances and Circular. Changes of Officers at Asylum. Gift of Rev. Dr. Worcester. A New Operating Theatre. Leave of Absence to Dr. Tyler. Gift from Rev. J. Spaulding. Legacy from Miss S. Pratt. Annual Meeting. Organization for 1867. Report for 1866. Generous Subscription. Debt paid. Dr. Tyler's Report . . 574

CHAPTER XVI.

February 22, 1867, to 1872.

Dr. Tyler's Absence in Europe. Gift through Dr. J. M. Warren. New Grounds at Asylum. Female Students at Hospital. Death of Dr. J. M. Warren. Dr. J. H. Denny, Assistant at Asylum. Legacy from Dr. J. M. Warren. Death of Dr. J. Jackson. Bequest from him. Religious Services at Asylum. Resignation of Mr. Whitney. Annual Meeting. Organization for 1868. Report for 1867. New Operating Theatre. Dr. Tyler's Foreign Observations. Death of the President of the Corporation, Mr. Hooper. Further Bequests. Changes in the Medical Staff. Annual Meeting. Organization for 1869. Report for 1868.

CONTENTS. xvii

PAGE

Dr. Tyler's Review. Lady Visitors at Hospital. New Officers. Gift from John C. Gray. Warren Prize. Appeal from Dr. Morton's Family. Annual Meeting. Organization for 1870. Report for 1869. Department for Skin Diseases. Post Mortem Register. Committee on Autopsies. Donations from Dr. H. J. Bigelow. Female Supervisor at Asylum. Changes of Officers. New Surgical Instruments. Legacy from Rev. Dr. Worcester. Experiment of a Skin Disease Ward. Annual Meeting. Organization for 1871. Report for 1870. Resignation of Dr. Tyler. Resignation of Dr. Whittemore. An Incident connected with the Asylum. Award of the Warren Prize. Proposals for a New Location for the Asylum. Resignation of Mr. Farnsworth. Donations received. Subject and Advertisement for the next Warren Prize. Dr. Ray in Temporary Charge of the Asylum. Statistics of Surgical Operations. Dr. Jelly chosen Superintendent of Asylum. Dr. H. P. Quincy, Artist of the Hospital. S. D. Warren, Trustee. Donation of James McGregor. The Nabby Joy Fund. Resignation of Dr. Shaw. Election of Dr. N. Folsom as Resident Physician of Hospital. Remarks on the Hospital and Asylum. Conclusion 627

STATISTICAL TABLES AT HOSPITAL AND ASYLUM 701
SUBSCRIPTIONS, DONATIONS, AND BEQUESTS, TO THE MASSACHUSETTS GENERAL HOSPITAL 710
OFFICERS OF THE INSTITUTION 731

HISTORY

OF THE

MASSACHUSETTS GENERAL HOSPITAL.

CHAPTER I.

URGENT NEED OF HOSPITAL. — BEQUEST OF WILLIAM PHILLIPS, 1804. — CIRCULAR LETTER, 1810. — CHARTER, 1811. — SUBSEQUENT ACTS TO 1851. — RIGHTS UNDER LIFE-INSURANCE CHARTERS. — GRANT OF PROVINCE HOUSE. — LEASE OF SAME FOR ONE HUNDRED YEARS, &C.

MORE than a third of a century* has elapsed since the establishment of the Massachusetts General Hospital. Its endowments amount to, and perhaps exceed, one million of dollars. Its building for the sick, erected in a spacious enclosure of four acres, is one of the most imposing edifices of the city of Boston. Its Asylum for the Insane is beautifully situated on a rising ground within the quiet precincts of the adjoining town of Somerville. Nearly fourteen thousand patients have received the benefits of the former department of the institution, and more than thirty-three hundred have been inmates of the latter. The

[* Written in 1851.]

greatest discovery of the age — the power of producing insensibility to pain — has gone forth from the one; while the like humane treatment, and the same high professional skill evinced in the other, have extended its reputation throughout the length and breadth of our land, and gathered within its walls sufferers alike from the frozen North and the sunny South. One generation has passed away, and a new one has arisen. The circumstances and instrumentalities connected with those early days have thus, to a considerable extent, already become matters of tradition. Many of the original patrons and officers of the Hospital have gone to their reward. A few, indeed, yet survive, to rejoice in the extensive usefulness of a charity which they contributed, in an eminent degree, to establish and perpetuate. May the services alike of its living and its deceased founders be ever held in grateful remembrance!

At the beginning of the present century, Massachusetts had no Hospital or Insane Asylum, though such institutions had been for many years established in the States of New York and Pennsylvania. There were various indications, however, that the want of such establishments was beginning to be felt in our community.* Thomas Boylston, Esq., by will dated

---

* Thomas Hancock gave a sum to the Town between 1760–1770. Rev. Frederick T. Gray shewed me a letter stating newspaper reports on the subject.

Nov. 12, 1798, proved in 1800, made the town of Boston his residuary devisee in trust, among other objects, to erect a small-pox hospital and a lunatic hospital. The testator was, unfortunately, a member of the firm of Lane, Frazier, and Company, of London, which became insolvent. Hon. William Phillips, by a codicil dated April 18, 1797, proved in 1804, bequeathed the sum of five thousand dollars to the town of Boston for this object.* In August, 1810, a circular letter was prepared by Drs. James Jackson and John C. Warren, addressed to several of our wealthiest and most influential citizens, for the purpose of awakening in their minds an interest in the subject. This circular letter may be regarded as the corner-stone of our institution.† On the 25th of Feb-

---

* "Fourthly, — I give to the town of Boston five thousand dollars, towards the building of a Hospital; and direct my executors to pay that sum to any person or persons whom the town shall appoint to receive the same, *as soon as they shall determine to begin the work.*"

† BOSTON, August 20, 1810.
Sir, — It has appeared very desirable to a number of respectable gentlemen, that a hospital for the reception of lunatics and other sick persons should be established in this town. By the appointment of a number of these gentlemen, we are directed to adopt such methods as shall appear best calculated to promote such an establishment. We therefore beg leave to submit for your consideration proposals for the institution of a hospital, and to state to you some of the reasons in favour of such an establishment.

It is unnecessary to urge the propriety and even obligation of succouring the poor in sickness. The wealthy inhabitants of the town of Boston have always evinced that they consider themselves as "treasurers of God's bounty;" and in Christian countries, in countries where Christianity is practised, it must always be considered the first of duties to visit and to heal the sick. When in distress, every man becomes our neighbour, not only if he be

ruary following (1811), the charter was obtained from the Legislature. It incorporates James Bowdoin and fifty-five others of the most distinguished inhabitants

of the household of faith, but even though his misfortunes have been induced by transgressing the rules both of reason and religion. It is unnecessary to urge the truth and importance of these sentiments to those who are already in the habit of cherishing them, — to those who indulge in the true luxury of wealth, the pleasures of charity. The questions which first suggest themselves on this subject are, whether the relief afforded by hospitals is better than can be given in any other way; and whether there are, in fact, so many poor among us as to require an establishment of this sort.

The relief to be afforded to the poor, in a country so rich as ours, should perhaps be measured only by their necessities. We have, then, to inquire into the situation of the poor in sickness, and to learn what are their wants. In this inquiry, we shall be led to answer both the questions above stated.

There are some who are able to acquire a competence in health, and to provide so far against any ordinary sickness as that they shall not then be deprived of a comfortable habitation, nor of food for themselves and their families; while they are not able to defray the expenses of medicine and medical assistance. Persons of this description never suffer among us. The Dispensary gives relief to hundreds every year; and the individuals who practise medicine gratuitously attend many more of this description. But there are many others among the poor, who have, if we may so express it, the form of the necessaries of life, without the substance. A man may have a lodging; but it is deficient in all those advantages which are requisite to the sick. It is a garret or a cellar, without light and due ventilation, or open to the storms of an inclement winter. In this miserable habitation, he may obtain liberty to remain during an illness; but, if honest, he is harassed with the idea of his accumulating rent, which must be paid out of his future labours. In this wretched situation, the sick man is destitute of all those common conveniences, without which most of us would consider it impossible to live, even in health. Wholesome food and sufficient fuel are wanting; and his own sufferings are aggravated by the cries of hungry children. Above all, he suffers from the want of that first requisite in sickness, a kind and skilful nurse.

But it may be said, that instances are rare among us, where a man, who labours, with even moderate industry, when in health, endures such privations in sickness as are here described. They are not, however, rare among those who are not industrious; and who, nevertheless, when labouring under sickness, must be considered as having claims to assistance. In cases of

of the various towns of the Commonwealth, by the name of the Massachusetts General Hospital, with power to hold real and personal estate of the yearly

long-protracted disease, instances of such a description do occur amongst those of the most industrious class. Such instances are still less rare among those women who are either widowed, or worse than widowed. It happens too frequently that modest and worthy women are united to men who are profligate and intemperate, by whom they are left to endure disease and poverty under the most aggravated forms. Among the children of such families also, instances are not rare of real suffering in sickness. To all such as have been described, a hospital would supply every thing which is needful, if not all they could wish. In a well-regulated hospital, they would find a comfortable lodging in a duly attempered atmosphere; would receive the food best suited to their various conditions; and would be attended by kind and discreet nurses, under the directions of a physician. In such a situation, the poor man's chance for relief would be equal perhaps to that of the most affluent, when affected by the same disease.

There are other persons, also, who are of great importance in society, to whom the relief afforded by a hospital is exceedingly appropriate. Such are generally those of good and industrious habits, who are affected with sickness, just as they are entering into active life, and who have not had time to provide for this calamity. Cases of this sort are frequently occurring. Disease is often produced by the very anxiety and exertions which belong to this period of life; and the best are the most liable to suffer. Of such a description, cases are often seen among journeymen mechanics and among servants.

Journeymen mechanics commonly live in small boarding-houses, where they have accommodations which are sufficient, but nothing more than sufficient, in health. When sick, they are necessarily placed in small, confined apartments, or in rooms crowded with their fellow-workmen. They are sheltered from the weather, and have food of some sort; and these must, in many cases, be the extent of their accommodations. Persons of this description would do well to enter a hospital, even if they had to pay the expense of their own maintenance. In most cases, they would suffer less, and recover sooner, by so doing. When, as sometimes happens, they have not the means of payment, they become objects of charity; and the welfare of such persons should be considered among the strong motives in favour of establishing a hospital.

Servants generally undergo great inconveniences, at least when afflicted with sickness, and oftentimes much more than inconveniences. With so

value of thirty thousand dollars. The Governor, Lieutenant-Governor, President of the Senate, Speaker of the House, and the Chaplains of both Houses, are

much difficulty is the care of them attended in private families, that many gentlemen would pay the board of their servants at a hospital, in preference to having them sick in their own houses. In some cases, however, neither the master nor servant can afford the expense of proper care in sickness. Not uncommonly, a young girl is taken sick in a large family, where she is the only servant. She lodges in the most remote corner of the house, in a room without a fireplace. The mistress is sufficiently occupied with the unusual labours which are thrown on her at a time perhaps when she is least fitted to perform them. Under such circumstances, how can the servant receive those attentions which are due to the sick? Of what use is it that the physician leaves a prescription to be put up at the Dispensary? He goes the next day, and finds that there has not been time even to procure the remedies which he had ordered; meanwhile, the period in which they would have been useful has passed by, and the incipient disease of yesterday has now become confirmed.

Persons of these descriptions would not be disposed to resort to a hospital on every trivial occasion. But, when afflicted with serious indisposition, they would find in such an institution an alleviation of their sufferings, which it must gladden the heart of the most frigid to contemplate.

There is one class of sufferers who peculiarly claim all that benevolence can bestow, and for whom a hospital is most especially required. The virtuous and industrious are liable to become objects of public charity, in consequence of diseases of the mind. When those who are unfortunate in this respect are left without proper care, a calamity, which might have been transient, is prolonged through life. The number of such persons, who are rendered unable to provide for themselves, is probably greater than the public imagine; and, of these, a large proportion claim the assistance of the affluent. The expense which is attached to the care of the insane in private families is extremely great; and such as to ruin a whole family that is possessed of a competence under ordinary circumstances, when called upon to support one of its members in this situation. Even those who can pay the necessary expenses would perhaps find an institution, such as is proposed, the best situation in which they could place their unfortunate friends. It is worthy of the opulent men of this town, and consistent with their general character, to provide an asylum for the insane from every part of the Commonwealth. But if funds are raised for the purpose proposed, it is probable that the Legislature will grant some assistance, with a view to such an extension of its benefits.

constituted a board of Visitors. The institution is placed under the care of twelve Trustees, of whom four are chosen by the board of Visitors. A grant

Of another class, whose necessities would be removed by the establishment of a hospital, are women who are unable to provide for their own welfare and safety in one of nature's most trying hours. Houses for lying-in women have been found extremely useful in the large cities of Europe; and, although abuses may have arisen in consequence, these are such as are more easily prevented in a small than in a large town.

There are many others who would find great relief in a hospital, and many times have life preserved when otherwise it would be lost. Such especially are the subjects of accidental wounds and fractures among the poorer classes of our citizens; and the subjects of extraordinary diseases, in any part of the Commonwealth, who may require the long and careful attention of either the physician or surgeon.

It is possible that we may be asked whether the almshouse does not answer the purposes for which a hospital is proposed. That it *does not*, is very certain. The town is so much indebted to the liberality of those gentlemen who, without compensation, superintend the care of the poor, that we ought not to make this reply without an explanation. The truth is that the almshouse could not serve the purpose of a hospital, without such an entire change in the arrangements of it as the overseers do not feel themselves authorized to make, and such as the town could not be easily induced to direct or to support.

The almshouse receives all those who do not take care of themselves, and who are destitute of property, whether they be old and infirm, and unable to provide means of assistance; or are too vicious and debauched to employ themselves in honest labour; or are prevented from so employing themselves by occasional sickness. This institution, then, is made to comprehend what is more properly meant by an almshouse, a bridewell or house of correction, and a hospital. Now, the economy and mode of government cannot possibly be adapted at once to all these various purposes. It must necessarily happen that in many instances the worst members of the community, the debauched and profligate, obtain admission into this house. Hence it has become, in some measure, disreputable to live in it; and, not unfrequently, those who are the most deserving objects of charity cannot be induced to enter it. To some of them, death appears less terrible than a residence in the almshouse.

It is true that the sick in that house are allowed some greater privileges and advantages than are extended to those in health; yet the general arrangements and regulations are, necessarily, so different from those required

was made of the Province-house Estate, so called, with authority to sell the same and use the proceeds at pleasure, provided that within five years an addi-

in a hospital, that the sick — far from having the advantages afforded by the medical art — have not the fair chance for recovery which nature alone would give them. Most especially they suffer for the want of good nurses. In these officers must be placed trust and confidence of the highest nature. Their duties are laborious and painful. In the almshouse, they are selected from among the more healthy inhabitants; but, unfortunately, those who are best qualified will always prefer more profitable and less laborious occupations elsewhere. It must, then, be obvious that the persons employed as nurses cannot be such as will conscientiously perform the duties of this office.

In addition to what has already been stated, there are a number of collateral advantages that would attend the establishment of a hospital in this place. These are the facilities for acquiring knowledge, which it would give to the students in the medical school established in this town. The means of medical education in New England are at present very limited, and totally inadequate to so important a purpose. Students of medicine cannot qualify themselves properly for their profession, without incurring heavy expenses, such as very few of them are able to defray. The only medical school of eminence in this country is that at Philadelphia, nearly four hundred miles distant from Boston; and the expense of attending that is so great, that students from this quarter rarely remain at it longer than one year. Even this advantage is enjoyed by very few, compared with the whole number. Those who are educated in New England have so few opportunities of attending to the practice of physic, that they find it impossible to learn some of the most important elements of the science of medicine, until after they have undertaken for themselves the care of the health and lives of their fellow-citizens. This care they undertake with very little knowledge, except that acquired from books; — a source whence it is highly useful and indispensable that they should obtain knowledge, but one from which alone they never can obtain all that is necessary to qualify them for their professional duties. With such deficiencies in medical education, it is needless to show to what evils the community is exposed.

To remedy evils so important and so extensive, it is necessary to have a medical school in New England. All the materials necessary to form this school exist among us. Wealth, abundantly sufficient, can be devoted to the purpose, without any individual's feeling the smallest privation of any, even of the luxuries of life. Every one is liable to suffer from the want of such a

tional sum of one hundred thousand dollars should be obtained by private subscriptions and donations. A further term of five years was allowed by an Act of June 14, 1813. The Charter imposed on the Corporation the obligation of supporting thirty of the sick and lunatic persons chargeable to the Commonwealth. This provision was modified by the additional Act, so as to make the number of patients to be thus supported depend on the actual income derived from the Province House. The tendency of any such provision, however, was considered disadvantageous, as

school; every one may derive, directly or indirectly, the greatest benefits from its establishment.

A hospital is an institution absolutely essential to a medical school, and one which would afford relief and comfort to thousands of the sick and miserable. On what other objects can the superfluities of the rich be so well bestowed?

The amount required for the institution proposed may, at first sight, appear large. But it will cease to appear so, when we consider that it is to afford relief, not only to those who may require assistance during the present year or present age, but that it is to erect a most honourable monument of the munificence of the present times, which will ensure to its founders the blessings of thousands in ages to come; and when we add that this amount may be raised at once, if a few opulent men will contribute only their superfluous income for one year. Compared with the benefits which such an establishment would afford, of what value is the pleasure of accumulating riches in those stores which are already groaning under their weight?

Hospitals and infirmaries are found in all the Christian cities of the Old World; and our large cities in the Middle States have institutions of this sort, which do great honour to the liberality and benevolence of their founders. We flatter ourselves that in this respect, as in all others, Boston may ere long assert her claim to equal praise.

We are, sir, very respectfully, your obedient servants,

JAMES JACKSON.
JOHN C. WARREN.

making the institution a merely pauper establishment; and it was virtually repealed by a resolve passed Feb. 13, 1816.

By this resolve of 1816, authority was finally granted for sale of the Province House, on the sole condition of giving bond to pay the proceeds of sale into the State Treasury, unless, within one year from such sale, said additional sum of one hundred thousand dollars should be obtained.

By a resolve passed June 12, 1817, it is provided that the stone for the erection of the Hospital should be hammered and fitted for use by the convicts in the State Prison. The work thus done is estimated at over thirty thousand dollars. And, by a resolve of Feb. 11, 1824, a bill due from the Hospital for stone work at the State Prison, for the use of the Insane Asylum ($4,176.33), was remitted, as coming within the resolve of 1817.

An Act passed June 18, 1819, points out the mode of filling vacancies in the Board of Trustees. An Act passed Feb. 15, 1821, exonerates from performance of military duty certain officers of the Hospital; and a like exemption is provided for by the Revised Statutes, passed in 1836.

By an Act passed Feb. 24, 1814, the Corporation was authorized to grant annuities on lives. In a charter, subsequently granted to the Massachusetts

Hospital Life Insurance Company, a proviso was inserted, by which one-third of its whole net profits from insurance on lives is made payable to the Hospital. An additional Act, passed Jan. 17, 1824, sanctions a most important agreement between these two Corporations, by which the Hospital, in lieu of all former rights, became entitled to one-third of all the earnings of said Insurance Company, over and above six per cent. Now, this Insurance Company has a capital of five hundred thousand dollars; and the chief branch of its business is the management of property deposited with it in trust, and for which a charge is made of one half per cent commission. The regular annual dividends for several years have been nine per cent, — say eight per cent to stockholders, and one per cent, or five thousand dollars a year, to the Hospital; and three *extra* dividends have also been received, making a total of $150,687. In all the charters subsequently granted for insurance on lives, similar provisions in favor of the Hospital have been introduced, viz.: the New England Mutual Life Insurance Company, April 1, 1835; State Mutual Life Insurance Company, March 16, 1844; the Bowditch Mutual Life Insurance Company, March 26, 1845. Little has yet been or ever can be realized under these latter charters, as the percentage of the Hospital is reckoned only on the *guaranty capital* of said companies, which is quite small. The granting of any such charter, without such a provision, would, however, exonerate the Massachusetts Hospital Life Insurance Company from all obligations in favor of the Hospital; or, in other words, would, as respects its sources of income, be a loss to the Hospital of more than a hundred thousand dollars. To prevent such a contingency, a bill was reported and discussed at the present session of the Legislature, in the words following : —

"Whenever any persons or corporation shall be empowered to make insurance on lives upon land, the right so to do shall be deemed subject to the same obligations for the payment of a certain share of the profit accruing therefrom, to the Massachusetts General Hospital, as are imposed on the Massachusetts Hospital Life Insurance Company, by the laws now in force, unless express provision to the contrary shall be made in the Act or Acts empowering any such persons or corporation to make such insurance on lives as aforesaid."

The passage of such a law was, of course, immaterial to the Hospital, if the Legislature, in each particular charter, should continue to insert the same provisions as had always heretofore been done. To show the importance either of such general or special legislation, the Chairman of the Trustees submitted a memorial to the Legislature, May 5, 1851, stating the exact amount which had been received from the Massachusetts Hospital Life Insurance Company, but expressing no wish for the passage of any general law. The proposed law was passed.

The above is a condensed view of all the legislative enactments respecting the Hospital from its foundation to the present time. The Province-house Estate, thus liberally given by the Commonwealth, embraced a tract of land measuring eighty-six feet six inches on Washington, formerly Marlborough Street, and extended back two hundred and sixty-seven feet to Governor's Alley or Province Street, where it measured in width seventy-six feet, being about half an acre of land. Stores have now been erected in front on Washington Street; and a block of brick houses, on the northerly side of Province-house Court, stand on the back part of the estate. The old Province House still remains, surmounted by its figure of an Indian, though the days of its glory have departed. In 1796 it had been sold to John Peck for $16,600, and in 1799 was reconveyed for the same price. At the time of the donation to the Hospital, it was valued at twenty thousand dollars. In the early accounts of the Hospital (1822), it is estimated as worth forty thousand dollars. It would now probably sell for at least one hundred thousand dollars, independently of all improvements. On April 1, 1817, the Hospital leased this estate to David Greenough, Esq., for ninety-nine years, at an annual rent of two thousand dollars, or an outright sum of thirty-three thousand dollars, at his option; and, on Oct. 1, 1824, he elected to pay this latter sum. The reversion of the estate (to come into possession in A.D. 1916) still remains in the Hospital. Its present value is small. But the Corporation will live for ever; and it is to be hoped that no future Board of Trustees will alienate this, the first donation made to the institution. Rather let it remain to the latest times an enduring monument of the liberality of the Commonwealth, as in times past it was the representative of its official dignity. And, in acknowledgment of this splendid gift, and of the many subsequent benefits derived from the same source, may our institution always preserve unchanged its corporate name of the *Massachusetts* General Hospital!

CHAPTER II.

1813–1817.

ORGANIZATION. — TRUSTEES ELECTED, 1813. — LIBERAL SUBSCRIPTIONS. — PURCHASES OF TWO ESTATES.—DEED OF ASYLUM ESTATE, ON CONDITION. — DEFECT OF TITLE IN HOSPITAL ESTATE, BUT CLAIM FAVORABLY COMPROMISED. — ITS GREATLY INCREASED VALUE. — CHOICE OF DR. JAMES JACKSON AND DR. JOHN C. WARREN AS PHYSICIAN AND SURGEON OF HOSPITAL. — LIEUTENANT-GOVERNOR WILLIAM PHILLIPS INCREASES HIS FATHER'S GIFT OF FIVE THOUSAND TO TWENTY THOUSAND DOLLARS. — COMMON SEAL.

A CHARTER had now been obtained, containing a liberal grant, made *on the condition that one hundred thousand dollars more should be subscribed by individuals.* The fifty-six persons named in the Act were the first members of the Corporation. By by-laws, subsequently adopted, all who are specially elected, all who have given one hundred dollars, and all who have served as Trustees, are made members of the Corporation. The first meeting of the Corporation was held on April 23, 1811, — Hon. John Adams, moderator, — at which Richard Sullivan was chosen Secretary, and a Committee appointed to prepare by-laws, which were adopted July 5, as reported by the Committee. They are recorded *in extenso*, occupying ten large folio pages. They have been since modified as convenience or necessity dictated; and, as a large edition has been printed of the present rules, &c., no analysis of these earlier regulations is thought necessary. At this last meeting, thanks were presented to Josiah Loring for the gift of an elegant record-book. It is still used, and will last fifty years more. Trustees were not chosen till Feb. 2, 1813. The Corporation was organized by a President and Vice-President, Treasurer and Secretary; the Secretary being, *ex officio*, Secretary of the Board of Trustees. At first, the President always attended the meetings of Trustees, and presided; but, since 1818, the Trustees have acted by a Chairman, who presides at all their meetings; the duty of the President or Vice-President being merely to preside at the annual meetings of the Corporation. The earliest record-book of the Trustees is a little volume, of about five inches by eight, of the poorest and cheapest paper and covers, containing a hundred and sixty pages. It forms an amusing contrast with its more brilliant successors. It embraces the period from 1813 to 1817 inclusive. The first Board of Trustees consisted of Messrs. T. H. Perkins, Josiah Quincy, Daniel Sargent, Joseph May, Stephen Higginson, jun., Gamaliel Bradford, Tristram Barnard, George G. Lee. Francis C. Lowell, Joseph Tilden, John L. Sullivan, and Richard Sullivan. Messrs. Quincy, Higginson, Lowell, and Tilden were chosen by the Board of Visitors; and, of the remaining eight, six were specially elected members of the Corporation, namely, all except Thomas H. Perkins and Richard Sullivan, who were named in the Act of Incorporation. No changes occurred in the Board, until the choice of Jonathan Phillips by the Board of Visitors, in place of Mr. Higginson, in February, 1816; and the choice of John Lowell and Joseph Coolidge, jun., by the same Board, in December of the same year, in place of F. C. Lowell and Joseph Tilden; — the others having resigned. At the first meeting of the Trustees, Feb. 23, 1813, held at the house of Colonel T. H. Perkins, the draft of an address to the public was read, adopted, and ordered to be printed, " with a suitable circular letter to every clergyman in the Commonwealth;" Colonel May and the Secretary being a Committee for that purpose. At the same meeting, Messrs. Barnard and Higginson were appointed a Committee as to selecting a site for the Hospital, either on the Almshouse land (in Leverett Street), or elsewhere. At the next meeting, March 9, the Committee reported unfavorably as to that site, and suggested for consideration the Winthrop Estate in Cambridge, or the made land at bottom of the Common, since known as the Public Garden. A plan was subsequently made of this last estate; and, at a meeting held May 14, several communications from physicians, Drs. Rand, Hayward, Warren, and Dexter (besides a special communication from Drs. Jackson and Warren), recommending it, were received and read; and Messrs. Perkins, Barnard, and Higginson were appointed a Committee to see gentlemen residing near the Common, to obviate objections, if any, to that location. On Nov. 22, the expediency of establishing a temporary Hospital in the Province House was discussed. On Jan. 9, 1814, an address to the public, having been approved by the overseers of the poor, was adopted, and Committees appointed to solicit subscriptions. This address is extant in a pamphlet form. It is drawn up with great earnestness, and is signed by the whole twelve Trustees. It is published with the following motto: —

> "As, in some solitude, the summer rill
> Refreshes, where it winds, the faded green,
> And cheers the drooping flowers, unheard, unseen,
> Such is this charity!" &c.*

The address shows the urgent need of such an institution for the relief both of sick and insane; that the Almshouse is in its nature a mere asylum for poverty; that indeed "the Almshouse in this metrop-

* On the publication of the first edition, I received a note from President Quincy, in which he informs me that his daughter reminds him of the fact that this address was written by himself, the motto having been selected by his late wife.

olis does not pretend to *cure;*" and that "*all it possesses are accommodations for eight patients.*" It then proceeds to show the safeguards as to the management of the proposed institution, — that "its conductors are responsible to the executive of the Commonwealth and to the subscribers by an annual election;" that it is designed to be a State establishment, extending its benefits to all; that, without the aid of all, the condition annexed to the grant of the Commonwealth cannot be complied with. The basis of the subscription is announced to be, that "no sum subscribed shall be demanded, unless, before Jan. 1, 1815, the sum subscribed by individuals to the institution shall amount to at least a hundred thousand dollars." The Trustees declare, that a liberal endowment at the outset is essential to the reputation, and therefore to the usefulness of the institution; and they conclude with the following paragraph : —

"Besides, the undersigned are willing to confess that they are not ambitious of being the guardians of a charity *merely nominal.* They are satisfied that the sum affixed by the Legislature as the condition of its grant, is so small, when compared with the wealth of individuals and the greatness of the State, that no plea arising from 'the hardship of the times,' 'the general embarrassment of affairs,' or 'the claims of other charities,' can or ought to avail the community. If such a proposal as this fail, it will be, in the judgment of the undersigned, decisive of the fate of the establishment. It will then be apparent that *the will is wanting* in the public to patronize such an undertaking; and that the honor of laying the foundation of a fabric of charity so noble and majestic must be left for times when a higher cast of character predominates, and to a more enlightened and sympathetic race of men."

On May 18, 1814, a communication from Dr. George Parkman was received as to a Hospital for the Insane, proposed to be erected by him for accommodation of such patients as shall be able to pay their own expenses. On Jan. 18, 1815, the proposed subscriptions were suspended. March 10, 1816, Messrs. Quincy, Tilden, and J. L. Sullivan were appointed a Committee on the subject of granting annuities, who reported at the next meeting. On March 25, a Committee was appointed to see if the estate of Jonathan Merry, near the North Church, can be purchased. Messrs. Quincy and J. L. Sullivan were appointed a Committee to draft a new address to the public. Colonel May was directed to confer with Dr. Bowditch, of Salem, respecting annuity tables, and the comparative duration of life in this country and Europe, &c.

On April 14, the address was ordered to be printed in pamphlet form; and, on April 21, a thousand copies of it were directed to be prepared for distribution. This second address is also extant. It is very short. It refers to the former one two years before, and states, that, owing to a modification in the terms of the gift of the Province House, the Board is ready to receive subscriptions, independently of any specific amount to be raised within any prescribed period; also that, to meet the existing diversity of views, subscriptions would be received generally or specially for either department of the proposed institution, and the sums subscribed be faithfully applied as requested. Appended to this address are letters directed to members of the Board, detailing circumstances showing the urgent need of such an institution. The Board resolved itself, at this last meeting, into Subcommittees for subscriptions: Colonel Perkins and Captain Barnard to call on all whose names begin with A, B, C. The remaining letters of the alphabet were distributed as follows: To Messrs. May and Phillips, D, E, F, G; Messrs. Sargent and Lowell, H to L; Messrs. Quincy and Lee, M to R; Messrs. Tilden and J. L. Sullivan, S to Z.

On April 15, 1816, authority was given to buy the Merry Estate at twelve thousand dollars. This estate was situate at corner of Salem and Charter Streets, and formerly belonged to Sir William Phipps. It was not purchased by the Hospital, but was subsequently (in 1820) bought by the Boys' Asylum. On April 28. a Committee was appointed to devise a plan of obtaining contributions from all the towns in the Commonwealth, who, on May 5, reported an address to individuals resident in such towns; of which six hundred copies were ordered. I have not seen any copy of this circular letter.

On Oct. 4, 1816, a communication from Dr. George Parkman was received, to the effect that the Magee Place and sixteen acres of land in Roxbury can be had for sixteen thousand dollars. "If the institution will pay five thousand dollars, *he will procure to be given to this institution the remaining eleven thousand.*" This proposal was accepted; a Committee appointed to complete the purchase; and Dr. Parkman was appointed Superintending Physician of said institution, "whenever the Magee Place shall be purchased, as provided in the preceding vote." At the foot of the page is the following memorandum: "The Board subsequently considered that it was inexpedient to purchase the Magee Place." Dr. Parkman, as I learn, then had a private institution for the insane on this estate, which is the same since occupied by the widow of Governor Eustis. Of the eleven thousand dollars promised by him, ten thousand was the amount agreed to be subscribed by friends of the institution, who at his solicitation were willing that their intended donations should be applied to this purchase. It was not, as the Board apparently supposed, a new donation of Dr. Parkman.

Dec. 15, 1816, Messrs. Lowell, Quincy, and Barnard were appointed a Committee to contract with B. Joy, Esq., for the purchase of the Barrell Place (or Joy Estate at Charlestown), to be paid for as soon as the state of the funds shall admit of it. A renewed attempt was also made to get the land west of the Almshouse for a Hospital. On Dec. 17, the Humane Society subscribed five thousand dollars for the Insane Hospital, and a suitable vote of thanks was passed. On Dec. 18, the Board decided to purchase part of Mr. Joy's land. Dec. 20, the several Ward Committees for collecting subscriptions were appointed, and were requested to commence proceedings on the 26th instant.* Mr. Lowell was appointed a Committee to prepare an address to the public. This address is drawn up with the characteristic fer-

---

* The following gentlemen composed these Ward Committees, viz. : —

WARDS 1, 2, 3. — Dr. Webster, Dr. E. Eliot, N. Webb, Esq., Gedney King, Henry K. May.

WARDS 4 and 5. — Joseph Coolidge, jun., Esq., William Mackay, Edward Tuckerman, jun., R. G. Shaw, Lynde Walter, John Osborn, George [W.] Lyman, Abraham Touro.

' WARDS 6 and 7. — Thomas Bartlett, Esq., Daniel Davis, Esq., Edmund Dwight, Gideon Snow, Nathan Appleton, Ebenezer Farley, E. Motley, Geo. Sullivan, James Prince, John Mackay, Thomas W. Sumner.

WARDS 8 and 9. — Joseph Tilden, Esq., Joseph May, John Tappan, Benjamin Russell, Josiah Bradlee, Francis Welch, Israel Munson, Samuel Parkman, jun.

WARD 10. — David S. Greenough, Benjamin Rich, George Trott, William Sturgis, William Ropes, Lewis Tappan.

WARDS 11 and 12. — Samuel May, Benjamin West, Joshua Davis, Joseph Richards, John D. Williams, William Brown.

vor of the writer. It is a pamphlet of eight pages. It is signed by eleven Trustees, — all except Mr. Lee, who had recently died. It shows that private charity cannot meet the evils which this public institution is designed to remedy. It announces the purchase of the Joy Estate as completed, of which it remarks: " The situation selected appears to unite every practicable advantage; we should almost say, the irreconcilable ones of propinquity and distance, being scarcely separated from the town by water, while its peninsular situation places it at the most desirable distance." It also adds, that the Trustees have " procured a grant of land west of the Almshouse [on Leverett Street], upon which they have voted to erect the General Hospital, as soon as the moneys, which they flatter themselves will be readily subscribed, shall have been collected."

On Dec. 29, the Ward Committees met with the Board of Trustees, and reported *that in three days the subscriptions were* $78,802. Committees for the towns of Salem, Beverly, New Bedford, Plymouth, Charlestown, Medford, Cambridge, Roxbury, and Newburyport,* were also appointed. Charles Bul-

---

* COMMITTEE FOR SALEM. — Hon. Benjamin Pickman, Hon. Joseph Story, N. Silsbee, Joseph Peabody, N. Bowditch, Nathaniel West, John Pickering, Dudley L. Pickman, Pickering Dodge, and Ezekiel Savage, Esqs.

FOR BEVERLY. — Dr. Fisher, Hon. T. Stevens, Moses Brown, Esq.

FOR NEW BEDFORD. — Wm. Rotch, jun., Samuel Rodman, James Arnold

finch, Esq., was employed to visit the Hospitals of New York, Philadelphia, and Baltimore. Meetings now began to be held at the Athenæum, having before been held at the houses of the officers.

In 1817, Ebenezer Francis and David Sears became Trustees, in place of George G. Lee and John L. Sullivan. On Jan. 5, the subscriptions had increased to $93,969. Authority was given to purchase more of Mr. Joy's land, not exceeding in all fifteen acres, or to cost over fifteen thousand dollars. The Hon. John Phillips was requested to examine the title. On Jan. 12, the Committee reported a purchase from Mr. Joy for $15,650; and the Board approved of their Committee's act, though they had somewhat exceeded their powers; and Mr. Lowell, with Mr. Phillips, was appointed a Committee to

Seth Russell, jun., Joseph Ricketson, John A. Parker, And. Robeson, Esqs.

FOR PLYMOUTH. — Hon. Joshua Thomas, Wm. Davis, Barnabas Hedge, Henry Warren, Esqs.

FOR CHARLESTOWN. — Hon. Josiah Bartlett, Joseph Hurd, Nathan Adams, Nathan Bridge, Ebenezer Breed, William Austin, Timothy Walker, Samuel Jaques, Seth Knowles, Nathaniel Austin, Esqs.

FOR MEDFORD. — William Ward, Abraham Touro, Dudley Hall, Isaac Brooks, E. Hall, Nathaniel Hall, Esqs.

FOR CAMBRIDGE. — James Winthrop, L. Baldwin, A. Bigelow, S. Bartlett, S. P. P. Fay, Tim. Fuller, Esqs., and Messrs. Hayden and Merriam.

FOR ROXBURY. — General H. A. S. Dearborn, Thos. Williams, W. Bosson, Charles Davis, George Zeigler, D. S. Greenough, Esqs., and Captain Charles Curtis.

FOR NEWBURYPORT. — William Bartlett, Moses Brown, J. B. Bannister, John Pettingil, Abner Wood, William Woart, Esqs.

procure the deed. Jan. 19, a salary was given to the Secretary of a hundred dollars. At the annual meeting of the Corporation, Jan. 21, Richard Sullivan declined a re-election as Secretary, and was thanked for his services. On Jan. 26, a letter was received from Hon. Benjamin Pickman, recommending a physician of the Asylum. This was a most important communication, as the nominee was Dr. Rufus Wyman; and, coming from one of so high standing, and who had had especial opportunities of learning Dr. Wyman's eminent qualifications, it had great weight. A final vote of thanks to the Ward Committees for their services in obtaining subscriptions was passed at this meeting.

Feb. 2, 1817, an address to the public was adopted to obviate an impression that the Insane Hospital was designed exclusively for the wealthy. I have not seen a copy of this document. On Feb. 16, Messrs. Lowell, Quincy, Francis, and Barnard, a Committee of the Board, with Nathaniel Bowditch, Francis C. Lowell, and Peter C. Brooks, not of the Board, were requested to consider the expediency of, and to report a plan for the granting of annuities. Feb. 23, thanks were given to Mr. Phillips for his services in examining the title of the Joy Estate. Public notice was ordered that all subscriptions were payable on March 1. It was also stated that the Province

House had been leased at public auction for ninety-nine years. March 2, Messrs. Lowell, Barnard, and Quincy were appointed a Committee to select a site for a Hospital on the town's land near Almshouse, or elsewhere. Mr Bulfinch presented a written report on his visits to other Hospitals. March 9, the Treasurer was invited to attend all the meetings. Public notice was ordered on selection of superintendent for Asylum. The Committee on the subject of granting annuities reported against the measure. On March 16, 1817, the deed of Benjamin Joy was produced, and the Secretary ordered to buy a tin case to keep it in. It is still extant, and used for holding the title-deeds. Mr. Bulfinch presented a ground-plan for an Insane Hospital. The Committee, on March 23, reported that they had examined several sites, and were pleased with one in North Allen Street, and arranged that the Board should visit it. Mr. Lowell reported the rules and regulations for an Insane Asylum. Dr. George Parkman offered himself as candidate for physician of that institution; whose communication, with a model and several documents, was placed on file. Charles Bulfinch sent in a plan for a General Hospital. March 30, each Trustee approved of the site in Allen Street. The Committee were authorized to buy it at not over twenty thousand dollars, provided the title be good, and the street now laid out through the same be discontinued. If it could not be had on these terms, they were to apply for land west of the Almshouse. April 6, Drs. Samuel Danforth, Isaac Rand, John Jeffries, Lemuel Hayward, David Townsend, Thos. Welsh, Aaron Dexter, and Wm. Spooner, were chosen consulting physicians; Dr. James Jackson, acting physician; Dr. John C. Warren, acting surgeon. Dr. Jackson, in the office of consulting physician, continues to manifest an undiminished interest in the prosperity of the institution. Dr. Warren, after thirty-four years, yet holds his office. He bears lightly the age of more than " three-score and ten," and, like England's " Iron Duke," is still at his post of duty and of honor.*

April 20, 1817, Messrs. Lowell, Francis, and Quincy were instructed to prepare alterations and additions to the by-laws. A letter from Hon. William Phillips announced his readiness to pay his subscription of twenty thousand dollars, as soon as the town would discharge him, as executor of his father's will, from the five thousand dollars given thereby. On May 4, the Committee for building an Asylum reported in favor of two wings or buildings, seventy-six feet by forty, three stories high instead of one, and of brick instead of stone. Authority was given to buy

---

* The year 1852 brought to a close the life of the Duke of Wellington and the official labors of Dr. Warren.

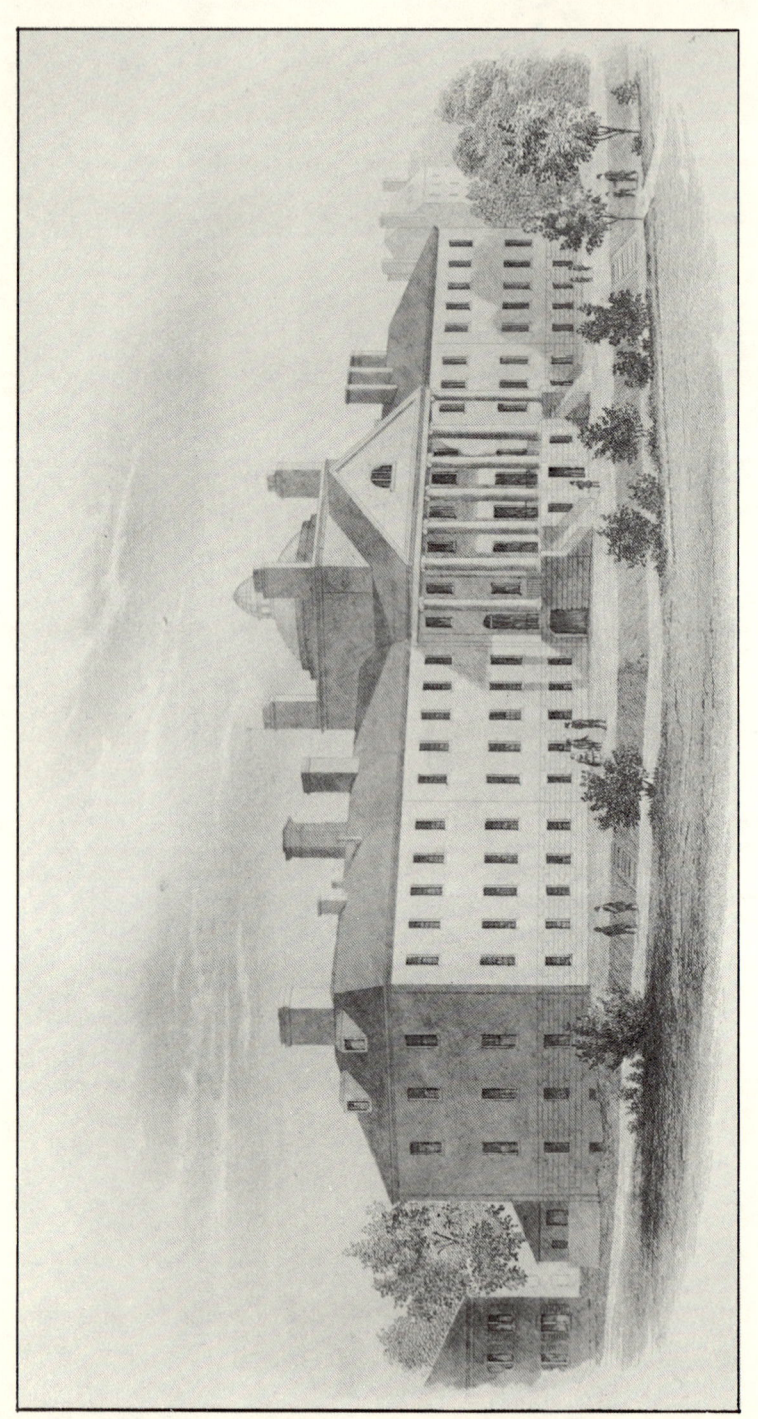

Massachusetts General Hospital, Boston

the Allen-street Estate at twenty thousand dollars, if the offer should be accepted in six days. On May 7, a Corporation meeting was held, at which rules and regulations were adopted for the Asylum for the Insane, which, as recorded, occupy ten large folio pages. At a Trustees' meeting, June 12, a letter from Mr. Quincy was received, with a written report from Benjamin Gorham, Esq., as to an uncertainty or defect in the title; and he was authorized to consult Hon. William Prescott. July 14, Messrs. Francis and Sears were added to this Committee with instructions; and, on Aug. 4, they were requested to apply to the city of Boston to close any streets which may pass through the land. Aug. 25, the Committee reported that they were informed that the street had not been legally laid out, and could be closed at any time; and they were authorized to buy the estate at a price not exceeding twenty-three thousand dollars. On Oct. 6, after various delays and negotiations, the Committee reported "the Allen-street purchase as substantially complete." Oct. 27, a Committee was appointed to apply to the selectmen to discontinue Bridge Street, laid out through this estate. Nov. 3, the Committee reported the draft of an advertisement, offering a hundred dollars' reward for a plan of a Hospital; also a circular letter to all the ministers of the gospel in the Commonwealth.

Nov. 24, a common seal was ordered to be prepared; and, on Nov. 30, Colonel May laid it before the Board, — the device being an Indian with his bow in one hand, and an arrow in the other; * and on his right a star, being encircled with the inscription, "MASSACHUSETTS GENERAL HOSPITAL, 1811;" and it was accepted accordingly. Dec. 7, it was ordered that the Hospital be " of stone, and *of that kind called granite.*" Jan. 4, 1818, several plans were received by the Board; and, on Jan. 11, referred to Messrs. Lowell, Quincy, and Francis.

The result of this period, then, was that subscriptions were secured to the amount required by the condition of the charter, and the estates were purchased where the two departments of the institution are now situated. The subscriptions had been extremely generous. William Phillips, as we have seen, increased his father's legacy of five thousand dollars to the sum of twenty thousand.† The importance of this donation can hardly be over-estimated. It encouraged the friends of the project, and awakened a corresponding liberality in others. It is not too much to say, that it was the one circumstance which insured the success of the undertaking. The

---

* This is the device of the seal of the Commonwealth.

† At the annual meeting of 1852, Dr. J. C. Warren mentioned that his father, Dr. John Warren, had written to Mr. Phillips on this subject, and had been consulted by Dr. James Jackson and himself, touching their circular letter of 1810.

Humane Society gave five thousand dollars; Messrs. James Perkins, Thomas H. Perkins, and David Sears, each gave the same sum.

There were in all one thousand and forty-seven subscribers, residing in Boston, Salem, Plymouth, Charlestown, Hingham, and Chelsea (including a few residents elsewhere); and 245 of this number, by giving one hundred dollars and upwards, became members of the Corporation. Several subscribed exclusively for the Hospital, and several exclusively for the Asylum, and some for both; and the amount actually expended on each separate branch of the institution subsequently exceeded the sum thus specially appropriated; so that the wishes of each donor have been complied with. A donation-book, prepared in 1828 by Colonel Joseph May, includes these subscriptions, and some subsequent ones, making in all the truly magnificent total of more than a hundred and forty thousand dollars.

The purchase of the Charlestown Estate was encumbered with divers conditions and provisions, a strict compliance with which is of the utmost importance. It is to be regretted that Mr. Joy should have deemed it necessary, for the adequate protection of his remaining adjoining estate, to impose these restrictions; *and it is unfortunate that the Committee should have accepted a deed with a condition capable of work-*

ing, in any possible event, a forfeiture of the estate. The lot is about five hundred feet wide by sixteen hundred feet in length, extending to the water, with the flats appurtenant. Upon it stood a dwelling-house, built by Joseph Barrell, Esq., a former owner, and which has been since enlarged and altered, and is now used as the residence for the Physicians and the Superintendent and their families. The two brick wings at first erected have since been enlarged by additions of the parts surmounted by domes, and constitute the present buildings used for the male and the female patients. The Building Committee, during this period, devoted much time and attention to the erection of these first edifices ; Mr. Francis visited the Hospitals of New York and Philadelphia. It was thought desirable that they should each communicate with the dwelling-house, and also that they should be as distant from each other as possible. They are therefore placed at diverging lines, which rendered the subsequent addition of the parts surmounted by domes extremely awkward; it being found impossible to continue them in the same direction, without interfering with the mansion-house. Mr. Barrell had planted two fine rows of elms, ranging from his mansion-house in the direction of the old wards. All of them were subsequently cut down at the suggestion of Dr. Wyman. It was once remarked in my hearing, that the buildings were erected to accommodate the trees, and then the trees cut down to accommodate the buildings. The ground falls off so rapidly that these wards are entered at the second story; and there are in them so many dark passages, so many ascents and descents, and so many turnings and twistings, that, should the oldest Trustee of the institution be suddenly left alone during a visit, he would probably be puzzled to know exactly where he was, or by what means he could best escape from the labyrinth around him.

The purchase of the land in Boston had been attended with great difficulties, and was a most fortunate arrangement for the institution. The five thousand dollars bequeathed by Mr. Phillips required that the Hospital should be within the limits of Boston, and would have been unavailable if the original requirement of the charter in that respect had not been repealed. Negotiations for the purchase of this estate were opened with James S. Colburn, Esq., acting for the Prince heirs, who were supposed to be sole owners; and he once or twice increased the price which he had originally demanded. It was then ascertained that certain others (heirs of the Wells family) had an interest which must be extinguished. A street which had been laid out for the benefit of the Canal Bridge, in continuation of Bridge Street, and respecting the laying out of which some informality had been discovered, was shut up. And still there remained a serious objection, that part of the land had been set off on execution in 1781, on a judgment for £741, against one Hezekiah Blanchard; the sheriff making a general return, that the appraisers were *appointed according to law*, instead of stating specially which of them was chosen by the creditor, debtor, and sheriff respectively. The land was appraised at only about half of the debt (£430). The debtor was for years afterwards supported by the creditor, and died a pauper, and was buried at his expense. Strong as was the equity of the case, the legal title of this lot (making an important part of the estate) was bad. Mr. Lowell, an excellent lawyer, and a most influential member of the Committee, was opposed to completing the purchase on the ground of this objection. Messrs. Francis, Quincy, and others of the Committee, were willing to take the risk. Mr. Lowell left for Europe, and his colleagues decided to buy. It is an interesting circumstance, that, just before the end of the forty years allowed by law, Charles G. Loring, Esq., was employed to institute a suit for Benjamin Gray and his sister, as the heirs of the old owner; which was favorably compromised, in part doubtless through Mr. Loring's good offices; the Hospital paying five hundred dollars, and an intervening warrantor paying five hundred more. This same demandant subsequently recovered an estate in Atkinson Street for breach of condition, under circumstances so inequitable, that the suit, as reported in the books (Gray *v.* Blanchard), is known as *the atrocious case ;* and the Court avowed that they intentionally postponed giving their opinion, in hopes that the delay would have led to a compromise. Mr. Gray knew no higher standard of right or of duty than " the statute in such case made and provided." He at first refused to accept the Hospital's offer of one thousand dollars. The case was opened to the jury; and Benjamin Gorham, Esq., counsel for the Hospital, began to exhibit him in so unenviable a light, that he intimated his readiness to take the sum offered. The case was thereupon withdrawn from the jury. But for this arrangement, the Hospital would have been put to great inconvenience, if not loss. This possible consequence certainly goes far to justify Mr. Lowell's objections, while the actual result fully warrants the decision of his associates.

This estate, independently of improvements, is now probably worth at least about three hundred thousand dollars. It cost less than a twelfth of that sum.

CHAPTER III.

1818–1822.

Thomas H. Perkins, Chairman.—Dr. Rufus Wyman chosen Physician of Asylum.—Corner-stone of Hospital laid, July 4, 1818.—Addresses on the Occasion.—Tax on Licenses asked for.—Colonel May, Chairman.—Address by Richard Sullivan, 1819.—Capuchin Chapel.—Death of James Prince, Treasurer.—Election and Death of William Cochran.—Election of N. P. Russell.—Death of James Perkins, Vice-President.—Tolls on Canal Bridge.—Nathaniel Fletcher, Superintendent of Hospital.—First Patient, Sept. 3, 1821.—Bequests of Thomas Oliver, Samuel Eliot, Beza Tucker, &c.—Donation of Horace Gray, &c.—Address to Public, 1822.—State of Finances, &c.

In 1818, the same Board of Trustees were re-elected; and at their first meeting, Jan. 25, Thomas H. Perkins was chosen Chairman. The Committee reported that the plan of a Hospital by Mr. Bulfinch deserved the premium; and the President and Vice-President were asked to attend at the next meeting, and give their advice as to the erecting at present a centre building and one wing. Messrs. William Phillips and James Perkins attended accordingly, Jan. 28, and signified their approval of this measure. On Feb. 1, Mr. Bulfinch's plan (with slight modifications suggested by the Committee) was adopted, and immediate measures were directed for getting stone hammered at the State Prison. A Committee was appointed to inquire as to insurance on the Asylum buildings, and also as to the powers of granting annuities. The Committee on this last subject reported on Feb. 15. Messrs. Lowell and Francis were appointed, March 1, to engage a person to superintend the erection of the Hospital. March 3, the Building Committee at the Asylum was ordered to have a foot-bridge constructed over the creek, in place of one recently destroyed by ice. Insurance against fire was ordered to the amount of ten thousand dollars. March 15, the Board decided that it is expedient to unite in one person the offices of Physician and Superintendent of the Asylum. March 22, it appeared that the Physicians and Surgeons of the Hospital recommended Dr. Rufus Wyman (Dr. George Parkman having withdrawn his application for that office); and he was nominated accordingly. Mr. Francis was appointed a Committee for erecting a wharf at the Hospital grounds. On March 23, Dr. Wyman was unanimously elected, and was authorized to visit New York and Philadelphia. March 29, the heirs of Hezekiah Blanchard made their claim for part of the Hospital land. On June 2, Dr. Wyman, having returned from his tour, made a verbal report. Messrs. Francis and Lowell, and the Treasurer, were appointed the Building Committee of the Hospital.

On July 1, the Treasurer, and Messrs. May and

Francis, were appointed a Committee to cause the corner-stone of the Hospital to be laid on July 4; and Mr. Quincy was requested to deliver the address on that occasion.

"On Saturday, the 4th day of July, the corner-stone of the Hospital in North Allen Street, in pursuance of the vote of the Trustees, was laid in Masonic form by the Grand Lodge of Massachusetts, in presence of his Excellency the Governor, his Honor the Lieutenant-Governor, the Honorable Council, many charitable societies, the Selectmen and Board of Health of the town of Boston, the members of the Corporation of the Massachusetts General Hospital, and a great concourse of citizens, who assembled to witness the ceremony.

"Under the stone was placed, in addition to a number of coins, a silver plate or tablet, whereon was engraved the following inscription: —

"The Corner-stone of this Edifice,
DESIGNED AS A GENERAL HOSPITAL, FOUNDED BY THE MUNIFICENCE OF THE COMMONWEALTH OF MASSACHUSETTS, AND OF MANY OF ITS LIBERAL CITIZENS, WAS LAID AT THE REQUEST OF THE TRUSTEES OF THE MASSACHUSETTS GENERAL HOSPITAL, BY THE GRAND LODGE OF MASSACHUSETTS,

FRANCIS J. OLIVER, Esq., Grand Master.
His Excellency JOHN BROOKS, Governor.
His Honor WILLIAM PHILLIPS, Lieut.-Governor, President of said Corporation, and a most munificent donor.
The Municipal and Military Officers of Boston assisting at the Ceremonies;
THIS FOURTH DAY OF JULY, A.D. MDCCCXVIII. AND OF THE INDEPENDENCE OF THE UNITED STATES, XLIII.
ANNO LUCIS, 5818."

The addresses of Mr. Oliver and Mr. Quincy were in every respect eminently appropriate to the occasion. That of the Grand Master, Mr. Oliver, was as follows : —

"In your hands [the Master-Builder] I now place these tools of your profession, and commit to your care the superintendence in erecting this edifice, whose foundation is now laid in the land of our fathers, in presence of sages and philanthropists, with their fervent prayers for a blessing on the work. Be cautious in selecting your materials, and use all your skill in putting them together, that your workmanship may endure like that of faithfulness and truth; for this building is not to be a temporary pavilion for the display of opulence, splendor, and pride, but a temple dedicated to humanity, a lazar-house built by enlightened Compassion, where CHARITY and PHILOSOPHY are to walk a perpetual round to alleviate misery, and to combat with and destroy disease and pain.

"To secure your constant attention and highest exertions in this undertaking, you must keep in mind the noble purposes to which it is to be appropriated. It will be a testimonial of the liberality of this Commonwealth and the munificence of opulent individuals, — a sort of mile-stone on the journey of civilization, to show how far the Christian spirit had advanced in this age, in ameliorating the condition of man.

"The golden age, when men were happy and free from crime, lives only in fable; but a religious and humane age, amidst crime and wretchedness, shall be matter of sober history.

"If he who gives a cup of cold water to the thirsty, with a charitable disposition, has already the promises of the gospel, how great will be the reward of those generous souls who create a perennial flow of all the healing balms and cordials that touch the lips or bathe the limbs of decrepitude and sickness.

"As this institution will long exist a proof of the liberality of feeling and purity of sentiment of the people of this day, and an example for future times, go on, Sir, and erect this building with taste, science, and fidelity, that it may be a model for the architects of a distant period; so that future master-builders may come and admire your work for its strength, beauty, and durability.

"If you commence your work in hope, and perform it with assiduity, prosperity will attend, and self-satisfaction, with the applauses of the wise and good, will crown your toils. Yours is no small or trifling trust; do your duty in this, and in all your hands find to do, in such a manner that the great Architect of time and eternity will number you among his master workmen who have happily toiled for the bread of life."

To which the master-builder replied: —

"Most Worshipful Sir,

"I accept these tools of my profession with diffidence but pleasure; and I promise to use my best endeavors to follow your advice and remember your instructions. The recollection of the importance of this institution, and the desire I feel to obtain the approbation of its patrons, will, I trust, stimulate me in the discharge of my duties. Whatever science or skill I possess shall be sedulously devoted to this work. As the corner-stone of the edifice is now laid in the full faith of the great advantages which are to flow from this institution, and with all holy and proper rites, it shall now be my earnest desire and constant exertion, that industry, harmony, and good fellowship shall prevail among the craftsmen, that the work shall proceed with despatch, and be finished in good time for the reception of such as it is intended to accommodate.

"The belief that the good feelings and wishes of the pious and benevolent are with me in this undertaking will strengthen my hands and encourage my heart, *for the prayer of the righteous availeth much.*"

The address of Mr. Quincy was as follows: —

"May it please your Excellency; — Gentlemen of the Masonic, Gentlemen of the Mechanic, Associations; — Fellow-citizens: — I am requested by the Trustees of the Massachusetts General Hospital to express to you, Sir, — to the officers and members of these respectable fraternities, — and to our fellow-citizens in general, their congratulations on this interesting occasion. You and they will be pleased to accept the thanks of the Trustees for the countenance and aid you have given this institution, by thus condescending to assist in laying its foundations, according to the rules of art, and with those solemn and mysterious forms and ceremonies which ancient wisdom has prescribed.

"Indeed, Sir and Gentlemen, the foundations of a noble charity have this day been laid; — a charity, destined to confer lasting blessings on future times, as it has already conferred immortal honor on the present; — a charity, of which it well becomes a citizen of Massachusetts to speak in the language of pride and exultation. For of what can the patriot be more justly proud than of witnessing in a community virtuous principles, emanating in generous efforts, and generous efforts crowned with resplendent success? When can exultation be more natural or suitable than on beholding the seed, which the common labor of the community has scattered, upspringing from the soil, bearing on its trunk and on its branches the pregnant promise of fruit and shade?

"In reference to this institution, it has been the happiness of the Trustees to witness among their fellow-citizens a zeal co-operating with its design and patronizing its establishment, as laudable as it has been exemplary, and not less encouraging than it has been honorable. They have seen individuals distinguished at once for wealth and liberality, surpassing all former records of benevolence in this country, and subscribing to their funds sums which in point of amount have seldom been equalled by individual subscription in any country, on any occasion. They have seen all classes of their citizens combining and concentrating their efforts, and the irresistible force of public opinion applied, not, as has happened in other countries, to destroy, but to found and erect institutions destined to be the refuge of the afflicted; and to provide relief and extend protection to those who labor under the most awful and humiliating misfortunes to which man is subject.

"These are efforts, of which he who loves his country may justly be proud. These are objects which the eye of the philanthropist delights to contemplate. These are scenes, amid which virtue and piety rejoice to dwell. These are honors which eloquence and history will not cease to celebrate, long after every other memorial of the present generation shall have passed away.

"But, may it please your Excellency, it ought not to be concealed on the present occasion, that, notwithstanding the donations on which this charity has been founded are great, yet that the necessities of the unfortunate and of this institution are still greater. It belongs to the occasion to state, that the funds already placed at the disposal of the Trustees will scarcely more than suffice to enable them to complete the Asylum for the Insane, and also two principal parts of the building destined for the General Hospital; leaving it to the sympathy of the Legislature and of the community to provide for the completion of the remaining third part of the building, and for the annual support of the establishment.

"Encouraged by the liberality and favor already displayed by their fellow-citizens and by the Legislature of the Commonwealth, and anxious, on their part, to fulfil the duties imposed on them in the spirit which the munificence of the public seemed to justify and to demand, the Trustees have deemed themselves compelled to commence their institution upon a scale and on a system coinciding less with the immediate state of the funds, than with the anticipated exigencies of society; assured that the liberality of the State and of individuals will not fail to complete an undertaking commenced under such honorable and happy auspices; relying that every want which shall occur will be supplied as well from the interesting and commanding nature of all the charities concentrated in their institution, as from the just and deep sympathies for its success which prevail in the community.

"To that sympathy, to the same noble and elevated sentiment, to which we are indebted for its conception, and, thus far, for its establishment, we confidently rely for its future support.

"To you, Sir, as the head and representative of this great Commonwealth, — to our fellow-citizens at large, — to all the wise, the liberal, the virtuous, and pious men of our country, we cheerfully commit its destinies; asking only of them, and of the Legislature of the Commonwealth, that the same munificent spirit which founded, may still preside over it, that it may thus be enabled to develop all its usefulness, and continue to be, what it now is, a monument of the wisdom, the liberality, and humanity of the rulers and citizens of Massachusetts."

The ceremonies were concluded by the following remarks from James Prince, Esq., the Treasurer of the institution: —

"Fellow-citizens, — The purposes for which we have assembled being accomplished, the moment of our separation from this now interesting spot has arrived. Let us, however, under those impressions which the occasion so forcibly inspires, in retiring, turn our thoughts from earth to heaven, and again implore the God and Father of all graciously to permit the top-stone of this intended edifice to be laid in love, in order, and without accident, as at this beginning; and to bestow the choicest of his blessings upon all those who have been, or who hereafter may be, donors to this humane establishment, not only in this world, but in that which is to come. Amen."

His Excellency, the Trustees, and other invited guests, then proceeded to the house of the Treasurer, Mr. Prince, and partook of a collation. The attendance was very numerous. Those who could not get into the house were accommodated in the garden. It was a scene of joyous festivity. "It was a great day," said one who was present, "for Marshal Prince," as it certainly was for the institution. Like the Union, with whose birthday its foundation is thus associated, may its benefits be ever more and more widely felt;

and may it continue to the latest times to afford its protection, and extend its welcome alike to the citizen and to the stranger who cometh among us!

On July 3, 1818, Joseph Head, Esq., one of the executors of Thomas Oliver, of Boston, merchant, announced that he had made this institution his residuary devisee. This bequest was gratefully accepted by the Trustees; and Messrs. Lowell and Francis were appointed a Committee on the subject.

This legacy exceeded twenty-four thousand dollars. A portrait of Mr. Oliver was subsequently given, which was placed in the Trustees' room at the Hospital. The institution is especially indebted to Mr. Head for this bequest, as the testator wished to bestow his property on him and his family; and it was solely in consequence of his truly disinterested advice, that Mr. Oliver made the Hospital the object of his bounty, after his wife's decease. The widow married again, and lived till July, 1835, enjoying till her death the income or interest of the estate. The Hospital received the property in 1826, and paid her from that time an annuity of thirteen hundred dollars.

On July 13, thanks were voted to the Grand Lodge of Massachusetts for their assistance at the ceremonies of the laying of the corner-stone. Sept. 1, Mr. Francis was appointed a Committee to advise with the Treasurer respecting the disposal of the funds. Detailed rules were adopted for admission of patients at the Asylum, and ordered to be printed. On Sept. 8, further rules and regulations for the general government of the Asylum were adopted. The Committee on Mr. Oliver's bequest reported that his widow is to have all the property, real and personal, for life; and consented to the immediate sale of land in Middle Street and Prince Street devised by him. On Sept. 15, 1818, Visiting Committees were arranged, each to be of three members, and to serve for three months; Messrs. Sullivan, Sargent, and Francis being the Committee for the next ensuing months of October, November, and December. Sept. 19, the Treasurer was authorized to borrow ten thousand dollars. Oct. 27, he was ordered, on account of the straitened means of the institution, to call in all debts due for subscriptions or otherwise. Nov. 15, the Visiting Committee were directed to hasten the delivery of the stone from State Prison, "that the roof of the Hospital may be covered in as soon as possible."

Nov. 23, the Visiting Committee report nine patients received at Asylum. Mr. Francis states that he well remembers the admission of the first patient. A father asked to have his son received as an inmate; and the Committee spent three hours in conversing with him, in order to learn all the particulars of the case. He informed them that he believed his son to be one of those spoken of in the Bible as "possessed with a devil;" and, when asked what remedial measures he had adopted, replied that he was in the habit of whipping him. The young man was entirely cured, and became subsequently a pedler, in which vocation he displayed so much Yankee shrewdness, that he acquired a property of ten or twelve thousand dollars. Three hours' deliberation on the admission of each patient would hardly be found practicable in these later times, when the institution numbers two hundred inmates. The Trustees, however, always scrupulously require a medical certificate as to the fact of insanity.

Dec. 20, voted that Messrs. Lowell, Quincy, and Coolidge be a Committee to wait on James Prince, Esq., Treasurer of the Corporation, to express the regret of this Board at learning his intention to resign, " their unanimous sense of his very able and zealous services," and their wish that he would consent to serve at least another year. With this request he complied, and remained in office till his death. The temperance reform had not as yet commenced, and a Committee was appointed to ask for a grant of " a tax on licenses to sell spirituous liquors." The Board of Visitors made a visit to the Asylum, by invitation of the Trustees, and are reported to the Board as having " expressed much satisfaction at the promising state of the institution." Messrs. Lowell and Quincy were appointed a Committee to confer with the Lechmere Point Corporation, on the subject of the " officers of the Hospital being permitted to pass their bridge free of toll." Dec. 27, the Treasurer furnished " a very judicious plan for keeping the accounts of the Asylum." Jan. 3, 1819, a Committee of five was appointed to get the signatures of individuals to the petition for a tax on licenses. Jan. 24, 1819, the Treasurer reported that he had borrowed a further sum of eleven hundred dollars, and was authorized to borrow five thousand more.

At the annual meeting, Jan. 19, Peter C. Brooks was elected a Trustee in place of Thomas H. Perkins, Esq., but declined serving. The thanks of the Corporation were presented to Colonel Perkins for his long and faithful services as Trustee. At this annual meeting, Mr. Francis, as Chairman of the Committee to examine the Treasurer's accounts, reported the property of the institution, exclusive of the Province House, at $4,188, " which would be far short of the sum necessary to complete the buildings." A Committee of seven was appointed to procure subscriptions for an historical picture, to be painted by Mr. Allston, and to be the property of the Hospital. No such picture was ever painted. Jan. 31, Colonel May was elected Chairman of the Trustees. Feb. 21, the town of Concord was thanked for its liberal donation. Feb. 28, Dr. Wyman's salary was fixed at fifteen hundred dollars. March 21, Mr. Francis was appointed a Committee to ascertain the cost of finishing the Hospital; and Messrs. Lowell, Sullivan, and Francis were appointed a Committee to arrange a plan for laying out the grounds at the Asylum. April 2, reports were presented of a very favorable character as to Dr. Wyman, and stating that his assistants had behaved "with all due humanity and attention." The whole number of patients was stated to be six females, nine males. April 4, the Acting Physician and Surgeon were re-elected. Of the eight Consulting Physicians, the only change was the election of Dr. James Mann, in place of Dr. Danforth, who, it is believed, was dead. April 11, Mr. Francis reported that $4,557.43 would finish the Hospital in a plain, simple style.

It was voted to apply to the Canal Bridge, "requesting such an extension of their order, as that the Trustees, Physicians, and all persons actually employed in the Asylum, when passing the bridge on the business of said institution, shall pass the same free of toll." May 2, the Treasurer was authorized to raise a sufficient sum to pay off the debts of the Corporation, by obtaining a loan, &c. May 18, a Committee was appointed to make arrangements for a public address to be delivered during the session of Legislature, on the progress and present state of the institution. A vote of the Directors of the Canal Bridge, relative to payment of toll by officers of the Asylum, was read and placed on file. It granted the privilege asked for, which accordingly has ever since been enjoyed, though of late years called in question.

June 1, 1819, the Committee reported that Thursday next, at 4 o'clock, was appointed for the delivery of an address by Richard Sullivan, Esq.; and that the Governor, Lieutenant-Governor, Council, Senate, and House of Representatives, had been invited to attend.

"On Thursday, June 3, the Trustees assembled at State House, where a procession was formed, consisting of the Civil Government of the Commonwealth, the Board of Visitors, Corporation, Trustees, Physicians, and Surgeons of the institution, reverend clergy, and citizens; who proceeded to King's Chapel, where, after appropriate prayers by Rev. Dr. James Freeman, and music by a select choir of amateurs, an elegant, feeling, and persuasive address was delivered by Richard Sullivan, Esq., on the utility and progress of the combined institution."

This address was published by order of the Trustees, and forms a pamphlet of twenty-one pages, containing, in an appendix of eleven pages, letters of physicians, &c., some of which had been published with the address of 1816.

July 1, Tristram Barnard having resigned, and Mr. Brooks declined, Joseph Head and Thomas W. Ward were elected by the Trustees to fill these vacancies. Thanks were presented to Mr. William H. Lane for the present of a mahogany medicine case, valued at two hundred dollars. July 6, a very cordial vote of thanks was passed, and ordered to be sent to Mr. Barnard. Depositions, in *perpetuance* of Mr. Prince and his sister Mrs. Tucker, were ordered to be taken as to the Allen-street Estate. Aug. 17, an invoice of medicines and shop-furniture ($111.20) was presented by Dr. Wyman, and suitably acknowledged. Oct. 7, the Treasurer was authorized to borrow one thousand dollars from Mr. Head, and five hundred each from Mr. Francis and Mr. Coolidge; and a Committee was appointed to solicit new subscriptions.

Oct. 19, David Sears resigned; and, on Nov. 2, Samuel Appleton was elected in his stead. The Committee on Subscriptions reported an address to the public, which was ordered to be printed. I have not seen a copy of this document. A bequest of four hundred dollars from Polly Russell, of Charlestown, is credited on the Treasurer's books. In November, the Treasurer was authorized to obtain a loan of six thousand dollars. Dec. 19, the Committee for subscriptions reported that " their success had been satisfactory." Benjamin Wiggin, Esq., offered a celebrated picture, " The Capuchin Chapel," to be exhibited for benefit of the Hospital, and was thanked for " his very generous offer." Jan. 6, 1820, Mr. William Hall presented " his patent for sweeping chimneys," to be used in the Hospital.

Jan. 23, the same Board of Trustees were re-elected on the part of the Corporation. Jan. 30, the munificent bequest of Mr. Samuel Eliot, of ten thousand dollars, for the use of the Asylum, was communicated by Mr. Lowell, one of the executors. Feb. 6, Messrs. Head and Francis made a detailed report on the accounts kept at the Asylum, recommending the employment of a person to post the books. On Feb. 20, John Belknap was elected a Trustee by the Board of Visitors, in place of Hon. John Lowell, resigned. March 19, a proposition to endeavor to effect a loan for finishing the Hospital was discussed. April 9, the Treasurer and Messrs. Francis and Coolidge were appointed a Committee " to proceed in finishing the Hospital." On April 18, a formal announcement of Mr. Eliot's bequest, and of the executor's readiness to pay the same, was received; and the donation was gratefully accepted by the Trustees. In amount it was surpassed only by the gifts of Mr. Phillips and Mr. Oliver. At this meeting a Committee was also appointed to thank Mr.

Wiggin for the $1,604, net proceeds of the exhibition of his picture.

May 2, Mr. Francis reported that the Committee had engaged workmen, procured materials, and employed James M'Allister to superintend the completion of the Hospital. June 6, the Trustees declined applying to the Legislature in aid of a project for a lottery, a portion of the profits of which were to be for the use of the Hospital. June 20, an extract from the will of Beza Tucker was read, giving a brick dwelling-house and land in a court leading from Boylston Street, now Boylston Place; and the Treasurer was ordered to receive the same, and to make suitable acknowledgments therefor. It was then worth about six thousand dollars, and was sold in 1827 for $5,350. Dr. Wyman was requested to assist the Building Committee of the Hospital. Mr. Francis resigned the office of Trustee, and, on July 19, his resignation was accepted; but he was requested still to advise and assist the Committee in finishing the Hospital. Oct. 5, it appeared that several elopements from the Asylum had occurred, and a Committee was appointed on the subject of measures proper to prevent the same. Oct. 22, the Building Committee were ordered to take measures to erect the western wing of Hospital in the ensuing spring. They reported that the centre and easterly wing were now nearly finished, but that it was inexpedient to open the Hospital immediately for the reception of patients. Nov. 19, blanks were ordered for admission of patients at Hospital, and a supply of necessary furniture.

Jan. 4, 1821, applications were received for office of Superintendent of Hospital, with recommendations. On Jan. 21, the existing Board of Trustees were re-elected; Mr. Francis being again chosen a member, notwithstanding his recent resignation. But, Mr. Quincy having declined, the Board of Visitors elected Daniel P. Parker, Esq. On Feb. 11, "the Chairman communicated to the Board, intelligence of the decease, yesterday, of James Prince, Esq., late Treasurer of the Massachusetts General Hospital and of the Provident Institution for Savings in the town of Boston, and Marshal of the District of Massachusetts. The exemplary zeal, activity, faithfulness, and punctuality, displayed by Mr. Prince in promoting the objects of this institution, were called to mind by the Trustees, and his disinterested exertions considered as entitling him to the grateful remembrance of the charitable and humane." Mr. Francis says that he was a most able and efficient officer, and that without his assistance the purchase of the Allen-street Estate could not have been effected.

At this meeting, Feb. 11, it was ordered that Visiting Committees should hereafter consist of two instead of three members, and the term of service of each Committee be two months instead of four. Feb. 25, William Cochran, Esq., the new Treasurer, elected on the 20th instant, was qualified. March 4, twenty-two applications were received and read for offices of Superintendent and Matron of Hospital. At the annual meeting, March 21, 1821, a new draft of by-laws, as reported by Colonel May and the Secretary, was adopted and recorded. March 21, Messrs. May, Sullivan, and the Secretary, were appointed a Committee on the rules and regulations for the Hospital. April 1, Capt. Nathaniel Fletcher and his wife were elected Superintendent and Matron of the Hospital. On April 29, it was voted to discontinue meetings on Sunday; which, however, were resumed in 1822. June 19, thanks were given to the Boston Manufacturing Company for a donation of three bales of sheetings. July 5, twenty-eight patients were reported as inmates of the Asylum; and rules and regulations were adopted for the Hospital, and recorded *in extenso*.

Aug. 21, notice was ordered to Drs. Jackson and Warren that the Hospital will be ready for patients on Sept. 1. On Sept. 3, one patient was admitted; and, until Sept. 20, not a single other application was made for admission. Sept. 4, Dr. Warren attended, and was requested to draft an address to the public.

A communication was received from Mr. Greenough, in regard to paying the capital sum as provided for in his lease of Province House. A Committee on the subject (Messrs. Francis, Sargent, and Sullivan) were appointed, who, at the next meeting, reported in favor of receiving the same. At a Corporation meeting, Sept. 21, N. P. Russell, Esq., was elected Treasurer, in place of Mr. Cochran, deceased. Oct. 4, Dr. Jackson nominated, as his assistant, Dr. Walter Channing. The Treasurer was authorized to borrow five thousand dollars. Oct. 11, Dr. Joshua Green was appointed Apothecary. Nov. 6, it appeared that ten patients had been received at the. Hospital, three discharged, one cured, and one relieved. Dec. 4, the title of the flats at the foot of Allen Street was ordered to be investigated, in reference to an alleged trespass by Charles Taylor, Esq. This strip of flats seems to have been conveyed to Mr. Taylor by the Hospital in 1822. On Dec. 23, a model of a machine, called a "gout-frame," invented by Mr. Joseph Trumball for the purpose of moving helpless people to and from bed, was presented. Messrs. Sullivan, Ward, and Bradford were appointed a Committee to prepare the annual report. Jan. 10, 1822, six free beds were established; three for medical, three for surgical patients.

At the Corporation meeting, Jan. 15, 1822, the Board of Trustees were thanked for their zealous and faithful services during the past year; and the same Trustees were re-elected, except that Theodore Lyman, jun., was chosen in place of Daniel Sargent, Esq. Drs. Warren and Jackson, Mr. Fletcher and Dr. Wyman, were severally re-elected to their offices. The Consulting Physicians were Drs. Isaac Rand, David Townsend, Thomas Welch, Aaron Dexter, William Spooner, James Mann; also, Drs. Joshua Fisher of Beverly, and Amos Holbrook of Milton. On Feb. 24, Mr. Sullivan, Drs. Warren, Jackson, and Wyman, and Mr. Lyman, were appointed a Committee to prepare a description and general account of the two departments of the Hospital; and it was ordered that one thousand copies be printed for distribution. On March 10, the same, as reported by Mr. Lyman, was, with some trifling amendments, accepted. On March 14, it was voted to be inexpedient *at present* to publish with said document a list of the subscribers and benefactors. Five strong rooms were ordered to be built " for raging female patients." March 24, the Committee reported that two thousand copies of their address had been printed.

April 21, a donation of a thousand dollars was received from Mr. Horace Gray, and three hundred from the Massachusetts Charitable Fire Society. The Building Committee were ordered to take measures for finishing the portico or pediment of the Hospital.

May 5, an anonymous letter, enclosing ten dollars, was received, and ordered to be published in the newspapers. May 19, notice was given of a bequest of Captain Seth Webber, who lately died in Liverpool, of one thousand dollars to the *Marine Hospital* in Boston, believed to be designed for this institution. Aug. 4, the Chairman stated the decease of James Perkins, Esq., " Vice-President of this institution, and one of its most munificent benefactors; " and that he, with others of the Board, attended his funeral yesterday. Sept. 1, a nomination of an Apothecary, as successor to Dr. Green, was made by the Physician and Surgeon ; and they were requested " *to withdraw the same, and to nominate some other person.*" The Treasurer was authorized to borrow five hundred dollars. Sept. 10, James M. Whittemore was nominated and appointed Apothecary. Oct. 10, twelve males, seven females, in Hospital. Dr. Jackson attended, and suggested certain regulations respecting nurses and attendants, with a view to the better preservation of order and quiet. The Visiting Committee were directed to inquire as to the expediency of excluding syphilitic patients. Nov. 3, the widow of Thomas Oliver being disposed to buy the furniture of her husband, of which she had the use for life, Mr. Head was authorized to do what he should " deem proper and liberal." He sold it to her for five hundred dollars. Nov. 10, a bedstead and other articles, made expressly for the late Abraham Touro during his illness, were presented by his sister. Dec. 1, the thanks of the Board were presented to the executors and residuary devisees of Captain Seth Webber, for their voluntary payment of his recent legacy of one thousand dollars; the same having been now received. Additional rules and regulations for the Asylum, &c., were adopted. Messrs. Coolidge and May were appointed a Committee to wait on Hon. William Phillips, to request him to sit for his portrait. This portrait by Stuart is, it is needless to say, a fine painting and an excellent likeness. Dec. 15, Samuel Appleton resigned his office of Trustee. On Jan. 7, 1823, Messrs. Sullivan, Phillips, and Coolidge were appointed a Committee to prepare the annual report.

The address to the public in 1822 is a pamphlet of thirty-four pages, signed by all the twelve Trustees, and is a very full and interesting summary of all that had been done for the institution, and its position and prospects at that time. It is believed to have been from the pen of Mr. Lyman. Letters from Drs. Jackson and Warren, and a report from Dr. Wyman, are embodied in it. The property of the institution is stated as follows: —

The Province House	$40,000.00
Boylston Place House	6,000.00
General donations in money	28,599.87
	$74,599.87
Donations specially for Hospital	73,809.29
„ „ for Asylum	53,997.47
Making the grand total of	$202,406.63
The cost of the Hospital-land and building being	$94,352.29
„ „ Asylum-land „ „ „	89,821.16
	$184,173.45

The debts of the institution being $19,850, and the income of its property not enough to pay the salaries.

The buildings of both departments had, however, been opened to patients; and they had been placed under the charge of two gentlemen, Dr. Wyman and Mr. Fletcher, who were admirably fitted for their respective posts. The one, indeed, was soon removed from us by a sudden and lamented death. The other, for many years afterwards, with an ever-increasing reputation and success, won for himself, while living, the most unbounded confidence and respect, and has left to his children an honored name, — the most precious of all legacies.

CHAPTER IV.

January, 1823, to June, 1827.

Mummy from Thebes. — Fifty Thousand Dollars invested in Massachusetts Hospital Life Insurance Company. — West Wing of Hospital finished. — Debt created. — Bequest of John M'Lean, over One Hundred Thousand Dollars. — Legacies of Abraham Touro, Eleanor Davis, &c. — Death of Mr. Fletcher — Nathan Gurney elected Superintendent. — Gift of a Sow. — Lafayette. — Annual Free Beds. — Portraits of Benefactors. — Col. May resigns. — Joseph Head Chairman. — Erysipelas at Hospital. — Patients removed. — Measures in Honor of John M'Lean. — Value of his Bequest as compared with Life Insurance Charters.

At the annual meeting in January, 1823, the Trustees reported that the funds had been increased $4,238.50 by donations; that the interior of the west wing of the Hospital was finished, and ready for occupation; and that the colonnade in front would be raised in the ensuing season. Three new Trustees were now elected; viz. Benjamin Guild and William H. Prescott chosen by the Corporation, and Gardiner Greene by the Board of Visitors, in the place of Richard Sullivan, Samuel Appleton, and John Belknap. Mr. Appleton had contributed two thousand dollars at the commencement of the establishment, and was thus one of the most liberal of its early benefactors. Mr. Belknap has taken great interest in the institution to the present time. He attends all the annual meetings; and, indeed, he and two or three others are generally the only representatives of the public on those occasions Mr. Sullivan, as Secretary and Trustee, had been connected with the Hospital from its foundation, and, as we have seen, had in 1819 delivered a public address in its behalf. The Board now consisted of Messrs. Joseph May, Chairman; Ebenezer Francis, Thomas W. Ward, Benjamin Guild, Gamaliel Bradford, Joseph Head, Theodore Lyman, jun., William H. Prescott, Joseph Coolidge, Daniel P. Parker, Jonathan Phillips, and Gardiner Greene. On Jan. 7, 1823, Messrs. Francis, Parker, and May, with the Treasurer and Secretary, were appointed a Committee on the subject of the Hospital's right to grant annuities, and at the next meeting reported the agreement with the Life Insurance Company, which was subsequently sanctioned by the Legislature in 1824. Feb. 2, Messrs. Head, Francis, and Greene were appointed a Committee to subscribe for stock in the Massachusetts Hospital Life Insurance Company, not exceeding fifty thousand dollars. The Committee subscribed for the whole sum named. It has proved a most fortunate investment, now yielding nine per cent interest.

Eight Consulting Physicians were chosen, — Drs. John G. Coffin, John Dixwell, and John Gorham, taking the place of Drs. Rand, Fisher, and Holbrook.

Feb. 23, the Treasurer was authorized to borrow ten thousand dollars. Messrs. Lyman and Guild were appointed a Committee for collecting a library for each department of the institution. March 9, a donation of three hundred dollars for the use of the Asylum was offered and accepted on condition, that, if the donor were ever subsequently to need it, the same should be repaid to him without interest. March 23, one hundred dollars more was offered and accepted on the same condition. Dr. Whittemore resigning, Mr. Benjamin Barrett was elected Apothecary. May 4, a mummy from Thebes was presented by Bryant P. Tilden and Robert B. Edes, in behalf of Jacob Van Lennep and Company, of Smyrna (the Hospital paying two hundred dollars out of the proceeds of its exhibition to the Boston Dispensary), which was gratefully accepted. This mummy is now an appropriate ornament of the operating room at the Hospital. May 18, Samuel Swett, Esq., was elected Trustee, in place of Gamaliel Bradford, who resigned. June 1. a donation of books, of the value of fifty dollars. transmitted through Dr. Warren, was presented, with a catalogue. July 8, Messrs. Francis and Guild were appointed a Committee to attend to the suit of Hezekiah Blanchard's heirs. This related to the claim before alluded to.

On July 23, the Treasurer was authorized to receive the legacy of Abraham Touro. It was the extremely liberal sum of ten thousand dollars. On Aug. 10, the donor of the four hundred dollars *on condition* was declared to be Mr. Lambert, of Roxbury, then deceased. Aug. 24, Charles W. Chauncey was chosen Apothecary, Mr. Barrett having resigned. A rule was adopted, which has since proved very salutary, to charge board for the whole quarter in all cases of insane patients removed by friends before the expiration of the quarter, and against the advice of the Physician. Sept. 9, a vote passed authorizing the borrowing of thirty thousand dollars, and, on Sept. 21, five thousand more, both on mortgage of the Province House Estate and Boylston Place House. Oct. 7, the Committee reported that they had *leased* the mummy one year for exhibition in other cities. The Chairman reported that the portrait of the President was finished; and, on Oct. 10, it was received. The west wing of the Hospital was now ready for patients.

Nov. 2, 1823, the gratifying announcement was made of a bequest from John M'Lean, of twenty-five thousand dollars, payable on death of his widow, and with the information that he had also made this institution his residuary legatee, by which " a much larger sum " would be secured. This residue proved to be over ninety thousand dollars. Mr. M'Lean was a truly noble specimen of a Boston merchant. Having many years before failed in business, he settled with all his creditors, and obtained a full discharge. Soon afterwards, by the safe arrival, as I believe, of a vessel supposed to have been lost, he retrieved his affairs. He forthwith called a meeting of his creditors, and paid to each of them the balance due, both principal and interest.

Nov. 23, Dr. John B. Brown was chosen Assistant Surgeon, on nomination of Dr. Warren. The office of Steward was created at the Asylum, to relieve Dr. Wyman of part of his duties; and John M. Goodwin was elected. A Committee was appointed to obtain a portrait of Mr. M‘Lean, and to report on the expediency of obtaining portraits of other liberal donors. Dec. 7, Messrs. May, Greene, and Francis, with the Treasurer and Secretary, were appointed a Committee to make a settlement with the executors of Mr. M‘Lean. The Secretary was subsequently discharged, and Mr. Guild appointed in his place. The Asylum was represented as being full, and several applications for admittance declined for that reason. The Committee for obtaining Mr. M‘Lean's portrait were also charged with procuring a portrait of the late Samuel Eliot. Jan. 6, the Treasurer was authorized to borrow six thousand dollars. Messrs. May and Francis were appointed a Committee to settle Mr. M‘Allister's accounts.

At the meeting of the Corporation in January, 1824, Mr. Lyman presented the report,* noticing in suitable terms the recent munificent bequest of John M'Lean, Esq. Dr. Jackson and Mr. Francis were appointed a Committee as to an alteration in the time of the annual meeting; and this Committee reported subsequently in favor of meeting on the second Wednesday of June, which report was accepted, so that the Trustees now chosen served a year and a half. Edward Tuckerman was elected Trustee in place of William H. Prescott. Feb. 1, a letter from Dr. Coffin was received, resigning his office of Consulting Physician, and making some observations on the offices of Attending Physician and Surgeon. Feb. 8, Messrs. Francis and Guild were appointed a Committee on the settlement of accounts by the executors of Mr. M'Lean, as to the amount charged for commissions, and the investment of the trust-fund.

In the ninth volume of Pickering's Reports, page 447, is a report of the suit brought by Harvard College and the Hospital, *v.* the surviving Trustee under Mr. M'Lean's will; in which the Court decided that the Trustees had the right to select any stocks they pleased for the trust-fund. They had appropriated to this object insurance stock, entitled to

---

* No copy of this Report was supposed to be extant; but one has been discovered.

large foreign claims, and manufacturing stocks, which shortly afterwards made large dividends for sale of patent rights and patterns and machinery. The two Corporations had offered to pay six per cent interest to the widow (three thousand dollars a year) in December, 1823; but their proposal was declined. The ultimate value of the trust-property received on the decease of Mrs. M'Lean, in the year 1834, was thus reduced to less than twenty thousand dollars for each of the two Corporations, while she herself received an income probably averaging twelve per cent per annum. It is believed that every Trustee of the Hospital and every Corporator of the College coincided in opinion, that this investment of the trust-funds, though adjudged to be legal, was not made in the exercise of a sound discretion, and with a due regard to the rights of all parties.

Feb. 20, a patient was dismissed by the Visiting Committee " for having introduced liquor privately." Feb. 24, Messrs. Francis and Head were appointed a Committee to advise and direct the Treasurer in the investment of sums of money he may receive. April 6, Messrs. Francis and Russell were appointed a Committee on the mode of keeping the accounts with the Superintendent. April 9, thanks were given to Gorham Parsons, Esq., "*for the present of a sow of an uncommonly fine breed.*" Her weight, in the Visiting Committee's records, is stated at 273 pounds. As this gift is noticed in both records, it evidently made a great sensation. May 2, notice was given of a settlement of Gray's suit by a judgment in favor of Hospital by consent, and a payment of five hundred dollars. June 6, a cold and warm salt-water bathing-house was ordered to be erected at the Hospital. Aug. 15, Dr. Henry Lane was elected Apothecary, in place of Dr. Chauncey, who resigned. The Humane Society announced their intention of giving enough annually to support six free beds; which generous proposal was gratefully acknowledged and accepted.

Sept. 26. the profits of the exhibition of the mummy are stated to be fifteen hundred dollars. The donation-book, probably deducting certain charges and the payment to the Dispensary, makes the sum but little less than twelve hundred dollars. Dec. 19, Messrs. Francis, Parker, and Lyman were appointed a Committee to consider the expediency of erecting an additional building at the Asylum. Dec. 31, thirty-two males and twelve females in Hospital: total, forty-four.

At the annual meeting of the Corporation, Jan. 7, 1825, no change was made in the Board of Trustees for this year. Jan. 7, Committees were appointed to procure portraits of Mr. Oliver and Mr. Touro.

The portrait of John M'Lean was brought in at this meeting. It is one of the happiest works of Stuart. The record says of this painting, "The resemblance is striking, and the expression characteristic." Feb. 20, a bequest of the late Mrs. Eleanor Davis, of nine hundred dollars, was communicated, with information that the amount had been paid by her executor, Dr. George C. Shattuck; and the Treasurer was directed to make suitable acknowledgments for the same. April 5, the subject of incurable patients at the Asylum was referred to Messrs. Francis, Prescott, and May.

May 1, Mr. Francis, of the Visiting Committee, stated the death of Capt. Nathaniel Fletcher this day, after an illness of less than a week; and that Dr. Lane, the resident medical officer, had been requested to act *pro tem.* The Chairman and the Visiting Committee were instructed to superintend the arrangements for the funeral. Mr. Francis says that Mr. Fletcher had always made a very exemplary officer, having given entire satisfaction to the Trustees. Messrs. Swett and Prescott were appointed a Committee to prepare the report, to be presented at the annual meeting, June 8 next, according to a late change in the by-laws.

At this annual meeting, Bryant P. Tilden, Esq., Captain Robert B. Edes, Jacob Van Lennep of

Smyrna, Rufus Wyman, and Samuel Swett, Esq., were elected members. The three first gentlemen had been instrumental in the late donation of the mummy. It was also voted, " That the Hon. William Prescott, Thomas H. Perkins, Josiah Quincy, John Lowell, Charles Jackson, Peter C. Brooks, and Dr. John C. Warren, be a Committee to devise the most becoming mode of perpetuating the memory of the late John M'Lean, Esq., as a munificent benefactor of this institution ; and that said Committee report to the Board of Trustees of this Corporation, whose decision thereon shall be final." May 29, 1825, fifteen applications for the office of Superintendent were considered; and, on June 12, Nathan Gurney, then of Abington, Mass., was unanimously elected. On Monday, June 20, General Lafayette, with his son and several gentlemen, accompanied by his Excellency the Governor and the Lieutenant-Governor, visited the Hospital. They were received by the President of the Corporation, the Board of Trustees, and the Physicians and Surgeons, and were conducted through the several wards and other parts of the building. The engagements of the General did not permit him to visit the Asylum for the Insane at Charlestown. July 2, the Board of Visitors made their visit at the Asylum. Mr. Gurney and his wife arrived, and commenced their duties.

July 24, a grant of one hundred dollars was made to Dr. Lane, for his services as acting Superintendent since the decease of Mr. Fletcher, " in which capacity his discreet and zealous performance of the duties of the office have met with the entire approbation of the Trustees." Sept. 28, plans were considered for an addition to the male wing at the Asylum, which, on Sept. 30, was ordered to be built; and Messrs. Francis, Parker, and Lyman were appointed a Building Committee to carry said vote into effect. Oct. 7, it was voted that the Visiting Committees should make their visits unattended by the superintendents, apothecaries, or nurses, probably in order that patients might more freely state any causes of complaint. Oct. 23, Dr. Lane resigned his office of Apothecary, and Mr. Joseph Reynolds was elected. An important vote was passed, placing a free bed for one year at the disposal of any one who should pay one hundred dollars. The result has been that more than sixty thousand dollars have been since received for free beds. Nov. 6, a quarterly analysis of the accounts, showing the cost of stores, &c., was ordered to be laid before the Board. Nov. 20, the last instalment of the fifty thousand dollars stock in the Massachusetts Hospital Life Insurance Company was paid in. Dec. 18, the subject of the admission of patients with syphilis and infectious disorders was referred to the

Visiting Committee and General Lyman. The fact that certain persons were in the habit of visiting the Hospital on Sundays, and having religious worship in the wards, often producing an unfavorable excitement in the patients, was communicated to the Board; and the subject was referred to the Chairman and Mr. Prescott, who, by a written report at the next meeting, put an end to the practice alluded to. Dec. 30, twenty-eight males and eighteen females in Hospital.

On Jan. 12, 1826, a Committee (by Mr. Francis, the Chairman) reported in favor of receiving actual possession now of Thomas Oliver's property ($24,138.70), and agreeing to pay his widow thirteen hundred dollars a year during her life; which report was accepted. Jan. 22, nineteen annual subscribers for free beds had been obtained. Feb. 5, a letter from Joseph Head, Sen. and Jun., executors of Mr. Oliver's will, was received and read, relinquishing twelve hundred dollars, the amount of their commissions; and the thanks of the Board were presented for this donation. An extra grant was made to Dr. Wyman of five hundred dollars for his services and aid in regard to the new building at the Asylum. Feb. 26, 1826, Dr. John B. Brown's resignation was accepted. March 19, Allen Crocker's bequest of one hundred dollars was received and acknowledged; and

Dr. George Hayward was chosen Assistant Surgeon. Dr. Hayward, after serving as a surgeon of the institution for twenty-five years, resigned in 1851; and his labors were so highly appreciated, that the Trustees, by a special vote, requested him to withdraw his resignation, and, on his final retirement, passed a highly complimentary vote, to which all the Board felt that he was fully entitled.

On April 7, a free bed for life was placed at the disposal of Mrs. Ann M'Lean, widow of John M'Lean, Esq. April 11, four incurable patients were removed from the Asylum, to make room for curable cases. May 21, Messrs. Head, Francis, and Prescott were appointed a Committee to prepare the annual report; and it was ordered that the rate of board, once fixed by the Visiting Committee, should not be altered, except by vote of the Trustees, — a rule still acted on. May 21, the Committee on Mr. Eliot's portrait reported that it was painted by Mr. Stuart, and had been placed at the Asylum. June 4, 1826, Mr. Goodwin resigned as Steward of the Asylum. As will be hereafter seen, he subsequently died holding the office of Superintendent of the Hospital. June 12, the Committee appointed at the last meeting of the Corporation, to take into consideration the best mode of perpetuating the memory of John M'Lean, recommended that the Asylum be hereafter known as " The

M'Lean Asylum for the Insane;" which report was accepted and ordered to be laid before the Corporation. The report itself is copied on the records of the Corporation. It closes as follows: " Your Committee have reason to believe, from the information of one of their number, that the proposed arrangement will be entirely satisfactory to the friends of the testator and benefactor."

At the annual meeting in June, 1826, considerable changes were made in the Board of Trustees. Messrs. William Sturgis and Edward H. Robbins, jun., were elected by the Corporation, and George Ticknor by the Board of Visitors, in the place of Messrs. Lyman, Prescott, and Daniel P. Parker, who had retired, and to whom the thanks of the Corporation were voted for their faithful services. Mr. Parker has lately died. He was one of the early liberal benefactors of the Hospital, having subscribed five hundred dollars to its funds. Mr. Lyman subsequently held the office of Vice-President, and at his death left a name indissolubly connected with the public charitable institutions of Massachusetts, one of the most important of which he had founded. His memory, as that of one of the purest and wisest of philanthropists, will be held sacred through all coming generations.

At a Trustees meeting, July 23, and five or six subsequent ones, various sums were placed at the disposal of Mr. Francis, as Chairman of the Building Committee. Oct. 6, John Welles, Esq., offered trees and shrubs from his place at Dorchester, for the use of the Hospital; also the loan of his teams, plough, and driver, to put the grounds in order. Oct. 10, Mr. Eliot's portrait was removed from the Asylum to the Hospital. Oct. 26, Mr. Phineas M. Crane was elected Apothecary, in place of Dr. Reynolds, resigned. Nov. 5th, Colonel Joseph May having tendered his resignation, " voted that this Board is desirous of expressing its regret that Colonel May, after twelve years of faithful and important services as a Trustee, and after having been many years the presiding officer of this Board, has found it necessary, from circumstances connected with his other duties, to resign his place; and they pray him on this occasion to accept the assurance of their respectful regard." Nov. 29, thanks were given to Hon. John Welles and Hon. Jonathan Hunnewell, for a large number of young trees and ornamental shrubs.

Dec. 3, Joseph Head was elected Chairman; and Amos Lawrence, Esq., was elected a Trustee in place of Colonel May. Dec. 29, forty males and sixteen females in Hospital. Jan. 9, 1827, erysipelatous inflammation having appeared at Hospital, the expediency of removing all the patients was discussed; and Messrs. Tuckerman, Sturgis, Phillips, and Guild were appointed a Committee on the subject. Jan. 14, Mr. Francis, Chairman of the Building Committee, reported $28,888.07 as expended at the Asylum to Jan. 10. The Committee reported that they had decided, after conference with the Physician and Surgeon, to make a temporary removal of all patients from the Hospital (as far as practicable), with a view to a " thorough purification by fumigation or otherwise ; " and that the Rev. Dr. James Freeman has very liberally and readily offered his dwelling-house in Vine Street, near the Hospital, for the accommodation of the patients. Jan. 21, twelve patients were reported as removed to Dr. Freeman's house, and twenty-one discharged. The Canal Bridge asked for a copy of their letter as to the immunity, granted to the officers of this Corporation in 1819, from paying toll; and it was sent. Jan. 28, the Hospital was reported to be entirely clear of patients, and " cleansing, fumigation, and alteration of fire-places, &c , in progress." Feb. 4, the patients from Dr. Freeman's house were received back into the Hospital. March 25, Dr. Robbins was appointed a Committee to return to Dr. Freeman the key of his house, with thanks. April 22, the house devised by Beza Tucker, in Boylston Place, was sold to Matthew M. Hunt, Esq., for $5,350 at auction. May 20, Messrs. Head, Ticknor, and the Secretary, were appointed a Committee to prepare the annual report. June 29, males twenty-six, females eighteen : total, forty-two in the Hospital.

This third period of five years was a very important one. The great event of the M'Lean donation served to relieve the institution from embarrassments, and insured its success. The contingency had now occurred, which was contemplated in the charter, of a donation greater than that of the Commonwealth. It was the feeling of Mrs. M'Lean, and also, at first, of others of the testator's connections, that the corporate name should be changed. There was an earnest desire to do all that could or ought to be done to express the high sense entertained of this act of munificence. The decision finally made was, it is believed, alike expedient for the Hospital, and just to the deceased. His name was given to one of the two great departments of the institution, on which a very large sum was forthwith expended for the erection of additional buildings, and where many expensive improvements have since been made, so that the actual cost of the establishment which bears his name is more than double the amount realized from his whole bequest. On the other hand, the corporate name remaining unchanged, many sons and daughters of Massachusetts have since contributed to it as a *State* institution, what perhaps they would have hesitated to bestow, if it had borne the name of a private founder.

None of the annual reports of the institution prior to 1826 have been preserved. This report is on one printed sheet. It states that forty-three free beds had been kept at the Hospital during the preceding year; that thirty-one males and twenty-six females were then in the Asylum under treatment. It estimates the value of the invested property of the Hospital at $96,694.06; and its annual expenses, for Hospital, $9,942.10, and for Asylum, $5,390.62: total expenses, $15,332.72. Total income, deducting Mrs. Oliver's annuity, $6,336.18. It mentions Mr M'Lean's donation, and alludes to the measures in progress in relation to a suitable testimonial of the gratitude of the institution. It states that the fifty thousand dollars invested in the Massachusetts Hospital Life Insurance Company had not yet begun to yield any income. No printed copy of the annual report prepared in 1827 has been preserved. Within this period of five years, a new west wing had been erected at the Hospital, completing that building as it stood down to 1844. A large and expensive addition was in progress at the Asylum to complete the buildings for male patients as they now are. The debts of the institution were all paid, and fifty thousand dollars had been invested in the Massachusetts Hospital Life Insurance Company; and the highly important arrangement before alluded to had been made with that Company. Mr. Francis was Chairman of the Committee of the Hospital for effecting this arrangement. He was also a member of the Committee of the Life Insurance Company, as well as its largest private stockholder; a circumstance which, of course, gave additional weight to his opinions and advice. Dr. Bowditch, the Actuary of that Company, had always felt an interest in the Hospital, having been a zealous and efficient member of the Committee for collecting subscriptions in its behalf in the town of Salem. Both these gentlemen believed that the true interests of the Insurance Company rendered a liberal arrangement with the Hospital highly expedient, even if viewed merely as a matter of policy. They felt convinced that the good-will universally cherished toward the Hospital would, in coming times, tend to protect the Insurance Company from that jealousy to which large moneyed institutions are naturally exposed. It should ever be remembered, then, that to the sagacity, intelligence, and liberal views of the Committees of the Hospital and of the Life Insurance Company, on this occasion, our institution is nearly, if not quite, as much indebted as it is to the noble munificence of John M'Lean.

CHAPTER V.

June, 1827, through 1832.

Bequest of William Phillips. — Varioloid at Hospital. — Domestic Coffee. — Donation Book. — New Building at Asylum. — Fire at Hospital. — Auditor of Accounts. — Silver Spoons. — Ebenezer Francis, Chairman. — Mr. Joy's Brick-kiln. — Death of Mrs. Gurney. — Wedding at Hospital. — Death of General Cobb. — Dr. George Hayward chosen Junior Surgeon. — Colored Patient. — Plank Sidewalk. — Bequest of Jeremiah Belknap. — Donation of Joseph Lee. — Lying-in Hospital. — Edward Tuckerman, Chairman. — Donations of John P. Cushing and John C. Gray. — Bequest of Isaiah Thomas. — Cholera Patients. — Dr. Wyman's Illness and Two Resignations. — Dr. Walker's Services. — Munificent Bequest of Miss Mary Belknap, One Hundred Thousand Dollars. — Services of Joseph Head. — Portrait of Mr. Belknap: how painted. — Bequest of Miss Margaret Tucker. — A Painted Letter. — Belknap Ward. — Prosperous Condition of the Institution.

At the annual meeting, June 13, 1827, Hon. Nathaniel Bowditch and Henry Codman, Esq., were elected members of the Corporation; and Patrick T. Jackson and Mr. Codman were elected Trustees, in place of Messrs. Swett and Sturgis, who declined election, and were thanked for their services. Amos Lawrence, Esq., who had been chosen by the Trustees to supply the vacancy at the resignation of Colonel May, was now elected by the Corporation. The officers at this period were Hon. Thomas H. Perkins, President; Hon. John Lowell, Vice-President; Hon. Nathaniel P. Russell, Treasurer; Nathaniel I.

Bowditch, Secretary; Joseph Head, Chairman; Ebenezer Francis, Edward Tuckerman, Benjamin Guild, Edward H. Robbins, jun., Amos Lawrence, Patrick T. Jackson, and Henry Codman, Trustees, chosen by the Corporation; Gardiner Greene, Joseph Coolidge, Jonathan Phillips, and George Ticknor, Trustees, chosen by the Board of Visitors. The Consulting Physicians, elected at the first meeting of the Trustees, July 1, were Drs. Thomas Welsh, William Spooner, John Gorham, John Dixwell, George C. Shattuck, and Jacob Bigelow, of Boston; and Drs. Abraham R. Thompson and William J. Walker, of Charlestown. On July 3, the annual visitation was made by the Board of Visitors. Two hundred copies only of the annual report being printed, it is not now extant. Of one later report, four thousand copies were printed: fifteen hundred is now the usual number. Aug. 20, the Massachusetts Humane Society were thanked for a renewal of their annual subscription for free beds during a further term of three years.

Sept. 2, a letter from Jonathan Phillips, Esq., was received, communicating a bequest from his late father, William Phillips, of five thousand dollars, as a fund, the income " to be applied for the relief of the sick poor of the city of Boston; " and this donation was gratefully accepted " as a new instance of the testator's munificence towards this institution." At the next meeting, the amount, having been received, was ordered to be placed in the Massachusetts Hospital Life Insurance Company during the life of the Secretary. The portrait of Mr. Phillips was at this meeting loaned to the Trustees of Phillips Academy. A vote was also passed, which is still acted upon, that all moneys received from patients by the Superintendent shall be placed at once to their credit on the books of the Hospital. On Sept. 12, the Treasurer was authorized to borrow of the Massachusetts Hospital Life Insurance Company twenty-five thousand dollars, on pledge of the shares in that Company. Oct. 5, Dr. John B. S. Jackson was elected Apothecary at the Hospital. Oct. 9, Henry Pierce, of Salem, was elected Steward of the Asylum, in place of G. W. Folsom, the late Steward, deceased. Dec. 16, the Board expressed to the late Apothecary, Dr. Crane, their sense of the satisfactory manner in which he had performed his duties. The Visiting Committee, appointed at the last meeting, reported on the subject of rates of board at the Asylum, that they should never be less than three dollars nor more than twelve dollars per week. By special vote, subsequently, some have paid at rates as low as two dollars, and as high as twenty dollars per week. A circular was directed to be prepared, soliciting free-bed subscriptions at the Hospital.

At a special meeting, Dec. 29, Drs. Jackson and Warren attended, and announced a case of varioloid in the Hospital (Dr. Crane, the late Apothecary), and the measures which they had taken to prevent infection, such as removal of the patient, vaccination &c.; and they were requested to publish a newspaper statement, " that no unnecessary degree of alarm may be excited in the public mind." Owing to the judicious measures adopted, no other case occurred. Jan. 11, 1828, the Superintendent was directed not to buy any more " domestic coffee." The nature of this " villanous compound " is not stated on the records; but it was probably a preparation of rye. Mrs. John C. Warren was thanked for " her friendly present of twenty-one volumes " to the Hospital Library. Jan. 27, forty free beds were established. There are now eighty.

On March 9, Colonel May was requested to prepare a list of all donations to the Massachusetts General Hospital, and one hundred dollars was appropriated to that object. This vote is the origin of the " Donation-book," decidedly the most important of all the records of the institution. It was completed down to this date in a beautifully neat style of penmanship, and has been since continued to the present time in an equally satisfactory manner by Henry B. Rogers, Esq. Thomas B. Wales, Esq., was thanked for his donation of $825 for the purchase of a free bed for life. March 23, Mr. Francis, from the Building Committee, reported that the whole expenses since May, 1826, at Asylum, were $64,166.57; of which fifty-eight thousand dollars had been paid by the Treasurer on orders of the Committee; — that the lodge (a separate brick building for violent patients) was now finished and occupied; the large building nearly finished, and in part occupied, &c. April 11, 1828, Dr. Wyman was authorized to procure a carriage and a pair of horses, to be used at the M'Lean Asylum for the Insane, for the purpose of giving air and exercise to the boarders. A grant of one hundred dollars was made to Mr. and Mrs. Gurney, "for their kind, assiduous, and faithful services as Superintendent and Matron of the Hospital." On April 27, Mr. Greenough applying to buy the reversionary interest of the Corporation in the Province House Estate, Messrs. Francis and Lawrence were appointed a Committee to ascertain its value. The Hospital declined making the proposed sale.

May 11, Messrs. Guild, Jackson, and Robbins were appointed a Committee to prepare the annual report. June 8, the mansion-house at the Asylum was ordered to be repaired, though it must be "at considerable expense." The annual report is signed by Joseph Head, Chairman of the Trustees. It occupies but two and a half octavo pages. It states the whole number of free patients discharged for the year ending April 1, 1828, to be 218. Appended to the report are tables, showing donations during the year: from a black woman, 50 cents; Samuel T. Armstrong, $100; Thomas B. Wales, $825; thirty-three free beds, $3,320; life-free beds of Jeremiah Belknap, $654, and Peter C. Brooks, $810; dividend of Massachusetts Hospital Life Insurance Company, $3,500, &c.; making in all, $14,473.64. The invested property of the Hospital was stated at $38,900. June 6, there were thirty-one males and twenty-eight females in the Hospital.

At the annual meeting, June 11, 1828, William H. Gardiner was chosen a Trustee in place of P. T. Jackson, Esq., who declined a re-election, and was thanked for his services. All the medical and surgical officers, &c., of the last year, were re-elected. July 3, the Board of Visitors visited. "His Excellency (Levi Lincoln) was pleased to express great satisfaction at the result of his visit." July 8, the Secretary was directed henceforth to audit the accounts of both branches of the institution, with a salary of one hundred dollars additional for that duty. This vote is still acted on, and has relieved the Trustees of a duty which had been gradually becoming very irksome and laborious. July 11, 1828, the cylindrical tin case, containing the title-deeds, &c., was deposited in the safe of the Massachusetts Hospital Life Insurance Company. [In March, 1844, it was again restored to the Treasurer's custody.] July 11, the Acting Physician and Surgeon were requested to nominate assistants; "the Trustees deeming it desirable that occasional changes should be made in those nominated, when consistent with the welfare of the institution." On Aug. 3, the number of assistants was restricted not to exceed three for each. Dr. Walter Channing was nominated and appointed Assistant Physician; and Drs. Edward Reynolds and George W. Otis, Assistant Surgeons. The Board declined, "though with sincere regret," loaning the portraits of their donors for an exhibition of "Stuart's Pictures." Sept. 7, the Apothecary was ordered to be styled the House Physician; and Dr. Augustus A. Gould was appointed for one year from Sept. 1.

Henry Codman, Esq., the late Secretary, having relinquished his salary for several years, was thanked for this donation; the Trustees acknowledging "the uniformly zealous and faithful discharge of his official duties, of which the records of this Board throughout afford such ample testimony." Oct. 26, the Treasurer was authorized to borrow ten thousand dollars more. Mr. Francis and the Visiting Committee were appointed to revise the rules and regulations for the

Asylum. On Nov. 11, they made a report, abolishing the office of Steward, and substituting a Clerk and Supervisor, with prescribed duties, with salaries of three hundred and four hundred dollars. Nov. 23, Mr. Oliver B. Bond was chosen Supervisor. Dec. 7, Dr. William Spooner resigned as one of the Consulting Physicians, and was thanked for his services.

On Sunday, Dec. 14, a special meeting of the Trustees was held; present, the whole Board, except Dr. Robbins, confined by illness. The record reads: "The present meeting was in consequence of a fire which broke out in the eastern wing of the Hospital, just before the morning service, and which, though at first threatening the destruction of the building, was happily subdued, after causing some injury to the roof and upper apartments." Messrs. Coolidge, Francis, and Ticknor were appointed a Committee to investigate the cause of the fire, and to make all repairs. Votes were passed, thanking the fire-department of this and the neighboring towns, which were ordered to be published, with a notice, "that the damage sustained by the building is not so great as to interrupt the reception of patients as usual." Thanks were also presented to individuals who had kindly offered the use of their houses, should the removal of the patients have become necessary. The Board expressed their sense of the zeal " manifested by the citizens generally on this occasion, and particularly by those who assisted in restoring the house to order, after the fire was extinguished." Hon. Josiah Quincy, the Mayor, attended at the meeting, " for the purpose of affording, on behalf of the city, any aid which might be required." Nathan Gurney, Esq., the Superintendent, was publicly thanked by the Board " for his care and attention to the patients, and generally for his considerate and judicious arrangements adopted on this occasion." It appears that ten convalescent patients were discharged, and all those in the east wards removed to the other part of the house, but without any great " suffering, either from the alarm or the removal."

A few weeks after this event, a patient, the nature of whose disorder required that he should be separated as far as possible from others in the house, was placed in the most remote apartment in the range of one-story wooden out-buildings, which then extended from the north side of the Hospital to Allen Street. It was an intensely cold night, and a large fire was made in the stove in his apartment, the funnel from which came out through the north side of the room into the open air. A watchman, going his rounds, had his attention attracted to a blaze, three or four feet in height, just kindled around this aperture, and extinguished it without any general alarm;

the slumbers even of the patient not being disturbed. A few days afterwards, as one of the medical officers was making a visit, attended by his students, a smell of smoke became perceptible; and an attendant came into the ward in an agitated manner, and mentioned something to him in an under tone. He turned round in a smiling manner to the students, and said, " Young gentlemen, *nothing unusual is the matter;* I am merely informed that the house is on fire." The beginnings of a fire from some combustibles in the cellar were speedily extinguished with no damage. Since these remarkable coincidences, we have enjoyed an entire immunity from any dangerous accidents of this sort.

Dec. 21, the Treasurer was authorized to borrow seven thousand dollars more. Mr. Francis presented a report as to the cause of the fire. The Committee " found on the north side of the chimney, between the ceiling of the upper story and the floor of the garret, a piece of timber and plank introduced into the chimney," which probably caught fire from the chimney having been burnt out that morning; — " that two years ago an alteration was made, and a flue heretofore used for ventilation was converted into a smoke flue by a person not acquainted with the original plan, and who had no knowledge that any wood was connected with the flue; " that no blame was attachable to the Superintendent, or those under his direction, for burning out the chimneys; that the day was favorable, and the hour proper; that the repairs had been nearly completed, and at much less expense than was expected. It did not exceed six hundred dollars. Dec. 26, there were twenty-three males and fifteen females in the Hospital: total, thirty-eight.

Jan. 22, 1829, an appeal was ordered to be taken from the probate-decree in the matter of Mr. M'Lean's trust-fund. Feb. 3, James S. Russell, of Dracut, was chosen clerk at the Asylum. Feb. 12, an additional House Physician was ordered to be appointed; and the Superintendent was ordered to purchase "a suitable number of silver spoons for use at the Hospital, instead of the present pewter ones." Feb. 16, Willard Parker was elected House Physician.

On March 8, the death of Mrs. Gurney yesterday, after a short illness, was announced; and a vote was passed, expressing the sense entertained by the Board of her "kind and careful services," and assuring Mr. Gurney of their sympathy "for his personal loss," and granting him leave of absence. March 22, Mr. Gurney becoming seriously ill, Dr. Gould was requested to act as Superintendent *pro tem*. April 7, Dr. Reynolds resigned his office of Assistant Surgeon. April 10, Mr. Coolidge was appointed a Committee to cause the grounds to be restored to as good order as before the late fire. April 26, Messrs. Codman, Francis, and Lawrence were appointed a Committee to prepare the annual report. This report is about four pages long. It presents an interesting view of what had been accomplished to that date. Total receipts of the year, $8,213.31. Cost of Hospital, $130,640.31; of Asylum, $187,326.70. May 24, the Treasurer was authorized to borrow three thousand dollars more. June 7, Dr. Hayward was requested to supply Dr. Warren's place during a temporary absence; the Board taking occasion " to express to Dr. Warren their high sense of the value of his services, and their belief that this interval of relaxation will enable him soon to resume his arduous duties with improved health."

At the annual meeting of the Corporation, June 10, 1829, Colonel Perkins, having declined a re-election, was thanked for " his faithful services in the office of President for five years last past, and for the interest which he has uniformly manifested in the concerns of this institution." Francis C. Gray, Esq., was elected a Trustee in place of Joseph Head, Esq., who also declined a re-election, and was thanked " for his long, zealous, and faithful services." Hon. John Lowell was then elected President; and Gardiner Greene, Esq., Vice-President. July 7, Ebenezer Francis was elected Chairman of the Trustees. All the medical and surgical appointments, &c., were the same as last year, except that Dr. John Randall was elected a Consulting Physician in the place of Dr. Spooner, who had resigned.

Joseph Sweetser, a lessee of Benjamin Joy, Esq., having erected a brick-kiln in and over the fifty-foot way adjoining the north side of the land in Charlestown, in violation of the rights of this institution, the Secretary was directed to request Mr. Joy to remove the same. Counsel was employed, and a hearing had before Chief Justice Parker at his chambers, July 20, on an application for a writ of injunction. The result was, that the burning of the kiln was permitted; Mr. Joy executing a bond in penalty of two thousand dollars, that no similar trespass should again be allowed, and conditioned to remove all obstructions, &c., in sixty days.

On Aug. 9, 1829, the same Clerk and Supervisor were re-elected. Aug. 23, Mr. Francis Dana, jun., was elected a House Physician of the Hospital for the ensuing year. Aug. 28, the Board of Visitors, his Excellency Governor Lincoln, &c., visited. His Excellency again "expressed his sense of the order and neatness, and the arrangements for the comfort, convenience, and safety of the patients, which were everywhere visible." Sept. 27, Drs. Walter Channing and

John Ware were appointed Assistant Physicians, on nomination of Dr. James Jackson; and Mr. Lucius W. Caryl, a House Physician, on nomination of Dr. Warren. Mr. Ticknor and the Secretary were appointed a Committee on the subject of rules and regulations. Messrs. Francis, Gray, Lawrence, Ticknor, and the Secretary were appointed a Committee on the accounts of repairs and expenditures at the Asylum. The Treasurer was authorized to borrow seven thousand dollars more.

John Williams, "a colored man," having been admitted into the Hospital, under permit of Dr. George W. Otis, dated Sept. 19, it was voted that Dr. Otis be requested to state in writing to this Board the circumstances which, in his opinion, constituted this a case of emergency within the meaning of second article of second chapter of the rules and regulations. Oct. 6, the Committee on rules and regulations reported certain provisions for officers to be known as House Physician, House Surgeon, and Apothecary, with a detail of the duties to be performed by each. Oct. 9, Dr. Otis's answer was received, stating that he had never before seen a copy of the rules and regulations, and that he did *not* think the case referred to was one of emergency within the meaning of those rules.

On Nov. 22, General Cobb being now a patient in

the Hospital, where he subsequently died, a bill of Dr. Channing for extra services rendered him was referred to the Visiting Committee, who, after consultation with Drs. Jackson and Channing, approved the same. General Cobb was an aid of Washington's in the revolutionary war. At the time of Shays's insurrection, he was Chief Justice of the Common Pleas, and Major-General of that division of the militia. The rioters assembled to prevent the opening of the Court. General Cobb addressed them, and closed his remarks as follows: "Please God, I will this day sit as a Judge, or die as a General."

Dec. 20, *five dollars* was contributed towards the new plank sidewalk in Blossom Street. There were, on Dec. 22, thirty-six males and fifteen females — total, fifty-one — in the Hospital. Jan. 8, 1830, the Committee report that the whole expenditures at the Asylum from 1826 are, for the wharf, $1,147.32; well, $215.75; and for "general improvements," $96,822.33; — that this expenditure has been "for the building called the lodge, or strong rooms; for the large building connected with the former building for males; a new roof to the dwelling-house, with the addition of another story to the centre of it, and great repairs, even to the foundation wall; the necessary alterations in the old building for males, caused by adding the new one; also new water-closets, and brick partition-walls, and other improvements in the former building for males; improvements in the ventilation of the buildings both for males and females; the addition of a large wash-room, new kitchen, and extensive cooking apparatus; for removing the earth, forming and laying out the grounds, erecting several buildings in the yard, and a great extent of fences in forming and dividing the yards." The buildings, even now, with this great expenditure, were not completed. It would seem probable, that at least sixty-five thousand dollars of the above must be assigned as the cost of the addition to the male building. Much of the work was varied from time to time when in progress, as important objections or improvements were suggested. A plan was ordered of this new building, with all its flues, &c. A precisely similar addition to the female wing was subsequently constructed; and, by means of the prior experience acquired, it cost but forty-three thousand five hundred dollars.

Feb. 7, the Treasurer was authorized to consolidate all former loans in a new loan of fifty thousand dollars, on pledge of the shares in the Life Insurance Company. Hon. Jonathan Phillips was thanked for a present of books for the library. John Braser Davis, Esq., editor of the " Patriot," was thanked for his paper furnished for the use of the patients. Feb. 21,

Mr. Gurney's intended marriage was announced, and the subject was referred to Dr. Robbins and the Visiting Committee. Dr. George Hayward was elected to the office of Junior Surgeon. March 21, Mr. Gurney announced that his intended wife had consented to reside at the Hospital. The wedding was subsequently celebrated in fine style; the House Physicians, &c., officiating as groomsmen. Many patients were present at the wedding visit. It was a gay scene, — one seldom witnessed in a Hospital. Messrs. Gray, Ticknor, and the Secretary were appointed a Committee to make an entirely new draft of the rules and regulations; whose reports were accepted, May 9 and 23, for the Hospital and Asylum respectively. They were prepared with great care and labor, each paragraph being discussed and considered, and the whole being finally read by the Trustees, and by the Physicians and Surgeons. These rules and regulations are recorded *in extenso*, occupying twenty pages. One important change introduced was, that, though each Trustee should serve for two months on the Visiting Committee, one Trustee should go out each month, so that there should always be one member of the Committee informed of the existing state of affairs. This arrangement has always since continued. May 9, Messrs. Gray, Greene, and Robbins were appointed a Committee to prepare the annual report. This report I have never met with. June 24, there were eighteen males and thirteen females — total, thirty-one — in the Hospital.

At the annual meeting, July 6, 1830, Hon. John Lowell retiring from the Presidency, Gardiner Greene was elected in his stead, and Joseph Head was elected Vice-President in place of Mr. Greene. Josiah Quincy, jun., was elected a Trustee in place of William H. Gardiner, Esq.; and the officers who retired were thanked for their faithful services. Benjamin D. Greene and James Bowdoin were new Trustees, chosen by the Board of Visitors in August. Mr. Bowdoin declining, Hon. Heman Lincoln was elected by that Board in January, 1831; and, he also declining, Mr. George Bond was elected in February, 1831. Aug. 27, the annual visitation was made, and Governor Lincoln again expressed "his entire satisfaction."

At a special meeting, Aug. 30, a bequest of the late Jeremiah Belknap, of ten thousand dollars, invested in an annuity in trust in the Massachusetts Hospital Life Insurance Company, was communicated by his sister and executrix, Mary Belknap; which was gratefully accepted, and a free bed for life was thereupon placed at her disposal. Dr. Henry I. Bowditch was chosen House Physician for the ensuing year, on nomination of Dr. James Jackson. Mr. Dana, the late House Physician, presented a written certificate of satisfactory deportment in office from the Acting Physician. A similar certificate from the Superintendent was held necessary before the Board felt authorized to vote the annual grant of fifty dollars, pursuant to the rules and regulations. Oct. 5, Mr. Bond resigned as Supervisor; and, on the 8th, Mr. Columbus Tyler was appointed his successor. After the lapse of twenty years, he is still one of the most valuable officers of the institution.

On Oct. 21, a letter from Thomas Lee, administrator of Francis Lee, a deceased patient, was received and read, communicating a gift from his father, Joseph Lee, Esq., sole heir of said deceased, of twenty thousand dollars for the use of the Asylum ($250 a year for four years to be paid to Dr. Wyman). The writer says: " In frequent visits to the Asylum, during nearly two years that the deceased was a patient, his friends having become acquainted with the admirable provision made for the alleviation and cure of one of the most severe afflictions that befall human nature, and appreciating the rare union of the requisite qualities possessed by the present Superintendent (Dr. Wyman), believe that a more appropriate or better use cannot be made of a portion of his estate, than by contributing to the support of this well-administered

JOSEPH LEE'S DONATION.

and most humane institution. They feel at the same time that they do but carry into effect what might have been the views of the deceased had the power been restored to him of acting for himself. That this may long escape the abuses to which the best public institutions seem so liable, and never want the means to accomplish its benevolent ends, under the guardianship of those whose characters are a pledge for the faithful application of the trusts reposed in them, is the wish of the donor, and, gentlemen, of yours," &c. It was thereupon voted to accept this munificent donation; and Messrs. Lawrence, Guild, and the Secretary were appointed a Committee to communicate to Mr. Lee " the grateful acknowledgments of the Board."

This donation consisted of twelve shares in the Eliot Manufacturing Company, and of eight shares in the Merrimack Company, under the restriction not to sell the same for ten years, except with the consent of Joseph Lee, Esq. On Oct. 23, a written answer, prepared by the Committee, was entered on the records, signed by all the Trustees, and sent to Mr. Lee. Messrs. Lawrence and Francis were appointed a Committee as to the investment or expenditure of the income of this donation. Dec. 5, a letter was received from Dr. Wyman, declining the donation of Mr. Lee, on the general and high-minded ground of the impropriety of receiving presents from any boarder or his friends. The Committee reported that a separate investment should be made of the income of this fund; and that, when it should be "sufficient to defray the expense of a solid, permanent building, the same shall be erected at the M'Lean Asylum for the Insane in Charlestown, and shall bear the name of the benevolent donor."

On Dec. 19, the Treasurer was authorized to borrow ten thousand dollars for four months. Dec. 31, thirty males, eighteen females — total, forty-eight — in the Hospital. Jan. 30, 1831, Messrs. Francis, Codman, and Lawrence were appointed a Committee respecting a Lying-in Hospital, in answer to a communication from the Trustees of the Humane Society. Feb. 13, at the request of Mr. Francis, he was discharged, and Mr. Quincy substituted on said Committee. At this meeting, Messrs. Francis and Lawrence were appointed a Committee to wait on Miss Mary Belknap, sister of Jeremiah Belknap, Esq., and on the relatives of Joseph Lee, Esq., to ask for their portraits; and said Committee, at the next meeting, reported that "no portraits of Mr. Belknap or Mr. Lee are in possession of their relatives." On Feb. 22, the executors and devisees of the late Joseph Lee presented five additional shares in the Eliot Manufacturing Company, to make up a depreciation in the ascertained value of the twelve shares in said Company originally given; which additional donation was gratefully received on the same conditions. These shares experienced a still further depreciation, and the amount finally realized from the whole seventeen thousand dollars of the Eliot shares was only one thousand and eight dollars. The Merrimack shares, however, paid very large dividends; the whole amount actually received, from both sources, taking the Merrimack shares at par, being $31,681.33. A separate account of this fund was kept till 1851, when, with allowance of interest on the dividends, it exceeded forty-five thousand dollars. A donation had meanwhile been received from Mr. Appleton, for the erection of a new building at the Asylum, so that it became impracticable to carry out literally the design of the preceding votes; and the Trustees proposed to give the name of Mr. Lee to the main building for male patients, that in which his son died. The whole subject was finally and satisfactorily arranged at that time.

On Feb. 27, 1831, the decision of the Supreme Judicial Court in regard to the M'Lean trust-fund was communicated; and on April 8, in reply to a request that the Board would consent that the fund should be managed by *one* Trustee, the Board say: " If the will of Mr. M'Lean requires the appointment of two Trustees, they cannot, consistently with their duty, acquiesce in the appointment of one." May 8, Messrs. Greene, Quincy, and Phillips were appointed to prepare the annual report; and on May 22, Gray and Lawrence were substituted for Greene and Phillips, who were absent. This report is believed not to be extant.

June 8, 1831, at the annual meeting of the Corporation, George Hallet was elected a Trustee in place of Ebenezer Francis, Esq., who was thanked for "his long, faithful, and peculiarly valuable services as a Trustee of this institution, to which office he has declined a re-election." July 3, the same immediate officers were all re-elected. July 5, Edward Tuckerman was chosen Chairman of the Trustees. July 8, Drs. Jacob Bigelow, John Randall, George C. Shattuck, and Abraham R. Thompson, were chosen Consulting Physicians; and Drs. William Ingalls, John B. Brown, John Dixwell, and William J. Walker, Consulting Surgeons. July 24, Thomas Sparhawk was elected House Physician; and on Aug. 21, Samuel Swett, jun., House Surgeon. Sept. 2, the annual visitation was made, nine Trustees being also present. His Excellency Governor Lincoln alluded to the appropriation for the Asylum at Worcester, as an unequivocal expression of public opinion that the M'Lean Asylum had been completely successful.

Sept. 20, a donation from John P. Cushing, Esq., of five thousand dollars, was received, and gratefully acknowledged. Rejoice Newton, Esq., was appointed agent to make any arrangement with the executors of Isaiah Thomas.

On Feb. 12, 1832, communications from Dr. Jackson and Mr. Gurney were received, stating seven cases of erysipelas in the Hospital, one of which had terminated fatally; and the subject was referred to the Visiting Committee, with full powers. They discontinued all new admissions till March 5. Feb. 26, a donation of one thousand dollars from John C. Gray was received, and suitably acknowledged. A letter from Amos Lawrence, Esq., resigning his office of Trustee in consequence of illness, was received; and a vote was passed, expressing the sense which the Board had of the value of his services, and their best wishes for his restoration to health. April 29, Messrs. Codman, Gray, and Hallet were appointed a Committee to prepare the annual report; but it has not been preserved.

On May 17, Dr. Wyman tendered his resignation on the ground of ill health. The Chairman, with Messrs. Hallet and Quincy, were appointed a Committee to confer with him, and make any arrangement. The Treasurer was ordered to pay five hundred dollars, voted Feb. 5, 1826, to Dr. Wyman, for his extra services, with interest; he having never yet received the same. May 20, a letter from Dr. Wyman thanked the Trustees for the regard and kindness manifested towards him and his family. The Committee reported that Dr. Wyman was to be for a time absent; and, " believing that the services of Dr. William J. Walker during that time would be highly valuable to the institution," they requested him " to visit it as often as he could, consistently with his other engagements."

At the annual meeting, June 13, 1832, Abbott Lawrence, Esq., was elected a Trustee in place of his brother, Amos Lawrence, who was thanked " for his zealous and faithful services during several successive years." The annual meeting was altered to the fourth Wednesday in January; so that the Trustees now chosen served only about six months. The Board of Visitors elected Thomas W. Ward in place of Jonathan Phillips; but, he not accepting, Samuel T. Armstrong was elected in August. The same Board of Physicians and Surgeons and the same officers were re-elected. July 12, Henry Codman, as Chairman of a Committee to reply to a communication received from Hon. Charles Wells the Mayor, reported in favor of receiving cholera patients in the Hospital, in case the City Hospital, specially prepared, should be filled, and not otherwise.

July 17, it was voted that a Matron be employed at the Asylum during the illness of Dr. Wyman. At a special meeting, Aug. 1, Dr. Wyman again requested the Trustees to accept his resignation; and the Visiting Committee were instructed to make a report on the next day. Mr. Lyman Bartlett was chosen House Physician; and Mr. James B. Gregerson, House Apothecary. Aug. 2, Dr. Wyman's resignation was accepted (with the view, doubtless, of relieving him from his feeling of responsibility); he still to reside at the Asylum. Dr. Walker was requested to continue his services. Aug. 23, the salary of the Physician and Superintendent at Asylum was to be henceforth twelve hundred dollars. Aug. 27, Mr. John Odin, jun., was chosen House Surgeon. Aug. 31, the annual visitation was made by his Excellency Governor Lincoln and the Board of Visitors. Sept. 19, the duties of Physician and Superintendent were ordered to be separated. Dr. Wyman was elected Physician, with a salary, fixed at the next meeting, of fifteen hundred dollars. In other words, he was so highly appreciated that the Board thought themselves fortunate in securing his services for one only of the offices, at a price greater than they believed those of any other person could be worth who should fill both situations.

And now was communicated to the Board the most

magnificent bequest, with one single exception, which has ever been bestowed upon it. Messrs. John and Andrew E. Belknap, and Joseph Head, jun., executors of the will of Miss Mary Belknap, then recently deceased, presented a copy of her will, making this Corporation her residuary devisee. This residue amounted to $88,602. It was most gratefully accepted by the Trustees.

The extent to which this Board is indebted to the good will and kind offices of the late Joseph Head, may be inferred from the following facts. There existed between him and the late Jeremiah Belknap, Esq., the most intimate friendship. He had unbounded influence over him, and gladly directed his bounty, and eventually that of his sister, towards this institution, as he had formerly done in the case of Thomas Oliver. There is no one, indeed, whose portrait is better entitled to a place at the Hospital, among the ranks of its chief benefactors and most faithful officers, than that of Mr. Head. It is a curious fact that a portrait of Mr. Belknap was painted for the Hospital by the late Henry Sargent, *from looking at Mr. Head.* Mr. Belknap and Mr. Head, at a certain hour of each day, often walked together; and Mr. Sargent, to refresh his recollection of how Mr. Belknap used to look, was in the habit of going out and meeting Mr. Head when he was walking alone, that his imagination and his pencil might be thus aided in recalling the features of Mr. Head's former companion. The likeness is by no means perfect; yet, I think, all who knew Mr. Belknap would feel sure that it was intended for him.

On Oct. 3, Captain Luke Bigelow, of Lancaster, was chosen Superintendent, with a salary of seven hundred dollars. Oct 9, Mr. Rufus Wyman, jun., was requested to act until his arrival. Oct. 21, an extra grant was made to Mr. Tyler for his services during Dr. Wyman's illness, and his salary was raised to a thousand dollars. On the nomination of Dr. Wyman, Miss Mary Sawyer, of Stirling, was appointed to the new office of Supervisor of the female department. She subsequently married Mr. Tyler, and is now the efficient, or I may rather say truly admirable matron of the establishment. New rules and regulations at the Asylum, as modified by the late changes of offices, &c., were adopted at this meeting, and recorded.

On Nov. 4, the executors of Miss Belknap transmitted a list of the residuary property, amounting to $72,852 in personal estate. Land and buildings, Nos. 26 and 28, Washington Street, then valued at $12,000; ditto, 73, Broad Street, valued at $3,750; making the total of $88,602. The Broad-street Estate was sold in 1834 to Samuel Sanford for $4,700.

The greatly increased value of the Washington-street Estate, which is still owned by the Corporation, makes the total bequest at least one hundred thousand dollars. The Board voted that a bond of indemnity should be delivered to the executors on the transfer of this property, and a full receipt and discharge given to their satisfaction. Nov. 18, Dr. Robbins was appointed a Committee of advisement for the Treasurer, in regard to the sale and disposition of the property thus received.

On Dec. 14, Dr. Robbins, as Visiting Committee, recommended greater vigilance in admitting as patients those persons who ought to go to South Boston, — a most important suggestion. Dec. 16, Dr. William J. Walker having "visited at the Asylum, during seven months, four or five times each week," the Trustees request his acceptance of six hundred dollars as a small acknowledgment, on the part of this Board, of the zeal and fidelity with which he discharged the duties of Physician and Superintendent during the illness of Dr. Wyman. One hundred dollars was also granted to Dr. D. Davis, the resident assistant, for his services at this period.

Mr. Francis informs me, that one of the young medical men selected to assist Dr. Wyman in keeping his accounts (several years before this period) received the appointment, principally because the Trustees were delighted with his letter of application, which was the most exquisite specimen of penmanship that they had ever beheld. He entered on his duties, and was found to write a most illegible hand. He was asked whether that letter was his own unaided composition. He replied that it was. " But," added he, " I did not *write* it, — I *painted* it." It was, indeed, the elaborate production of an *artist*, executed with great delicacy by means of a *hair-pencil*.

The Treasurer presented the following exhibit of the property of the institution: —

Turnpike shares	$200.00
Life-office stock	50,000.00
Trust-policy under will of William Phillips	5,000.00
„ „ „ „ Jeremiah Belknap	10,000.00
Joseph Lee's donation, estimated at	20,000.00
Mary Belknap's legacy	88,602.00
A note	167.91
	$173,969.91
Debts due	61,000.00
Leaving	$112,969.91

The general receipts are stated as follows: —

Donations and legacies	$411,927.73
Thomas Oliver's legacy (subject to $1,300 annuity)	22,938.70
Donation of Joseph Lee and accumulation of do.	22,140.00
Received on account of Isaiah Thomas's bequest	1,307.00
	$458,313.43

The permanent expenditures, as follows : —

Land and buildings of Hospital in Boston	$144,498.91	
„ „ „ of M'Lean Asylum	188,422.22	
		332,921.13
Balance		$125,392.30
Board of free patients from 1822 to 1832, estimated at $3 per week		$36,590.25
Donations for free beds, including income of the bequests of Wm. Phillips and Jeremiah Belknap for that object, since 1822		29,405.94
Balance		$7,184.31

Income for 1833 estimated at $12,547.
Expenditures „   „   at 11,040.

On Dec. 30, Messrs. Greene, Quincy, and Bond were appointed a Committee to prepare the annual report. Jan. 8, 1833, a bequest of Miss Margaret Tucker of $2,600, for perpetual support of a free bed at the Hospital, was announced and gratefully accepted. It was not paid over till 1842.

Jan. 11, it was ordered that no free beds should be occupied by the same persons over three months, except on special vote of the Trustees.

Jan. 20, a letter from Dr. William J. Walker was received and read, expressing his gratitude for the favorable opinion entertained by the Board and for the liberal compensation voted him, and requesting their acceptance of a donation of four hundred dollars. The Secretary was directed to assure Dr. Walker of the high gratification afforded to the Trustees by this new proof of his regard for the institution.

The annual report for this year, signed by Mr. Tuckerman the Chairman, also by the Committee, is about six pages long. It states the interesting fact, that Dr. Wyman had for fourteen years passed only five nights away from the Asylum, and the measures taken to lighten his duties, and thus restore his health; alludes to the numerous recent proofs of public confidence, and the noble donation of Miss Belknap; and suggests (what has since been executed) that, whenever an additional wing shall be erected for female patients, "it would be a compliment signally appropriate to give the name of this great benefactress to that part of the establishment which is particularly devoted to the benefit of her sex;" but states that the erection of such a building now would absorb the whole funds of the institution. It speaks of the valuable services and the gratifying donation of Dr. Walker.

The result of this period is, that during no previous term of five years had the donations been more numerous or munificent. There had been received bequests from the late William Phillips, Jeremiah Belknap, and his sister Miss Mary Belknap, Joseph Lee and his devisees, Miss Margaret Tucker, and Isaiah Thomas; and donations from John P. Cushing,

John C. Gray, Thomas B. Wales, Henry Codman, Dr. William J. Walker, &c., — which, in the aggregate, amounted to nearly a hundred and fifty thousand dollars.

A hundred thousand dollars had been expended in improvements at the Asylum, and a debt of sixty thousand dollars contracted in making these improvements. But it was forthwith to be paid off out of the more recent of the donations just received. The pecuniary position of the institution at this time is exactly stated in the summary in the preceding page. The institution still retained, at the head of its two departments, the services of Dr. Wyman and of Mr. Gurney. Mr. and Mrs. Tyler had become officers of the Asylum. The same medical and surgical staff continued to discharge their duties. The narrow escape of the Hospital from destruction by fire was not the least of the fortunate events of this period.

The number of patients in the Hospital was, at the close of this year, thirty-two males, twenty females, — total, fifty-two; and, at the Asylum, twenty-seven males, twenty-four females, — total, fifty-one. Thus the usefulness and reputation of the institution had continued steadily to increase; and it had attained to a degree of prosperity which must have been highly gratifying alike to its original founders and to those who now had its management and control.

CHAPTER VI.

1833–1837.

DEATH OF GARDINER GREENE, PRESIDENT. — RESIGNATION OF MR. GURNEY. — CHOICE OF GAMALIEL BRADFORD. — FINAL RESIGNATION OF DR. WYMAN, AND CHOICE OF DR. THOMAS G. LEE. — COLUMBUS TYLER ELECTED STEWARD OF ASYLUM. — SERVICES OF MRS. TYLER. — BEQUEST OF JONATHAN MOSELEY. — PORTRAIT OF THOMAS OLIVER. — RESIGNATION OF JOSEPH HEAD, PRESIDENT. — GEORGE BOND, CHAIRMAN. — DIET AT HOSPITAL. — FREE BEDS FOR LIFE. — BEQUEST OF MISS SUSAN RICHARDSON. — PIANO-FORTE AND BILLIARD TABLE AT ASYLUM. — TRUSTEES' MEETING : NOBODY PRESENT. — DEATH OF DR. LEE, AND VOTES OF TRUSTEES. — DR. LUTHER V. BELL ELECTED HIS SUCCESSOR. — COLORED PATIENT. — INTERESTING REPORT OF S. A. ELIOT ON OCCASION OF NON-OBSERVANCE OF RULES AND REGULATIONS. — RESIGNATION OF DR. JAMES JACKSON : HIS CHARACTER AND SERVICES. — RESIGNATION OF MR. RUSSELL THE TREASURER, AND CHOICE OF HENRY ANDREWS. — SUMMARY. — GREAT CHANGES OF THE OFFICERS. — DONATIONS ONLY A THOUSAND DOLLARS FOR THE FIVE YEARS.

AT the annual meeting, Jan. 23, 1833, it was voted, " That this Corporation entertain a grateful recollection of the zealous and faithful services of the late Gardiner Greene, Esq., in the offices of a Trustee and President of this institution ; " also voted, " That the thanks of this Corporation be presented to Joseph Coolidge, Esq., who, for many successive years, from the first establishment of the institution to the present time, has held the office of a Trustee, discharging his duties with the utmost zeal and fidelity, and to which office he has declined a re-election." Francis J. Oliver, Esq., was elected by the Board of Visitors a Trustee in the place of Mr. Coolidge, and the Board was organized as follows: Joseph Head, President; Ebenezer Francis, Vice-President; Nathaniel P. Russell, Treasurer; Nathaniel I. Bowditch, Secretary. Henry Codman, Francis C. Gray, Benjamin Guild, George Hallet, Abbott Lawrence, Josiah Quincy, jun., Edward H. Robbins, and Edward Tuckerman, Trustees, on the part of the Corporation; and Samuel T. Armstrong, George Bond, Benjamin D. Greene, and Francis J. Oliver, Trustees, on the part of the Board of Visitors. Feb. 17, all the medical and other officers of the last year were re-elected.

Richard S. Roberts applied for leave to remove a blind placed against the window of his house in Fruit Court, overlooking the Hospital Garden. March 3, William B. Shaw was appointed Apothecary, and Rufus Wyman, jun., Clerk at the Asylum. July 5, Mr. Roberts was allowed to have a window with a reversed blind. Aug. 11, Dr. F. H. Gray was appointed House Physician; and, on Sept. 8, Dr. Henry Tuck, House Surgeon; Mr. Benjamin F. Parker, House Apothecary.

On Sept. 13, Nathan Gurney, Esq., tendered his resignation as Superintendent of the Hospital, to take effect in November next. This resignation was accepted; and it was voted, "That, in accepting this resignation, the Trustees would express to Mr. Gurney their sense of the zeal and ability with which he has discharged the duties of his office, and their regret that his valuable services must cease in so short a time. They have seen his energy, decision, and good judgment; his kindness and attention to the patients; his skill and economy in managing the concerns of the establishment, and the order, regularity, and neatness which have always been preserved there; and they have esteemed themselves fortunate in the selection of one who united in so high a degree the various qualifications for the situation, and who, with the power, possessed also the disposition, to promote the best interests of the department of the institution confided to his care. The trustees would therefore assure Mr. Gurney, that they have always been entirely satisfied with his efforts in their cause, and that he will retire from office with their best wishes for his future happiness." Mr. Gurney subsequently became an alderman of the city of Boston, and died, not long since, one of our most highly-respected citizens.

On Oct. 8, Benjamin D. Greene, Esq., resigned his situation as a Trustee, in view of an intended absence in Europe. He was, however, re-elected the ensuing year. Oct. 11, all the Board were present except Mr. Codman, who was ill. Gamaliel Bradford, M.D., was unanimously elected Superintendent of the Hospital. The Belknap Estate in Washington Street was leased for ten years at a rent of nine hundred dollars. It was at first rented for seven hundred dollars. It has since been rebuilt, and rents for fifteen hundred dollars. Dec. 1, where a patient remains less than one day, one dollar is to be charged. Dec. 15, the Chairman, Messrs. Oliver, Codman, and the Visiting Committee, were desired to consider the expediency of erecting a new building at the Asylum. Dec. 23, Messrs. Gray, Quincy, and Bond were appointed a Committee to draw up the annual report.

This report was prepared by Josiah Quincy, jun., as Chairman, and occupied nine pages; and, with the documents annexed, makes a pamphlet of twenty-three pages. It gives a detailed and very interesting and satisfactory account of both departments of the Hospital; states the invested property of the institution to be $113,750, — including, however, the Eliot shares of seventeen thousand dollars, which realized but a thousand and eight, so that the actual amount is a hundred and two or a hundred and three thousand dollars; shows that its annual expenses render it still in need of continued assistance and support; alludes to the prominent events of the year; speaks of the "universal satisfaction" given by Mr. Gurney; and mentions the election of Dr. Bradford, "who has given pledges of being entitled to the high praise of fully supplying the place of his predecessor." The number of patients in the Hospital at the close of the year were twenty-seven males, twenty-four females, — total, fifty-one; in the Asylum, forty males, twenty-four females, — total, sixty-four. It contains a table of all the admissions at the Asylum, viz.: In 1818, nine; in 1819, twenty-six; 1820, twenty-eight; 1821, thirty-three; 1822, forty-five; 1823, thirty-nine; 1824, thirty-three; 1825, twenty-nine; 1826, twenty-three; 1827, thirty-one; 1828, forty-eight; 1829, thirty-seven; 1830, forty-seven; 1831, forty-five; 1832, sixty-five; 1833, sixty-six: total, 1,015, with various tables, showing proportions of recoveries, &c.; the total of those removed in that period being 948, out of which 362 were recovered.

Jan. 8, 1834, the Board express great satisfaction with the services of Miss Sawyer [Mrs. Tyler], and raised her salary to two hundred dollars. A memorial from the Physicians and Surgeons as to a new building or wing at the Hospital was received and referred. Eleven years afterwards, such a building was erected. Jan. 19, Mr. Hallet resigned his seat as a Trustee.

At the annual meeting, Jan. 29, Charles G. Loring and Samuel A. Eliot, Esqs., were chosen Trustees in place of George Hallet and Benjamin Guild, Esqs., who had resigned, and who were thanked for their zealous and faithful services. Jan. 23, the Board of Medical and Surgical Officers, and the heads of the two departments, were re-elected; Henry A. True being Apothecary at the Asylum. On March 9, Mr. Luke Bigelow resigned his office as Superintendent of the Asylum. April 16, Messrs. Tuckerman and Quincy were appointed a Committee on the subject of any new arrangements at that institution, who on May 18 made a report, which was accepted. This directs that the head of the institution be known as the Physician and Superintendent; that an Assistant Physician be chosen, with a salary of seven hundred dollars; and likewise a Steward, having the salary heretofore paid to the Superintendent. Luke Bigelow was then elected Steward; and Dr. Thomas G. Lee, of Hartford, Assistant Physician.

On July 8, the Secretary was appointed a Committee to look into the title of the Corporation to land bought of Mr. Joy, and to confer with Mr. Loring respecting measures which may be thought necessary to procure a release of the condition contained in the deed. It was found impracticable to get a release executed at this time. July 11, the application of Eliza Bryant for leave to erect a building on Fruit Street, with windows opening on the Hospital-ground, was declined. A copy of the will of Jonathan Moseley, making this Corporation residuary legatee, was received; and a legacy, informally given by a codicil, was confirmed. July 11, Lieutenant-Governor Armstrong resigned his office of Trustee, and was thanked by the Board for his valuable services.

On July 20, a very elaborate and excellent report from Mr. Eliot was entered on the records, defining the relative duties of the Superintendent and of the Physicians, &c., of the Hospital. It concludes thus: " Much must be left to the discretion of those who hold responsible stations; and, having expressed their general views of the subject, — having stated, as it were, their theory of the government of the institution, — the Trustees must leave the application of them to the good sense and good feelings of the present incumbents, with the single intimation, that they consider harmony of action in the officers essential to the prosperity of the Hospital." Copies of this report were ordered to be transmitted to the Superintendent and to the Medical and Surgical Officers.

On Aug. 17, Mr. Estes Howe was elected House Physician, and Aug. 31, Mr. Stephen Salisbury, House Surgeon for the year ensuing. Oct. 10, Mrs. Lee, the widow of the late John M'Lean, having deceased, the Treasurer was authorized to receive a transfer of the property now belonging to the Corporation, which had been held in trust during her life. Nov. 23, Luke Bigelow resigned the office of Steward at the Asylum. Dec. 21, Messrs. Greene, Codman, and Oliver were appointed a Committee to prepare the annual report. Of this report I do not possess a copy. Mr. William Wyman was elected Steward of the Asylum. Mr. Wyman was a very intelligent man and efficient officer. He has since been a representative from the town of Cambridge. He has always taken great interest in the institution. The estate in Broad Street, devised by Miss Belknap, was ordered to be sold by the Treasurer.

On Jan. 9, 1835, — " whereas Dr. Wyman has repeatedly and earnestly requested to be relieved from his arduous and responsible duties as soon as the interests of the M'Lean Asylum will admit, and the Trustees feel it a duty to him to fix a time for his retirement, in order to give him an opportunity to make suitable arrangements for the future, — voted, that his resignation be respectfully accepted, to take effect on May 1 next. Voted, that, in consideration of his long, zealous, and unwearied exertions during sixteen years, — in the commencement of an institution then novel in this part of the country, and in conducting it to its present prosperous state, — the sum of one thousand dollars be granted to him and paid by the Treasurer : " and, on Jan. 16, Dr. Thomas G. Lee, Assistant Physician, was promoted to his post, with the same salary and privileges as had been enjoyed by his predecessor; and he was requested " not to confine himself too strictly to his duties, or debar himself from the enjoyment of social intercourse with his friends, or to neglect that occasional relaxation by which his health may be improved and preserved." Mr. Columbus Tyler was promoted to the office of Steward, which he still so acceptably continues to hold.

At the annual meeting, Jan. 28, Henry Andrews, Esq., was elected Treasurer. It was voted, " That the thanks of this Corporation be presented to Hon. N. P. Russell, who, for fourteen years past, has gratuitously discharged the duties of Treasurer of this institution, with great zeal, ability, and usefulness; he having declined a re-election to that office." It was also voted, " That the thanks of this Corporation be presented to Henry Codman, Esq., who has declined a re-election as Trustee; he having, in that office and in the office of Secretary, been connected with the institution for eighteen years past, and having always promoted its interests with the greatest zeal and fidelity." Dr. Wyman was then elected a Trustee in the place of Mr. Codman; but, he being present at the meeting and declining, Thomas B. Curtis, Esq., was elected. John P. Thorndike, Esq., was elected a Trustee by the Board of Visitors, in the place of Mr. Armstrong. It was also voted, " That the thanks of this Corporation be presented by their Secretary to Dr. Rufus Wyman for the zeal, ability, and faithfulness with which, from the establishment of the M'Lean Asylum for the Insane, he has filled the office of Physician and Superintendent, with the assurance that this Corporation feel bound to declare that these qualities have mainly contributed to raise the reputation of the institution to its present respectable standing, and have equally elevated his own character in his profession and as a philanthropist."

On Feb. 8, the same officers of the two institutions, and Visiting Physicians and Surgeons, were re-elected; Drs. George B. Doane and Solomon D. Townsend being elected Consulting Surgeons in place of Drs. Ingalls and Dixwell. March 22, certain changes were made in the duties of the Physicians and Surgeons, in accordance with a report of Messrs. Quincy, Eliot, and Robbins, a Committee to whom had been referred a communication from Dr. James Jackson. April 26, the Treasurer was authorized to overdraw one thousand dollars at the Suffolk Bank. Renewed discussions were had, as to a new building at the Hospital and at the Asylum, at this and the next meetings. May 17, Charles K. Whipple was chosen Apothecary at the Hospital; and Dr. J. B. S. Jackson, Assistant Physician.

On July 7, the widow of Mr. Oliver being deceased,

certain final payments of legacies were ordered, and a full discharge directed to be given to his executors. Oct. 4, Mr. Eliot was requested to report plans and estimates of a new building at the Asylum; and, on the 25th, he was authorized to engage the services of Mr. M'Allister for the erection of the same. Nov. 8, it was voted that the thanks of the Board be presented to the executors of Mrs. Prescott for the portrait of their late distinguished benefactor, Thomas Oliver, Esq. Mrs. Prescott was his widow; and the portrait thus given is in the Trustees' room at the Hospital. It is not a fine painting, and is said not to be a very good likeness. It is, however, valuable as being a portrait taken from life, of and for himself, and the only one which has been preserved.

Nov. 22, Mr. Homer Goodhue was chosen Supervisor, of which post he has always continued to discharge the duties in a most acceptable manner. Messrs. Eliot and Thorndike were appointed the Building Committee for the new building at the Asylum, and twenty-eight thousand dollars placed at their disposal. Dec. 6, the salary of the Superintendent of the Hospital was increased from five to six hundred dollars; this arrangement to include the present year. On Jan. 8, 1836, Messrs. Gray, Eliot, and Quincy were appointed a Committee to draw up the annual report.

The report, as prepared by Mr. Gray, had in a striking degree the merit of brevity. It was one sentence of six lines, purporting, without any comment, to present certain annexed reports from the two departments of the institution. Among these documents, however, was a very important and valuable one from Dr. Lee, describing minutely the system of occupation, diversion, and moral management at the Asylum; the Belknap Sewing Society; the weekly dancing parties; the religious service on the Sabbath, &c. Of his assistants he says: " We will not continue any male or female attendant whom we cannot invite into our family, seat at our table, and with whom we could not confidently place our own wives, sisters, and brothers. We do not consider their service as servile: they are the companions of the unfortunate, engaged in the same employments as ourselves; they shall command our friendship and respect." He adds, " I ask not for the institution or myself more devoted fellow-laborers." The whole forms a pamphlet of twenty-seven pages, twenty-three of which relate to the Asylum. It is one of the most important publications ever issued by the Trustees; and it will be a lasting monument to the memory of Dr. Lee, who, before the close of the coming year, was summoned from the eminently faithful and successful discharge of one of the most responsible of all earthly trusts to the presence of that Heavenly Father, whose word had ever been his delight, and by whose precepts his steps had ever been guided.

There had been discharged from the Hospital, during the year, one hundred and thirty-two males, sixty-one females, — total, one hundred and ninety-three; in the Asylum, May 1, fifty males, thirty-one females, — total, eighty-one.

At the annual meeting, Jan. 27, 1836, " Joseph Head, Esq., having declined a re-election to the office of President, — voted, that the thanks of this Corporation be presented to him for the performance of those personal services, and the exercise of that influence with the community in favor of the institution, to which it is so largely indebted for its present state of prosperity." Abbott Lawrence and Edward H. Robbins, Trustees on the part of the Corporation, and Benjamin D. Greene and Francis J. Oliver, Trustees chosen by the Board of Visitors, having declined a re-election, were severally thanked for their services. Charles Amory and Samuel Lawrence were then elected by the Corporation, and Henry Edwards and Robert G. Shaw were subsequently chosen by the Board of Visitors to be Trustees; and the Corporation was now organized by the choice of Ebenezer Francis, President, and Samuel Appleton, Vice-President; and, at the meeting of the Trustees, Feb. 7,

George Bond, Esq., was made Chairman. Dr. Winslow Lewis, jun., was appointed a Consulting Surgeon in place of Dr. John B. Brown. No other change was made in any of the appointments.

Mr. Hallet made application to purchase a free bed for life; and, on Feb. 21, a Committee was appointed to consider that general subject. On March 6, the Physicians and Surgeons were requested to report a system of diet for the patients; and, on March 20, their report was presented accordingly. Messrs. Eliot and Thorndike were then appointed a Committee to make an additional purchase of land near the Asylum, for a price not exceeding twenty thousand dollars. April 8, it was " voted that the sum of one hundred and fifty dollars be paid to Dr. Augustus A. Gould, in full for his services as Superintendent of the Hospital in the year 1829; and that the Secretary transmit to Dr. Gould a copy of this vote, with the assurance that it has been through inadvertence only that no earlier action has been had on the subject." April 24, certain new rules were adopted as to the admission of patients at the Hospital. May 8, Mr. Bowditch resigned the office of Secretary, which he had held during nine years; and, May 22, William Gray, Esq., was elected his successor.

On June 5, the price of free beds for life was fixed at such a sum as would be required by the annuity tables to purchase an annuity of one hundred dollars. In July, a bequest of Susan Richardson was received, for the support of female free patients, amounting to $250. July 5, Mr. Eliot was appointed a Committee to confer with Dr. Lee, " to hire or purchase a pianoforte for the Asylum, with appropriate music." Mr. Eliot and Mr. Lawrence were chosen a Committee to purchase a billiard table for the Asylum, if they should consider it expedient. Both were purchased. July 8, Dr. John Ware tendered his resignation as a Physician of the Hospital, which was accepted, — the Board taking occasion to express their high sense of the value of his services; and Dr. Jacob Bigelow was appointed his successor, and has been annually re-elected to the present time. August 7, Morrill Wyman was chosen House Physician; and Samuel Parkman, House Surgeon of the Hospital. Aug. 21, six thousand five hundred dollars was appropriated for rebuilding the lodge for female patients at the Asylum; and the subject of erecting a dome on the new building at the Asylum was referred to Messrs. Gray and Quincy; and, on Sept. 4, six thousand dollars was appropriated for the same.

At a quarterly meeting, Oct. 7, *no member of the Board made his appearance.*

On Oct. 23, a special meeting was called, in consequence of the illness of Dr. Lee. Ten members were present. Dr. Jackson was requested to visit Dr. Lee at Worcester, accompanied by the Chairman and Mr. Tuckerman. He died there, Oct. 29, at Dr. Woodward's. On the 30th, another special meeting was called, announcing Dr. Lee's death, at which a vote was adopted for attending the funeral; also the following, prepared by Mr. Eliot, viz. : —

"Voted, that the Board, while submitting in sorrow to the dispensations of Providence, cannot but feel deeply the loss which the institution under their care, and the public, have suffered in the lamented death of Dr. Lee. They had known him long enough to appreciate his talents, his attainments in his profession, his remarkable and entire devotion to the pursuit in which he had engaged, the beautiful purity of his character, the elevation of his views, and the propriety of the means by which he sought to attain the most worthy objects. They have often been struck with the soundness of his judgment and the kindness of his manners, and have perceived, in the institution of which he was the Superintendent, the happy influence of his professional skill, combined with the cheerfulness and gentleness of his deportment, and the piety which was the habitual guide of his life. After an association of nearly two years of an intimate character, they can say with truth that they have nothing to regret in their intercourse with him but its premature close. They had hoped to see the M'Lean Asylum long increasing in usefulness under his care, and to witness the extension of his well-earned reputation for many years; and they cannot suffer him to pass to the grave, without paying a just tribute to his many admirable qualities, and his peculiar fitness for the station in which he was placed."

A vote was also adopted, expressive of their sympathy for his widow, and for defraying all expenses of his last illness, and payment of his salary to April 1; also a vote inviting the widow to remain at the Asylum as long as she might think proper. And it was voted, " That the thanks of the Board be presented to Dr. Woodward and his family, for their kindness and assiduous attention to Dr. Lee during the illness which terminated in his death."

This just and beautiful tribute to the memory of Dr. Lee renders any remark of mine unnecessary. He died at the early age of twenty-eight years, after an illness of only a few days.

Francis C. Gray, Esq., resigned the office of a Trustee, and was thanked for his services. Nov. 6, the subject of an additional building at the Hospital was discussed, and deferred for the present. The Superintendent was directed " to call on Mr. Tappan, and inform him that it will not be convenient to receive into the Hospital the colored man proposed to be sent by him." Nov. 13, the rules as to the admission of patients were modified, and a salary of $150 established for the office of Assistant Physician.

On Dec. 11, Dr. Luther V. Bell was unanimously elected Physician and Superintendent of the Asylum, " provided a Committee then appointed, consisting of Messrs. Eliot and Quincy, shall be satisfied that he will pursue the course of moral and religious treatment of patients adopted by Dr. Lee, and they shall be so satisfied before communicating the appointment." By requiring this pledge from Dr. Bell, the Trustees paid the highest possible compliment to his lamented predecessor. How fully and admirably that pledge has been redeemed by Dr. Bell it is needless to mention in a community where his character and ability are so well known. It is praise enough to say, that the mantle of Dr. Wyman and Dr. Lee could not have fallen on a more worthy successor. The Treasurer was authorized to borrow fifteen thousand dollars. Dec. 15, his Excellency Edward Everett and the Board of Visitors made the annual visitation. Dec. 16, the Committee reported the acceptance of Dr. Bell. Jan. 1, 1837, Messrs. Loring, Amory, and Tuckerman were appointed a Committee to prepare the annual report. Jan. 13, the Treasurer was authorized to renew a loan of twenty thousand dollars.

At the annual meeting, Jan. 25, Ebenezer Francis, President, and Samuel Appleton, Vice-President, and Edward Tuckerman, Francis C. Gray, and Josiah Quincy, jun., Trustees, severally declined a re-election and were thanked for their services. Edward Tuckerman, Esq., was chosen President; Jonathan Phillips, Esq., Vice-President. Robert Hooper, jun., Martin Brimmer, and Nathaniel I. Bowditch, were elected Trustees in the place of those who had retired. The Corporation fully concurred in the votes of the Trustees, expressive of respect for the memory of Dr. Lee, and of sympathy towards his widow, and directed that those votes should be published in the annual report. A highly complimentary vote was passed respecting Mr. Columbus Tyler, the Steward, for the performance of his increased duties since Dr. Lee's death; and the Trustees were instructed to grant him a suitable compensation. The Corporation also declared the high estimation in which they held the services of Mrs. Lee and of Mrs. Tyler in the female department, and ordered that "their interesting report of the organization and proceedings of the Belknap Sewing Society" should also be published.

On Feb. 5, one thousand copies of the annual report were ordered to be printed. This report is drawn up by Charles G. Loring, Esq., and occupies six pages, with an appendix of twenty pages more.

It states a necessity (to this day still existing) of a further ward at the Hospital for the accommodation of patients affected by fevers, erysipelas, &c. ; — speaks of the erection of the new Belknap Ward as reflecting great credit on the architects, and on Mr. M'Allister, who superintended its construction ; — that its estimated expense will not exceed forty thousand dollars ; — mentions a purchase of six acres of land for about six thousand dollars. It pays a truly feeling tribute to the memory of Dr. Lee, and makes most honorable mention of Mr. and Mrs. Tyler's services, under their increased and arduous duties, resulting from his sudden decease. It mentions the fortunate selection of Dr. Bell as his successor. It is throughout one of the most able and beautifully written reports ever submitted to the Board. It closes with the following paragraph : —

"The Trustees feel that there is cause for great gratitude, that this institution enjoyed so long the talents and services of the honored individual (Dr. Rufus Wyman) whose fortune it was to lay the broad and deep foundations of its usefulness and reputation, and whose invaluable services shed so bright a lustre upon its early history ; and that, when he retired, exhausted by the toils and responsibilities of seventeen years devoted to its arduous duties, a successor was given to follow out his designs, to raise still higher this fabric of benevolence, and institute further inestimable improvements for the accomplishment of its great design.

And, commending its destiny to the same Beneficence which raised and has hitherto sustained it, they rely with confidence upon the ability and devotion of him to whose direction it is now mainly intrusted, that he will prove himself worthy the responsible station to which he is called; and that, when his labors shall be ended, his name shall be numbered with those of his predecessors, among the benefactors of his race."

The patients at the Asylum were forty-seven males, thirty females: total, seventy-seven. There had been discharged from the Hospital, during the year, one hundred and fifty-eight males, sixty-six females: total, two hundred and twenty-four. The documents appended to this report are also unusually interesting. Many details and anecdotes are given in Mr. Tyler's report in relation to the Asylum.

The same Medical and Surgical Staff and heads of departments were re-elected, except that Dr. John Jeffries was chosen in the place of Dr. Winslow Lewis, jun., as one of the Consulting Surgeons. Dr. John R. Lee was elected Assistant Physician and Apothecary at the Asylum. Feb. 19, Dr Walker declining to act any longer as Consulting Surgeon, Dr. A. L. Peirson, of Salem, was appointed. Mr. Bowditch and the Secretary were appointed a Committee to revise the rules and regulations of both institutions for publication. The thanks of the Board were presented to Dr. Abraham R. Thompson, " for his services as Physician at the Asylum during the illness and since the death of Dr. Lee," with the request that he would accept three hundred dollars. A grant of $250 was also made to Mr. and Mrs. Tyler for their extra services, as recommended by the Corporation. April 2, the Treasurer was authorized to borrow twelve thousand dollars. Messrs. Amory, Brimmer, and Bowditch were appointed a Committee to inquire into the increased expenditures at the Hospital and at the Asylum. On April 12, the Committee reported a *printed pamphlet* of rules and regulations, which was adopted, having been carefully read and examined by the Board, and also by the Physicians, &c., while in manuscript. April 19, a correspondence ensued between Dr. Lewis and the Trustees, in respect to the change in the Board of Consulting Physicians. The reply of the Trustees states, that they felt no doubt that his skill and attainments in his profession were such as would qualify him for the place; and expresses the hope that no injurious consequences would follow from the manner in which they had exercised their discretion.

April 23, the Visiting Committee, Messrs. Lawrence and Eliot, reported the following vote, drawn up by Mr Eliot, which was adopted: " Voted that the Trustees have recently seen, with great pain, that a violation of the rules of the institution by one of its officers has become the subject of newspaper animadversion. In an institution like this, to which it is so difficult to attract, and in which it is so important to command, public confidence, the strictest and most scrupulous adherence to rules, of which the propriety is unquestioned, is required by a just regard as well to its usefulness to the public, as to the character of those who have any agency in its direction and control. Where many persons are connected in different departments, the reputation of all is more or less affected by the conduct of each; and all are therefore bound, by respect for others as well as themselves, to conduct in such a manner as to give no reasonable ground of complaint. The Trustees have felt unlimited confidence that no officer of the institution would expose himself to just censure, and they have on all occasions been but very slightly affected by remarks which they have had reason to believe were founded on jealousy or misconception. But it is with very different feelings they regard an accusation of violation of rule, which, on inquiry, proves to be true; and they think it due to themselves to take serious notice of it, and to put on record their denial of all knowledge of the circumstance at the time of its occurrence, and to express their hope that nothing may ever again require a similar expression of their feelings. Lest, however, the breach of confidence may be imagined to be of a more serious character than it really was, they think proper to state, that the circumstance to which they allude was the employment of Dr. J. Mason Warren, a young man not connected with the Hospital, during the absence of his father, whose turn it was to officiate;" and a copy of this vote was sent to all the Surgeons of the Hospital.

When it is remembered, that Dr. John C. Warren had been Surgeon of the Hospital from its foundation, — that the Board had not the slightest distrust of the capacity of his son to perform the duties alluded to, it must be admitted, that the preceding vote is an honorable proof of their vigilance and independence. This son was a few years afterwards appointed one of the Surgeons of the Hospital, the duties of which station he has discharged with signal ability and success. A reply from Dr. Warren, which was of the most candid, manly, and appropriate character, was received at the next meeting. This censure, alike given and received in a proper spirit, did but tend thenceforth to strengthen and confirm between both parties feelings of mutual confidence, regard, and respect.

May 14, Dr. Warren announcing his intention of going to Europe, the surgical department of the Hospital was intrusted to Dr. Hayward. Aug. 13, William Church was chosen House Surgeon, and Joseph Sargent House Physician, for the ensuing year. Sept.

10, the wages at the Hospital were ordered to be reduced by the Superintendent. Sept. 24, the Treasurer was authorized to borrow twelve thousand dollars.

On Oct. 13, a communication from Dr. James Jackson, by which he resigned his situation as one of the Physicians of the Hospital, having been read, the following votes, submitted by Mr. Bowditch, were unanimously adopted; viz., "Voted that the Trustees have learned this determination of Dr. Jackson with the utmost regret. Connected as he has been with the institution from its first establishment, they are well aware how much he has always done to raise and maintain its reputation, and to extend its usefulness. Possessing the purest and most exemplary private character, with talents and attainments which have placed him at the head of the profession, and with kind and affable manners which have won the affections of his patients and conciliated the esteem and good-will of his associates, the Trustees cannot but regard his retirement from the Hospital as a most severe and serious loss. While they accept his resignation, therefore, they avail themselves of the opportunity publicly to acknowledge that he was among the most active and influential of the original founders of the Hospital; that, by an uniform course of disinterested professional and personal service, he has ever been one of its ablest officers and best friends; and that he is thus, in their opinion, entitled to the lasting gratitude of the institution and of the community. Voted also, that, as a testimonial of the respect of the Trustees for Dr. Jackson, a free bed in the Hospital be placed at his disposal during life." Dr. Enoch Hale was then elected to fill the situation thus vacated.

A successor of Dr. Jackson (Dr. O. W. Holmes) closes a humorous poem on the difference between being a patient and a physician, with a most feeling tribute to his predecessor. He had been describing what a physician ought to be, — one

> "Whose genial visit in itself combines
> The best of cordials, tonics, anodynes.
>   Such is the visit that, from day to day,
> Sheds o'er my chamber its benignant ray.
> I give *his* health who never cared to claim
> Her babbling homage from the tongue of fame:
> Unmoved by praise, he stands by all confessed
> The truest, noblest, wisest, kindest, best!"

On Nov. 5, the Treasurer was authorized to borrow eighteen thousand dollars, in part to pay existing loans, and in part, six thousand dollars, to defray current expenses. Messrs. Brimmer, Thorndike, and Loring were appointed a Committee on the subject of the Charlestown Branch Railroad, and also on the subject of removing the hill of gravel at the Asylum. Nov. 19, Mr. Bowditch was added to this Railroad Committee.

VOTE RESPECTING DR. JACKSON.

Messrs. Brimmer and Eliot were appointed a Committee " to consider and report what further marks of respect should be paid to Dr. Jackson." On Dec. 3, this Committee presented the following report: " The Trustees of the Massachusetts General Hospital, having received from Dr. Jackson the resignation of the office he has held since the first establishment of the institution, cannot suffer a circumstance of so much interest in the history of the Hospital to occur, without special notice of it on their records. It was, in great measure, owing to the active efforts of Dr. Jackson, and to the general knowledge of the fact that *he* would interest himself in its success, that this great charity was founded among us. So strong and just was the confidence of the community in his personal and professional character, that all suspicions of possible abuse in an institution of the kind under *his* care were speedily overcome, and liberally disposed persons were readily found to intrust to his integrity and skill the necessary funds for the foundation of an establishment which should do honor to the city. From its earliest existence to the present time, the Hospital has been watched over by Dr. Jackson with a zeal and fidelity which could not be surpassed, and has acquired a reputation, and been conducted with a success, highly honorable to him and to the other distinguished professional gentlemen with whom he has been associated. While his direct influence on the welfare of the institution has been thus decided and beneficial, the Trustees cannot but consider as equally valuable the indirect influence of the example of disinterested and faithful labor for the general good which he has given to the profession and the public. Under his constant attention, together with that of the professional friends assembled around him, the system on which the Hospital is conducted has been perfected, till it seems, at length, admirably adapted to the purposes for which the institution was founded, and promises to insure its utility during all its future existence. Long may it continue, by doing good to all classes, to embalm the memory of one who had so large a share in its foundation, and in conducting it to its present high rank; and long may this community enjoy the benefit of the direct and indirect influence of the pure, benevolent, and elevated character of Dr. Jackson! The Trustees, in communicating this copy of their record, take the occasion to request Dr. Jackson to sit for his portrait to some artist of talent, that it may adorn the walls which have so often been the witnesses of his disinterested labors." And this report was unanimously accepted.

A strong protest was, at this meeting, taken against the proposed location of the Charlestown Branch Railroad.

Dec. 17, a letter from Dr. Jackson was received, and the Chairman and Mr. Eliot were appointed a Committee to procure his portrait or bust as they may see fit. Dec. 21 and 22, his Excellency Mr. Everett and the Board of Visitors made the annual visitation. Messrs. Hooper and Bowditch were appointed a Committee to prepare the annual report. Jan. 12, 1828, the Treasurer was authorized to borrow twenty thousand dollars, as a substitute for loans formerly authorized. Jan. 17, leave of absence was granted to Dr. Bradford to visit Philadelphia.

The annual report at the close of this period notices the proceedings on the retirement of Dr. Jackson, and speaks of him as " one who, in the discharge of his official duties, has left a bright example to all who may succeed him, and whose name will never be mentioned by the friends of the Hospital but with affection and gratitude ; " mentions the completion of the Belknap Ward at a cost of $43,500, the estimates being forty thousand dollars, — that the institution is thus enabled to accommodate fifty additional boarders, and can therefore, to a certain extent, hereafter receive such as are known to be incurable. It states the measures adopted to oppose the location, &c., of the Charlestown Branch Railroad; the creation of a debt of forty thousand dollars; the diminished income of the institution ; and the need of a separate ward for fever-patients at the Hospital. It closes thus: "We do not think it expedient to make any actual call for subscriptions at the present time; but we feel the utmost confidence that such a call, when made, will be answered with that liberality which our institution has already experienced upon so many former occasions." Six years afterwards, such a call was made, and it was nobly answered. This report occupies five pages, and with its appendix thirty pages. From this pamphlet we learn that at the Hospital there were discharged one hundred and thirty-six males, seventy females, — total, two hundred and six; and that there were received at the Asylum, during the year, sixty-three males, fifty-seven females. The first report ever presented by Dr. Bell is one of the accompanying documents. It gives a very able, interesting, and satisfactory view of his department of the institution. It contains a table of all the patients received and discharged annually, from the very commencement of the Asylum, with the results of the cases.

SUMMARY. — This period of five years was a remarkable one in many respects. It embraced very numerous changes among the officers of the institution. The truly momentous event of the resignation of Dr. Wyman, the fortunate selection and premature decease of his successor, Dr. Lee; and the appointment of Dr. Bell, who has so successfully matured and perfected the admirable system of both his predecessors; the resignation of Mr. Bigelow; the temporary tenure of his successor, Mr. Wyman, ending in the auspicious selection of Mr. Tyler, the present incumbent, — mark this as a most important era in the History of the M'Lean Asylum. In the Hospital, also, the long-tried and valued services of Mr. Gurney had ended, and his place was filled by Dr. Bradford. The retirement of Dr. Jackson was indeed a loss which the Trustees felt could never be adequately supplied, so entirely had he identified himself with the institution from its very commencement. One President of the Corporation had died; and two others, Mr. Head and Mr. Francis, who had each been Chairman of the Board of Trustees, and among the ablest and most efficient officers of the institution, had now finally retired. Mr. Russell, after rendering the most valuable gratuitous services during fourteen years as Treasurer, had been succeeded by Mr. Andrews. Mr. Bowditch, in the office of Secretary, had been succeeded by Mr. Gray. Of the entire Board of Trustees at the beginning of this period, none remained except Mr. Bond, the Chairman; among those who had retired being Mr. Codman, whose services in the capacities of Secretary and Trustee had been of longer duration than those of any of his associates.

The general control of the institution, and the management of both its departments, had thus, as it were, passed into entirely new hands.

Only two donations, together amounting to but one thousand dollars, seem to have been received during this whole period of five years. A new building had been erected at the Asylum, finishing the female ward, to correspond precisely with that for male patients; and, pursuant to a previous suggestion of the Board, it had been appropriately named the Belknap Ward, in honor of that munificent benefactress of the institution, Miss Mary Belknap. In the erection of this building, a debt of forty thousand dollars had been contracted, for the payment of which, however, ample means existed. The M‘Lean Asylum continued to be conducted in such a manner as to deserve and receive the entire approval of the Trustees and of the public. The Hospital in Boston was, during this period also, conducted on the same general system as in former years. It would seem, indeed, from incidental notices in the records, that there had been occasionally some little temporary differences of opinion between the Medical Officers and the Superintendent; but the Board were satisfied that both parties were alike actuated by a sincere desire of doing their duty, and of most effectually promoting the welfare of the institution; and some slight and temporary inconveniences were, it is believed, the only result of the occasional want of harmony among its officers in this department. And it is due to Dr. Bradford to remark, in this connection, that his health, both of body and mind, was gradually becoming somewhat impaired by an alarming, and, as it proved, a fatal disorder, whose periodical attacks tended to render him unduly sensitive to the annoyances incident to his position. An occasional irritability, the natural result of his disease, from time to time manifested itself, and was a source of sincere regret to those who never ceased to respect and regard him, and to none more sincerely than to the Board of Trustees.

CHAPTER VII.

1838–1842.

DEATH OF DR. BRADFORD. — CHARLES SUMNER ELECTED SUPERINTENDENT. — HIS RESIGNATION. — JOHN M. GOODWIN CHOSEN HIS SUCCESSOR. — INDEX TO MEDICAL AND SURGICAL RECORDS. — RAILROADS AT THE ASYLUM. — PITIFUL LAND DAMAGES. — A WATER BED. — MISS BRIMMER'S BEQUEST. — JOHN M'LEAN'S PORTRAIT. — WARREN FUND. — SMALL POX AT HOSPITAL. — DEATH OF GEORGE BOND, CHAIRMAN OF TRUSTEES: HIS CHARACTER AND SERVICES. — ROBERT HOOPER, JUN., CHAIRMAN. — BUST OF DR. JAMES JACKSON.

AT the annual meeting of the Corporation, Jan. 24, 1838, Edward Tuckerman, President; Jonathan Phillips, Vice-President; Henry Andrews, Treasurer; and William Gray, Secretary, were severally re-elected. William Appleton was elected by the Corporation a Trustee in place of Charles G. Loring; and Thomas Lamb was subsequently elected by the Board of Visitors a Trustee in the place of John P. Thorndike. Both these gentlemen had declined a re-election, and were thanked for their services. The Board now consisted of Charles Amory, William Appleton, Nathaniel I. Bowditch, Martin Brimmer, Thomas B. Curtis, Samuel A. Eliot, Robert Hooper, jun., and Samuel Lawrence, Trustees on the part of the Corporation; George Bond, Henry Edwards, Thomas Lamb, and Robert G. Shaw, Trustees on the part of the

Board of Visitors. It was voted, "That the Corporation entirely concur in the sentiments expressed by the Board of Trustees in their votes adopted upon the resignation of Dr. Jackson;" and the same were ordered to be printed with the annual report.

Drs. James Jackson, George C. Shattuck, John Randall, and John Ware, were chosen Consulting Physicians; Drs. George B. Doane, John Jeffries, Abel L. Pierson, and Solomon D. Townsend, Consulting Surgeons. Drs. Jacob Bigelow, Walter Channing, and Enoch Hale, were re-elected Physicians; Drs. John C. Warren and George Hayward, Surgeons; and J. B. S. Jackson, Assistant or (since called) Admitting Physician. Feb. 18, Mr. Homer Goodhue was chosen Male Supervisor at the Asylum, and Miss Relief R. Barber, Female Supervisor; of which posts they have always performed the duties in a most exemplary manner. Miss Barber, indeed, is a second Mrs. Tyler. March 18, the Treasurer was authorized to borrow six thousand dollars. April 13, the free beds were reduced to twenty-four. April 18, a billiard-table was ordered for the female patients at the Asylum. April 22, Dr. J. B. S. Jackson resigning his office, Dr. Henry I. Bowditch was, at the next meeting, May 6, elected his successor. July 3, further loans of four thousand and six thousand dollars were authorized. Aug. 9, Henry

J. Bigelow was elected House Physician; and John B. Johnson, House Surgeon, for the year ensuing. Sept. 16, Mr. Lawrence resigned his office of Trustee. Messrs. Lamb and Bowditch were appointed a Committee on the subject of a bequest of the late Ambrose S. Courtis; to whom was also referred, on Sept. 30, a proposal of the heirs at law for a compromise. Pursuant to a subsequent report of this Committee, one quarter part of the bequest was accepted in full (two thousand five hundred dollars), provided no greater percentage be paid to any other legatee. Dec. 16, Messrs. Edwards and Brimmer were appointed to prepare the annual report.

This report is a pamphlet of seven pages, with documents annexed, making ten pages more. It states the illness of Dr. Bradford, and his temporary absence from that cause; — "the unexampled difficulties of the times;" — the embarrassed state of the finances; — total receipts (of which $6,740 was capital), $16,081; current expenses, $17,506.24; excess of expenditures, $1,425.24; due to Massachusetts Hospital Life Insurance Company, $50,000; — and the completion of the Belknap Ward. One sentence was destined to be strikingly verified a few years afterwards, viz.: " The Massachusetts General Hospital has always aimed to adopt and introduce the most recent improvements and discoveries in medicine and surgery." It mentions the increased number of inmates at the Asylum:— the cure of all the recent cases, excluding deaths and patients prematurely removed. It contains a very curious table, showing the occupations, &c., of all the male patients at the Asylum for twenty years. Remaining in the Asylum, Jan. 1, fifty-eight males, thirty-five females: total, ninety-three.

Dec. 30, thanks were voted to Dr. Warren " for his attention in procuring instruments and medicines."

At the annual meeting of the Corporation, Jan. 23, 1839, Samuel A. Eliot, Thomas B. Curtis, and Samuel Lawrence, having declined a re-election as Trustees, were severally thanked for their services; and George M. Dexter, Francis C. Lowell, and Henry B. Rogers were chosen in their stead; all three of whom still continue to be members of the Board. Mr. Eliot had been a very efficient officer. Many of the ablest reports of Committees were from his pen. In his relations to this institution, he always displayed his characteristic energy and independence, both of thought and action. At this meeting was passed the vote by which all persons who have served, or shall hereafter serve, as Trustees, are to be considered members of the Corporation. A remonstrance was ordered against the attempt of the Charlestown

Branch Railroad to connect with the Worcester Railroad.

On Feb. 10, one thousand copies of the annual report were ordered to be printed. Drs. Bigelow and Hale were re-elected Physicians; and Dr. Ware was chosen in place of Dr. Channing, who was thanked for his long and faithful services. To the two surgeons of last year was now added a third, Dr. Solomon D. Townsend. Dr. James Jackson and Drs. Shattuck and Randall were re-elected Consulting Physicians; and Dr. Homans was substituted for Dr. Ware. On the Board of Consulting Surgeons, Dr. Edward Reynolds was elected in place of Dr. Townsend. Messrs. Bond and Brimmer were appointed a Committee to procure the portrait of Dr. Jackson. March 24, measures were ordered to protect the Hospital-garden against claims of air and light from windows opening thereon. July 12, Dr. Henry J. Bigelow resigned as House Surgeon, and Mr. John F. Eustis was appointed to take his place at present, and was chosen House Physician; and Dr. Christopher C. Holmes was chosen House Surgeon for the year ensuing. At this time, Messrs. Bond and Bowditch were on the Visiting Committee; and there were but three foreigners in the House, one paying and two free.

On Oct. 11, Messrs. Shaw and Brimmer were instructed to report as to the expediency of rejecting syphilitic patients, or of charging them extra board; and this Committee subsequently reported, that such patients should be received only in urgent cases, and should always be charged double the usual rates of board; and this rule has ever since been acted on. Messrs. Bond and Bowditch were appointed a Committee to consider the expediency of applying to the Surgeons for the records, or for leave to copy the same, who at a subsequent meeting reported in favor of such an application. The Physicians had always regarded their records as the property of the institution. Dr. Warren, on the contrary, considered the surgical records as his own private memoranda. The appointment of this Committee, however, and their suggestions as to the importance of the institution's possessing either the originals of these records or copies of them, induced him very cheerfully to yield up any private claim.

On Wednesday, Oct. 23, a special meeting was held; and the following votes, prepared by Mr. Bowditch, were adopted: "It having been announced to the Board, that Gamaliel Bradford, M.D., Superintendent of the Massachusetts General Hospital, died on Tuesday forenoon, after an unusually violent attack of epilepsy, to which disorder he had been for some time subject, — Voted, that the Trustees would express to Mrs. Bradford their sincere and respectful sympathy upon an event which has thus suddenly taken from her and her young children an affectionate husband and father, and deprived this institution of the services of a zealous and faithful officer." By another vote, six months' additional salary was granted to Mrs. Bradford; and she and her family were invited to remain at the Hospital till the choice of a new Superintendent. And it was further voted, that the Trustees will attend the funeral of the deceased " as a tribute of respect for his private character, and a public acknowledgment of his official fidelity." Dr. Parker, of Roxbury, was requested to act as Superintendent *pro tem*. Mrs. Bradford was, by a special vote, subsequently continued in the office of Matron till the first of April following; and it may be truly said, that, from the moment when she first entered the Hospital until she left it, the Trustees felt the most entire satisfaction with the mode in which she had performed all the arduous and responsible duties of her post. And when she at last departed, a widow, with an interesting family, which had been growing up around her, she carried with her the respect and regard of all the members of the Board, and their most sincere good wishes, which have since been happily realized.

Nov. 3, at this meeting, the Committee upon the

records of cases made their formal report, which was accepted; and the House Physician and Surgeon were directed, for the future, to record all cases in volumes to be prepared for that purpose. A perfect index has been since made, both to the medical and surgical records, so that their entire contents and results are rendered at once accessible. Nov. 17, all moneys received by the Superintendent are ordered to be deposited in some one bank, in his name "as Superintendent." Dec. 15, Messrs. Shaw and Lowell were appointed a Committee to prepare the annual report. This report is very brief, about five pages, but contains at the end a report of Dr. Bell, eighteen pages in length, and other documents, making together a pamphlet of thirty-six pages. It mentions the death of Dr. Bradford, — " a man equally remarkable for strict integrity of purpose, and great independence of judgment;" states that " Mrs. Bradford continues, for the present, her valuable though unostentatious services, which have heretofore contributed so much to the success of the establishment." It shows that the number of patients treated this year at the Hospital (three hundred and sixty-nine) has been less than usual. Of the M'Lean Asylum it remarks, that "it continues to improve;" and the Committee add, "It would be difficult to find language that would imply greater praise to those who have the care of it." In this department there were remaining, Dec. 31, sixty-two males, forty-six females: total, one hundred and eight. It mentions by name all the free-bed donors of the year. Dr. Bell's report is very able, interesting, and important. I will not do him the injustice of making any analysis of it, or giving any extracts from his statements and views. It ends with the following sentence: " In closing this third year of his labors in a field of duty which to him has been one of unmingled enjoyment, the Superintendent cannot deny himself the satisfaction of bearing his testimony to the devoted, intelligent, and conscientious co-operation which he has uniformly had from all those associated with him."

Dec. 17, Mr. Charles Sumner was chosen Superintendent. Dec. 27, there were twenty-nine males, sixteen females, in the Hospital: total, forty-five. The number in July previous had on one occasion been reduced to twenty-one. Dec. 29, the Visiting Committee were authorized " to procure a water-bed, if they think proper." Jan. 10, 1840, the number of free beds was raised to thirty-two. On the 18th, the Visiting Committee were instructed to make arrangements for Dr. Bell's absence, and to continue his salary. John C. Gray, Esq., was thanked for a donation of three hundred dollars.

At the annual meeting, Jan. 22, 1840, the same Board of Trustees were re-elected, except that Ebenezer Chadwick took the place of Mr. Rogers, then absent in Europe. Feb. 9, one thousand copies of the annual report were ordered. Dr. Ware was thanked for his valuable services as Physician during the past year, his extensive private practice preventing him from being able to hold his office any longer; and Dr. J. B. S. Jackson was chosen in his stead. The Consulting Physicians were all re-elected, as were also the Consulting Surgeons, except that Dr. O. W. Holmes took the place of Dr. Doane, deceased. March 22, Mr. Cogswell's application for a loan of the portrait of Lieutenant-Governor Phillips, for the purpose of taking an engraving, was granted.

On April 15, the following vote was passed, which is still acted upon: "That any patient sent by a subscriber for a free bed at the Hospital shall be admitted, provided the subscriber's free bed be not pre-occupied by his order, notwithstanding the vote fixing the number of free beds." May 17, the rules as to the admission of students at the Hospital were modified; and it was made henceforth the duty of the Physicians and Surgeons to nominate two persons as House Physician and two as House Surgeon, one of these nominees to be subsequently chosen by the Trustees. This rule of a double nomination is also still acted on. June 14, the Treasurer and Messrs. Dexter and Bowditch were appointed a Committee respecting a new lease of the Belknap Estate in Washington Street. June 28, the Treasurer was authorized, with Mr. Lamb's concurrence, to make investments, or to pay off part of the existing debt. July 10, Messrs. Brimmer, Lowell, and Bowditch were appointed a Committee to examine reports of French and English Hospitals, sent from Europe by Mr. Brimmer. July 15, the officer called House Apothecary at the Asylum was ordered to be known as the Assistant Physician; and a grant was made to Dr. Fox of five hundred dollars, for the " highly satisfactory manner" in which he had performed his duties during the absence of Dr. Bell.

Aug. 16, 1840, William A. Davis was elected House Physician, and Elijah R. Mears, House Surgeon of the Hospital, for the year ensuing. Aug. 30, the Committee reported, as the result of their examination of foreign reports, that a comparison be instituted of the prices paid at the Hospital, at the Asylum, and at the Worcester Institution, for stores, &c. Sept. 13, it was voted that the portrait of Mr. M'Lean be removed to the M'Lean Asylum, and placed in the oval room. It now hangs there. The room thus designated was the dancing-hall in the days of the old owner, Mr. Barrell, and is now the room occupied by the Trustees, and for the reception of visitors. On Nov. 22, the claim against the Charlestown Branch Railroad was referred. Dec. 20, Messrs. Dexter and Lamb were appointed to prepare the annual report.

This report is only three pages long; yet with its accompanying documents it forms a pamphlet of no less than forty-three pages. It mentions the increased subscriptions for free beds, for which it says " the Hospital is greatly indebted to the personal exertions of the Assistant Physician, Dr. Bowditch." The subscribers are also especially thanked, and a list of their names is appended to the report. The bequest of Miss Brimmer for this object is gratefully acknowledged. The receipt of a dividend of one third of the profits of the Life Insurance Company ($20,000) is announced, and the fact that it was applied in part payment of the debt due that institution; the dividend from the stock in that institution being $7,825. The total receipts of the year were $41,471.24; total expenditures, $37,185.26. The report of Mr. Sumner, the Superintendent of the Hospital, contains various interesting statistics and analyses. Dr. Bell's report is sixteen pages long, besides eleven pages of republication of extracts from, and documents appended to, his report of two years before. Number of inmates, Dec. 31, seventy-four males, fifty-one females: total, one hundred and twenty-five. Total expenses, $20,919.63. It contains various tabular statements, showing the results for the preceding five years. It contrasts the slight personal restraint found necessary in our institution with that resorted to in similar establishments in Great Britain, &c.; the abuses of private mad-houses in that country, and the safeguards against like abuses here. This report of Dr. Bell will be found no less interesting and instructive than its predecessors. Dec. 25, twenty-two males, twenty-five females, — total, forty-seven, in the Hospital.

Jan. 15, 1841, the number of free beds for the quarter was fixed at thirty-five, and for the two next quarters was to be reduced to twenty-five. A letter from William D. Sohier, Esq., was received and read, giving notice of a bequest of five thousand dollars on certain trusts, in the will of Miss Mary Anne Brimmer, which was referred to Messrs. Bowditch and Lowell; and at the next meeting, on report of this Committee, it was voted to accept said legacy, " upon the trusts prescribed by her will, and with the wish to carry into full effect the benevolent intentions of the donor." The purchase of certain lands near the Asylum was referred to the Visiting Committee.

At the annual meeting of the Corporation, held Jan. 27, the same eight Trustees were re-elected. The

Board of Visitors elected Ignatius Sargent in place of Robert G. Shaw, who had resigned. Mr. Shaw, notwithstanding his numerous private engagements, had zealously discharged his duty as one of the Board for the preceding five years. Feb. 14, the Committee were authorized to publish what number of copies they saw fit of the annual report. All the Medical and Surgical Officers and heads of departments in office at the close of the year were re-elected. Feb. 28, Rejoice Newton, Esq., was requested to take steps for collecting the amount due from Isaiah Thomas's legacy. Mr. Bowditch, Chairman of the Committee on the subject of Miss Brimmer's legacy, made a detailed report, which was accepted, — to the end, first, that a separate investment and account of the fund should be kept by the Treasurer, and the income yearly paid to the Superintendent; second, that, as there were twenty-four free beds in the Hospital when Miss Brimmer died (Oct. 18, 1839), the Board must never establish a less number, as in such case the bequest would be forfeited; and, third, that on Jan. 1, 1842, two permanent free beds should be established, to be called the Brimmer Free Beds, to be for ever maintained by the income of said fund.

March 21, 1841, Captain Sumner having decided to resign his situation as Superintendent, Mr. John M. Goodwin was unanimously elected. Mr. Goodwin, it will be remembered, had been, several years before, an officer at the Asylum. April 4, Mr. Dexter was authorized to buy eight acres of land, at four hundred dollars per acre, near the Asylum, or to hire the Joy Farm at five hundred dollars a year for five years. April 16, the Brimmer bequest the Treasurer was authorized to invest in any mode sanctioned by her will. The thanks of the Board were presented to Dr. John C. Warren for " his donation to the Hospital of the records of surgical cases, which have been kept by the Surgeons of the Hospital." April 21, Mr. Dexter reported that he had bought the eight acres of land of the Lowell Railroad, at five hundred dollars per acre. This is the lot at the entrance of our avenue on the right-hand side, and is now probably worth five times as much as it cost.

May 9, Messrs. Bowditch and Dexter were appointed a Committee to settle the northerly line of the Belknap Estate in Washington Street, with Mr. Gibbs, the adjoining proprietor. June 6, the Visiting Committee, with Dr. Bowditch the Assistant Physician, were directed to take measures for preserving the medical and surgical records, and for bringing to the notice of the Trustees all cases of patients who had been over three months in the Hospital. Aug. 8, Ezra W. Fletcher was elected House Physician, and George Hayward, jun., House Surgeon, for the year ensuing.

Oct. 20, 1841, Mr. Bowditch, from the Committee on the Charlestown Branch Railroad, reported that the referees, Judge Fay and Messrs. Fletcher and Parker, had awarded *six hundred* dollars for damages which the Committee thought really amounted to *five thousand*. Nov. 7, Dr. Warren transmitted a letter enclosing one thousand dollars as a fund for the pnrchase of religious and moral books to be given to patients on leaving the Hospital. This donation was accepted; and Dr. Warren was thanked " for his early, efficient, and continued interest in this institution;" his letter being recorded *in extenso*.

Dec. 5, Mr. Ignatius Sargent resigned his office of Trustee, and transmitted a donation of four hundred dollars, which was suitably acknowledged by the Board, who expressed their great regret at losing him as an associate. Dec. 19, Messrs. Appleton, Bond, and Edwards were appointed a Committee respecting a fund in aid of poor, insane patients who are deemed curable. Messrs. Amory and Chadwick were chosen to prepare the annual report. This report is only four pages long, but, with the accompanying documents, makes a pamphlet of forty pages. It mentions the resignation of Mr. Sumner; that Mr. John M. Goodwin " entered upon his duties early in April last, and has since performed the same in a manner so satisfactory as to give every reason to believe that the Board made the best choice in their power." It mentions certain statistics, as to free beds for the past three years, furnished by Dr. Bowditch, " our most indefatigable Assistant Physician." It commends " Dr. Bell's most able and elaborate report" to " the careful perusal of all." It states the present property of the institution, deducting its debt of twenty thousand dollars to the Life Insurance Company, as about ninety thousand dollars; total receipts of the year, twenty-four thousand dollars; expenses, twenty-three thousand six hundred dollars. Dr. Bell's report fully justifies the commendation bestowed on it by the Committee. It is twenty-two pages long, exclusive of an appendix of forms of admission. It states that the patients, Dec. 31, were seventy-nine males, sixty-three females: total, one hundred and forty-two. Messrs. Bond and Bowditch were desired to consider the appointment of an Assistant Surgeon, and, on Jan. 14, were discharged from that duty. On Dec. 31, nineteen males, thirty females, — total, forty-nine, — in Hospital.

At the annual meeting of the Corporation, in January, 1842, Marcus Morton, jun., Esq., was elected Secretary in place of Mr. Gray, who had declined a re-election. All the Trustees on the part of the Corporation were re-elected; and Mr. Henry B. Rogers was again chosen by the Board of Visitors a Trustee in place of Mr. Sargent. Feb. 20, all the Medical and Surgical Officers, and heads of the two departments, were severally re-elected. April 21, the salary of the Male Supervisor, Mr. Goodhue, was raised to five hundred dollars, and of the Female Supervisor, Miss Barber, to two hundred and fifty dollars, in acknowledgment of their faithful and efficient services.

At a special meeting, May 3, it was voted, that the Trustees, under " their feeling of great anxiety from the introduction of the small-pox and varioloid into the General Hospital, hereby recommend, that, until these diseases are expelled, as few patients as possible be admitted into the Hospital; and that all patients who are admitted shall be first informed of the condition of the house; and that the Visiting Committee be requested to inform the Physicians and Surgeons of this opinion of the Trustees, and to urge upon them to give such care and directions as shall in their judgment be most effectual to prevent these diseases from spreading among the patients." The Visiting Committee and Mr. Dexter were appointed a Committee to cleanse, whitewash, and paint the Hospital.

On June 5, we find the following record, viz.: " Mr. Bowditch proposed the following votes, which were read and adopted: — George Bond, Esq., Chairman of this Board, having died May 23, aged fifty-four years, voted that this event has closed a life of honorable usefulness, depriving the community of one of its most upright, active, and intelligent citizens, who, in his better days, was among the foremost in all acts of private liberality and of public enterprise, and who bore adversity with a manly firmness which won universal sympathy and respect. Voted, that by this bereavement this institution has lost one of its best friends and benefactors, one who has ever manifested an untiring zeal in promoting its interests and objects, — devoting himself to his official duties with an assiduity and fidelity worthy of all praise and imitation. Voted, that a copy of these resolutions, expressing the sense which this Board entertain of the exemplary character and important services of their late associate, be transmitted to his widow and children."

Mr. Bond had been Chairman of the Board for seven years. By recent reverses in business, he had become bankrupt, and had been prevented by illness from attending any meeting since Jan. 29. He was particularly instrumental in the fortunate selection of Dr. Bell, and had always taken an especial interest in the affairs of the Asylum. He often made visits there in company with Mrs. Bond, and ever showed a deep interest in the welfare of its inmates. In the transaction of business, he was uniformly prompt and attentive; in his intercourse with the Board, courteous and affable. All its members cherished towards him a strong feeling of personal regard. I trust that it will not be deemed a violation of confidence, if I mention, in this connection, the interesting fact, that his associates sent him, shortly before his death, a letter expressive of these their sentiments, and enclosing five hundred dollars to defray his expenses during a journey to the South, in the hope that his health might thus be restored. He died among strangers; but none can doubt that this mark of attention and friendship, slight as it was, must have been beyond measure grateful to him, as he was leaving those familiar scenes to which he was never to return.

At this meeting, May 23, renewed admissions into the Hospital were recommended. June 3, two foreigners paying, two free; two Americans paying, eight free: total, fourteen.

June 19, Mr. Robert Hooper, jun., was elected Chairman. July 15, the Superintendent was directed to prohibit the use of tobacco *by the patients within the house.* It has been since much more stringently and generally excluded. Aug. 7, a permanent free bed was established, called the Tucker Free Bed, to be for ever maintained out of the income of the bequest of Miss Margaret Tucker, which had just been received. William Henry Thayer was elected House Physician, and Edward B. Pierson House Surgeon, for the year ensuing.

On Aug. 21, 1842, the Treasurer was authorized " to reimburse Mr. Brimmer the cost and expenses incurred by him in procuring the marble bust of Dr. Jackson." This bust is now in the Trustees' room. As a work of art, it is truly admirable. It is the most speaking likeness that can be conceived. It will transmit to coming times the calm and benignant countenance of the first Physician of the Hospital. Sept. 18, " George Washington " was placed on a free bed from his admission, probably on account of his name. Dec. 4, Messrs. Rogers and Andrews were appointed a Committee to prepare the annual report.

This report is about twelve pages in length, and, with the documents appended, forms a pamphlet of exactly the length of its immediate predecessor, — forty pages. It states the cost of the Hospital at $145,069.44, and of the Asylum, $245,845.98 : in all, $390,915.42. It states the various sources of income of the institution, and the expense of each department; that the Asylum will henceforth defray its general current expenses [it has done so]; that, on April 8, a case of small-pox occurred in the Hospital, and two others in the same ward were attacked by it, one of whom died ; that sixteen cases of mild varioloid occurred to June 1; that the number of patients was reduced from sixty-one to thirteen, the Directors having forbid all admissions during this period. It mentions, with suitable expressions of gratitude, the generous donation of one thousand dollars by Dr. John C. Warren. In regard to the Asylum, it states that the patients, on Dec. 31, were eighty-one males, fifty-two females: total, one hundred and thirty-three. It concurs with Dr. Bell in the opinion, "that in general health and peace, in freedom from every painful accident, and in its curative results, the year now completed will compare favorably with any former period." It especially commends the views embraced in his report, and refers to the interesting circumstance that it includes the results of a period of exactly twenty-five years. This report of Dr. Bell is sixteen pages long, besides an appendix of five pages. The Committee close with the following beautiful tribute to the memory of the late George Bond, Esq.: "Ever ready to devote his time, talents, property, and influence to all objects of public utility, he was the early friend of this institution, and by his faithful services and prudent counsels, contributed essentially to its present prosperity and success. A man of lofty principles, sterling integrity, sound judgment, and generous impulses, his memory is entitled to the respect of all who honor virtue, or love practical benevolence. May we not hope that his example will be duly appreciated and extensively followed?"

Dec. 30, thirty-one males, nineteen females, were in Hospital. Jan. 18, 1843, Mr. Brimmer declined a re-election as Trustee. An engraving was ordered of the Asylum Buildings. Messrs. Lamb and Bowditch were appointed the Free-bed Committee.

But two donations to the institution were made during this period of five years: Mr. Courtis's bequest, compromised at two thousand five hundred dollars, and Dr. Warren's donation of one thousand dollars. Miss Tucker's legacy, though now received, had been made many years previously. At the Hospital, the death of the Superintendent, Dr. Bradford, and the short term of his immediate successor, Mr. Sumner, had been followed by the appointment of Mr. Goodwin. The lamented decease of Mr. Bond had been followed by the selection of a most worthy and able successor. The small-pox, which had been introduced, fortunately proved fatal, as is believed, in only one instance. The pitiful amount received, under award of referees, for land at the Asylum taken by the Charlestown Branch Railroad, was more than compensated by the judicious purchase of other additional land in the vicinity. Both departments of the institution were successfully accomplishing the objects for which they were founded.

CHAPTER VIII.

1843–1847.

DONATION BOOK COMPLETED BY MR. ROGERS. — VARIOLOID AGAIN IN HOSPITAL. — MR. APPLETON'S DONATION, TEN THOUSAND DOLLARS. — ISRAEL MUNSON'S BEQUEST, TWENTY THOUSAND DOLLARS. — SEARS FREE BEDS. — LANDS IN SOMERVILLE TAXED. — TWO WINGS ADDED TO HOSPITAL: SUBSCRIPTION OF SIXTY-TWO THOUSAND FIVE HUNDRED AND FIFTY DOLLARS. — SERVICES OF MR. ROGERS. — MISS TAYLOR'S ILLNESS. — DR. BELL'S VISIT TO EUROPE AT REQUEST OF BUTLER HOSPITAL, OF RHODE ISLAND. — BEQUEST OF JOHN PARKER, TEN THOUSAND DOLLARS. — STATUE OF APOLLO. — LYING-IN DEPARTMENT DISCUSSED. — DANIEL WALDO'S BEQUEST, FORTY THOUSAND DOLLARS. — DEATH OF MR. GOODWIN. — ANECDOTE OF HIM. — RICHARD GIRDLER ELECTED. — TOMB OF THOMAS OLIVER. — NEW KITCHEN AT HOSPITAL. — ENLARGED MEDICAL AND SURGICAL STAFF. — MEDICAL COLLEGE. — JOHN REDMAN'S BEQUEST, ONE HUNDRED THOUSAND DOLLARS. — WILLIAM OLIVER'S, FIFTY THOUSAND DOLLARS. — OUTDOOR PATIENTS. — HOSPITAL FENCE. — MONUMENT TO JEREMIAH AND MARY BELKNAP. — ADDITION TO DWELLING-HOUSE AT ASYLUM. — BEQUEST OF SARAH CLOUGH, A DOMESTIC. — ETHER DISCOVERY. — SICKNESS AT ASYLUM. — DEATH OF SEVERAL PATIENTS, AND OF TWO CHILDREN OF DR. BELL.

AT the annual meeting, Jan. 25, 1843, the following officers were re-elected: Edward Tuckerman, President; Jonathan Phillips, Vice-President; Henry Andrews, Treasurer; Marcus Morton, jun., Secretary. The eight Trustees elected by the Corporation were Charles Amory, William T. Andrews, Nathaniel I. Bowditch, George M. Dexter, Robert Hooper, jun., Francis C. Lowell, Jonathan Chapman, and William F. Otis; the two last in the place of Messrs. Brimmer and Chadwick, who had resigned, and were thanked for their services. Messrs. Henry Edwards, Thomas Lamb, and Henry B. Rogers were re-elected by the Board of Visitors; and John A. Lowell, Esq., was chosen in place of Mr. Bond, deceased. All the Medical and Surgical Officers, and the heads of the two departments, were re-elected. Two thousand five hundred copies of the annual report were ordered to be published.

Messrs. Bowditch and F. C. Lowell were appointed a Committee respecting an application for a new Life Insurance Charter, now before the Legislature. Feb. 19, Mr. Bowditch was appointed to advise with the Treasurer as to investment of funds now in his hands. March 5, the Visiting Committee were ordered to confer with Dr. Bell as to procuring a clergyman to officiate at the Asylum. The House Apothecary at Hospital was ordered to be chosen annually, at the time of the choice of Physicians and Surgeons. March 19, the Visiting Committee and Mr. Bowditch were appointed a Committee to have tablets prepared with names of the donors, to be placed over such free beds as are supported from their funds, as in the case of the Brimmer and Tucker free beds. This was subsequently found to be very distasteful to patients, as making an odious discrimination between free and pay patients, and was rescinded.

On April 2, Mr. Rogers was appointed a Committee " to complete the list of subscriptions, donations, and legacies, commenced by Col. Joseph May." April 19, Dr. Chauncey Booth was chosen Assistant Physician and Apothecary at the Asylum. Messrs. Dexter and F. C. and J. A. Lowell were appointed a Committee on the subject of ventilation, warming, &c., of the Hospital; who subsequently reported plans, with estimates, and were instructed to execute the same. May 7, Messrs. Bowditch, Otis, and Amory were appointed a Committee on the house-diet and general discipline of the Hospital; and Mr. Bowditch was asked to ascertain the boundary of the Hospital flats, and to take measures to prevent encroachments.

On May 12, a special meeting was held, on information that one of the patients was believed to be ill of varioloid; and the Visiting Committee were requested to wait on Dr. Warren, ascertain facts, and act as they shall judge best. May 21, the Committee on diet, &c., made a report, which was accepted, and ordered to be communicated to the Superintendent, and by him to all the other officers; and it was " voted, that, whenever the Medical and Surgical Officers shall think there is any reason to suppose that a patient is ill of varioloid or small-pox, it shall be their duty forthwith to inform the Superintendent, to the end that he may take immediate measures to remove such patient from the institution, if he can be removed with safety;" and a copy of this vote was sent to all the officers. July 2, a box was ordered at the Hospital for preservation of valuable papers. It is now kept in the Trustees' room. Aug. 20, John Frasier Head was elected House Physician; William E. Townsend, House Surgeon; Charles K. Whipple re-elected Apothecary. Oct. 18, Mr. Dexter was appointed to express to Mr. George Taylor " the unanimous and decided opposition of the Trustees " to his project of laying out a new street through the Hospital-grounds.

Mr. Rogers, the Committee on the Book of Donations, reported that he had completed the same. His interesting letter, stating the difficulties of the task, and showing how successfully they were overcome, is recorded in full; and it occupies five pages of the record. He details the various services of Col. May; and of the early donors he says: " They belonged to every rank and condition of life; their subscriptions far exceeded in amount and number any thing of the kind which, even to this day, has been known in New England; and Mr. May seems to have taken a pride in recording their names, as alike honorable to themselves and to the social and political institutions under which they lived." It closes with the following interesting summary: —

TOTAL DONATIONS AND SUBSCRIPTIONS.

From the record as now made up, it appears that 1,191 persons subscribed to the Hospital and Asylum	$131,269.21
There had been received from public exhibitions, concerts, and incorporated bodies, among which are comprised twenty-four religious societies, twelve towns, and five benevolent associations .	15,723.36
Making a total	$146,992.57
Of which amount, $45,373.34 was specially subscribed for the Asylum.	
There had been bequeathed, devised, or given . . .	388,098.68
Received from annual donations to free beds . . .	46,657.00
Thus raising the gross amount received in various ways from the public, from the commencement to this date, and without including the right of the Corporation to the profits of the Massachusetts Life Insurance Company, to the magnificent sum of	$581,748.25

The task thus completed by Mr. Rogers was most ably and satisfactorily accomplished. No report, indeed, had ever been made to this Board either more gratifying in itself, or which more entitles the Committee by whom it was submitted, to the sincere thanks of the Trustees and of all friends of the institution.

At the same meeting, it was voted " that the subject of Mr. Lee's bequest to the Hospital be referred to Mr. Bowditch, with full powers." This, it is believed, related only to certain restrictions originally imposed by Mr. Lee, as to selling the stocks which he gave.

Dec. 3, a communication having been received from William Appleton, enclosing a check for the sum of ten thousand dollars, as a donation for the purpose of affording aid to such patients in the M'Lean Asylum as from straitened means might be compelled to leave the institution without a perfect cure, — it was " voted that the Trustees appreciate highly the liberality and wisdom of this act of charity, and accept this donation to be held sacred for the special purpose designated by the donor." Mr. Appleton's communication was ordered to be recorded, and the amount deposited in the Massachusetts Hospital Life Insurance Company, as " the Appleton Fund for the Relief of the Insane ; " Messrs. Hooper and F. C. Lowell being appointed to carry these votes into effect. On Dec. 17, Messrs. J. A. Lowell and Otis were appointed a Committee to prepare the annual report.

Of this document the unprecedented number of four thousand copies was published, — a compliment to which it was well entitled. It is twelve pages long, and contains an elaborate report of Dr. Bell, of forty-two pages, making in all a pamphlet of sixty-three pages. The report gives a very satisfactory view of the property of the institution. The donations of the year were $10,762.37 ; the payment of ten thousand dollars on the note to the Life Insurance Company leaving only a balance of ten thousand dollars due,

ENLARGEMENT OF HOSPITAL. 175

probably to be paid before the report shall be read It extracts from the donation-book the summary of all the donations, $581,748.25. It especially notices the welcome gift by Mr. Appleton of the fund of ten thousand dollars. Dr. Bell's report is one of the most valuable of his satisfactory annual communications. Appended to it is a table, showing all the results of the Asylum from its commencement. Eighty males and fifty-four females remained in that institution at the close of the year. A brief report from Mr. Goodwin, the Superintendent of the Hospital, is published, with the usual analyses. Dec. 29, thirty-three males, twenty-two females, in the Hospital.

Dec. 31, notice of annual meeting was ordered to be sent by the Secretary to all the members of the Corporation, so far as he can ascertain them. Voted " that the present and past Physicians and Surgeons of the institution be requested to suggest to this Board any changes in the management or arrangements of the Hospital, which in their view would increase its usefulness, and also to express their opinion of the necessity of enlarging the buildings." The result of this vote was the enlargement of the Hospital by the addition of two wings, each fifty feet square. Jan. 12, 1844, the Superintendent was authorized to buy a vapor-bath now at the Hospital; and grants were made of two hundred dollars to Dr. Bell, and one hundred each to Mr. and Mrs. Tyler.

At the annual meeting, Jan. 24, 1844, William Appleton, Esq., was elected President in place of Edward Tuckerman, Esq., deceased; and Charles S. Storrow and Edward Wigglesworth, Trustees in place of Messrs. Chapman and Otis, who had declined a re-election, and were thanked for their services during the past year. Feb. 4, on the Board of Consulting Physicians, Joseph Roby took the place of Dr. John Randall, deceased. There were no other changes of officers. Two thousand five hundred copies of the report were ordered to be printed.

On Feb. 18, Mr. Bowditch presented a remonstrance against a new railroad, prayed for near the Asylum, which was adopted, and ordered to be laid before the Legislature; and Messrs. Bowditch and Edwards were appointed to appear before the Committee of the Legislature in support of the same. This was the Maine Railroad, which the Trustees succeeded in keeping off at a *respectful* distance. March 3, fifteen hundred additional copies were ordered of the report, making in all four thousand.

On March 17, Messrs. Amory and Rogers were appointed a Committee to inquire into the facts relative to a donation of five thousand dollars made to this institution by David Sears in 1817, and to report. Certain alterations proposed in the female "lodge" at the Asylum, by Dr. Bell, were agreed to; and the Steward was authorized to make the same. The Treasurer, and Messrs. Bowditch and Dexter, were appointed a Committee to rebuild the Belknap Estate on Washington Street. A report of the Physicians and Surgeons was received, and a future meeting ordered, at which their attendance was requested; Messrs. Rogers and Dexter being requested to bring the title-deeds, plans, &c. March 26, the proposed meeting took place, the Visiting Physicians and Surgeons being present; and Drs. James Jackson and John Ware, past Physicians. Messrs. Amory and Bowditch were appointed a Committee on the subject of visits at the Hospital. The Chairman, J. A. Lowell, and the Treasurer, were appointed a Committee respecting a legacy of the late Israel Munson. This Committee reported at the next meeting, that they had received the same in United States six per cent stock.

On March 31, Messrs. Rogers and Andrews were appointed a Committee to expend fifty dollars for the formation of a permanent library at the Hospital. "It appearing, by report of the Committee, that in the year 1817 the sum of five thousand dollars was given to this institution by David Sears, Esq., with the wish and intent on his part that the same should be specially applied to the relief of surgical patients; and whereas two free beds are established in the Hospital, specially for cases of accident, — voted that the said two free beds be henceforth known as the Sears Free Beds." The Committee on Visits at the Hospital made a detailed report, recommending alterations in the rules and regulations, which were adopted. All title-deeds, &c., were ordered to be deposited with the Treasurer. All papers and plans as to enlargement of the Hospital were referred to Messrs. Amory, Dexter, and Storrow.

On April 12, a vote was passed, expressing the gratitude of the Trustees for the munificent bequest of Israel Munson, and also presenting their sincere thanks to Charles Barnard, Esq., the executor, for the prompt and satisfactory manner in which he carried into effect the testator's provisions in favor of this institution. Dr. Hale was permitted to erect a pole in the Hospital-grounds for the purpose of a rain-gauge. Messrs. Rogers, Bowditch, and Wigglesworth were appointed a Committee to consider the subject of procuring tablets of the names of benefactors of this institution, and to report thereon to this Board. This Committee have never yet acted. April 17, Mr. Benjamin Cushing was elected Apothecary at the Hospital. Messrs. Rogers and Amory were appointed a Committee as to

Physicians charging fees to patients able to pay, who subsequently reported in favor of the same in case of out-door patients. Messrs. Bowditch and J. A. Lowell were appointed a Committee to sue the town of Somerville, to recover back a tax paid under protest.

Messrs. Rogers, Amory, Edwards, and Andrews were appointed a Committee to solicit subscriptions for enlarging the Hospital. At the next meeting, May 19, this Committee reported an address to the public, which was adopted; and the President and other officers were requested to aid the Trustees in regard to this proposed appeal; and the address was ordered to be signed by all the officers and the Trustees, and recommitted, with authority to publish and circulate the same.

This address was accordingly published in a pamphlet of fourteen pages, and is a beautiful specimen of typography. It commences with the following account of the original subscriptions: —

"In the year 1816, the Trustees of the Massachusetts General Hospital, who, as early as 1811, had received a charter from the Commonwealth, accompanied by the liberal grant of the 'Old Province House' Estate valued at forty thousand dollars, upon condition that the sum of one hundred thousand dollars should be raised by private subscriptions; and who, in the hope of better things, had struggled patiently on through the long period of non-intercourse, war, and commercial disaster that had intervened, — determined to make an appeal in behalf of the institution over which they nominally presided. They laid their case before the public. They maintained that an establishment for the alleviation and cure of 'the sick and insane' was needed; and they appealed to the intelligence and humanity of a Christian people to supply the want. By able statements and addresses, which were extensively published, and by letters and circulars to clergymen of all denominations, and to private individuals of wealth and character throughout the Commonwealth, they informed and awakened the general mind, and created a strong and widely extended sympathy for their cause.

"All things having been thus prepared, they divided themselves into four Committees; and, abandoning their private affairs for a season, they went through our streets, day after day, soliciting subscriptions from all; for they deemed it important that every individual in the community should have an opportunity to contribute to a charity in which each was interested.

"They were greeted everywhere with smiles and kind expressions; and, in the course of a very few days, their books exhibited subscriptions to the amount of one hundred and ten thousand dollars, which were afterwards increased to over one hundred and forty-six thousand dollars. So great a result was worthy of the intelligence and public spirit of Boston and of Massachusetts. As a voluntary subscription from individuals, it is the largest that the statistics of charity in our country can furnish; and, taken in connection with the losses and embarrassments which had preceded, it may be regarded as extraordinary.

"As a noble tribute to a work of great utility and benevolence, we delight to record it for the praise and honor of the men who made it, and for the just consideration and imitation of their children and descendants. It was made by persons of all conditions of life, and in sums varying from twenty thousand dollars to twenty-five cents, — the gift of a poor black, whose name, as it deserves, is recorded with others on the books of the donors. With the proceeds of this munificent subscription, the Trustees laid the foundation of the Hospital in Allen Street, and of the Asylum at Somerville. The original contributors to this fund have, most of them, gone to render up their account; a few honored names only remain; but the fountain which their benevolence caused to gush forth still continues to flow on in an uninterrupted stream of health and comfort to many a suffering being. Since the commencement of the first buildings, many noble bequests and donations have been received from various public-spirited individuals, which have added greatly to the size and utility of the institution."

The address states ably and conclusively the insufficient accommodations of the Hospital, which, by reason of the great increase of the population of Boston, only provides one bed for every 1,666 individuals, while Paris provides one for every 250 persons, and London for every 500; — that the wealth of Boston has kept pace with its population. It mentions the intention of enlarging the Hospital, by wings fifty feet wide, fifty-seven feet deep, estimated to cost fifty thousand dollars; notices the recent bequest of Mr. Munson of twenty thousand dollars; and ends with the following fervent and eloquent appeal: —

"Upon the principles and for the reasons now explained, the Trustees invite subscriptions in behalf of the Hospital. The existing edifice bears honorable testimony to the virtue and philanthropy of our fathers; and the Trustees will not suffer themselves to doubt that the result of the present effort will prove equally honorable to their sons and successors.

"To found and maintain institutions for the relief of the sick and afflicted is not only the mark but the privilege of civilization; and he who gives evidence of his faithful discharge of duty in this regard will leave a memento of himself, that shall outlive his generation, and be dear to the hearts of his children and of every true man."

A letter of the six attending Physicians and Surgeons, addressed to the Trustees, in favor of this project, is appended to the report.

On June 2, 1844, Mr. Dexter was asked to prepare plans of the proposed addition to the Hospital with detailed estimates of the expenses. June 16, Messrs. Bowditch and Dexter were appointed with full powers to settle the south boundary of the Belknap Estate. June 23, Mr. Dexter reported plans of two additional wings; the Subscription Committee reported progress; and a Building Committee of five was appointed, — viz. Messrs. J. A. Lowell, Amory, Andrews, Rogers, and Storrow.

On Aug. 18, Henry Sargent was elected House Physician; George H. Gay, House Surgeon; Benjamin Cushing re elected Apothecary. Five new rules and regulations were adopted, one of which was, " The smoking of tobacco is prohibited in the premises of the Hospital." The Committee on enlarging the Hospital presented their report by H. B. Rogers, Chairman; and the same, with the appeal to the public, was recorded *in extenso*, occupying twenty pages of the records. It details in an interesting manner the circumstances which led to a conviction of the necessity of additional accommodations; the first intention to apply for one new wing, to cost twenty-five thousand dollars, and finally for two, to cost fifty thousand dollars; the publication in several newspapers, and in a pamphlet-form for distribution, of an appeal to the public; a meeting held, at which Thomas H. Perkins was Chairman, and J. Ingersoll Bowditch Secretary; resolutions offered by William Gray, and cordially supported by Drs. James Jackson, John C. Warren, and Hon. Abbott Lawrence; resulting at last in the noble contribution of $62,550, a result far exceeding the most sanguine expectations of the Committee, being $12,550 more even than was solicited. And it should always be remembered, that it was in an especial manner to the personal influence and exertions of Mr. Rogers, the Chairman, that the Hospital is indebted for this brilliant result. He was truly indefatigable, and displayed throughout on this occasion most conspicuously the same zeal and good judgment which had heretofore so essentially promoted the interests and welfare of the institution.

On Sept. 15, Messrs. Andrews and Lamb were appointed a Committee, with full powers, to obtain an engraving of the Asylum. It was executed accordingly. Sept. 29, Mortimer B. Tappan was chosen Apothecary in place of Mr. Cushing, who resigned; and a purchase, for five hundred dollars per acre, of land adjoining Woodworth's house by the Asylum, was authorized. Oct. 11, Henry A. Barrett was elected House Physician in place of Henry Sargent, who had resigned. William P. Gibbs's request for leave to open a window upon the yard of the Belknap Estate was refused. Nov. 3, certain changes were adopted in the rules and regulations of the Hospital respecting the attendance of students on clinical lectures or surgical operations and the issue of tickets of admission.

On Dec. 1, a letter from Dr. James Jackson, recommending that Miss Rebecca Taylor be continued at the Hospital during her sickness, on account of her long and valuable services to the institution, was read; and it was thereupon voted, " that the Trustees, entirely concurring with the opinions expressed by Dr. Jackson, expect that Miss Taylor will make the Hospital her home during her sickness; and that the Visiting Committee communicate to her Dr. Jackson's letter, and the action of the Board thereon." Miss Taylor is still with us, having been in the institution twenty-five years.* The highest praise that could be bestowed on an attendant at the Hospital would be, that she was as good a nurse as Miss Taylor. Dec. 1, the Butler Hospital, of Rhode Island, asking permission to send Dr. Bell to Europe for some months, Mr. Bowditch was requested to send an answer acceding to their request, and to make the necessary arrangements with Dr. Bell for that purpose. The compliment thus paid to Dr. Bell was truly gratifying, both to him and to this institution. On Dec. 15, he was authorized to engage Dr. Fox to assist Dr. Booth during his absence in Europe. Messrs. J. A. Lowell and Dexter were appointed a Committee, with full powers, for insuring the buildings, both of the Hospital and Asylum. A communication from John D. Williams, as to the construction of a reservoir at the Hospital, was referred to Messrs. Rogers and Dexter, with full powers. The interest thus manifested by Mr. Williams was at a later day displayed in a munificent bequest to the institution. Messrs. Wiggles-

* On June 30, 1851, I asked Miss Taylor how long she had been connected with the Hospital, and she told me that it was just twenty-five years *that very day*.

worth and Andrews were appointed to prepare the annual report.

This report is a brief one of four pages. It mentions the payment of the only remaining debt of the institution, — viz. the ten thousand dollars due to the Massachusetts Hospital Life Insurance Company; the number of patients at the Asylum, seventy-five males and seventy-seven females: total, one hundred and fifty-two. The prompt receipt of Mr. Munson's legacy of twenty thousand dollars from Charles Barnard, Esq., his executor, was suitably acknowledged. It gratefully announces the entire success which had attended the application for the enlargement of the Hospital, and subjoins an extract from Mr. Rogers's report, showing the particulars of the noble subscription which had been obtained. Dr. Bell's report of the preceding year having been unusually full and minute, his present one is more concise and general. It occupies ten pages. The whole forms a pamphlet of twenty-five pages. Dec. 27, twenty-five males, twenty-eight females — total, fifty-three — in the Hospital.

At the annual meeting, Jan. 22, 1845, no changes were made in the Board of Trustees. At this meeting was communicated an extract from the will of John Parker, Esq., by which, after the decease of his widow, a ten thousand dollars' fund is given for the support of free beds, with conditions similar to those in the will of the late Miss Brimmer, viz., that the number of free beds in the House at his decease (*i.e.* thirty-seven) should never be diminished; which bequest was gratefully accepted. Motions were then successively made and rejected, to communicate to the executors of Mr. Parker the number of said beds, and to instruct the Trustees never to diminish that number. On Feb. 2, all the Medical and Surgical Officers, and those of the two departments, were re-elected. Two thousand five hundred copies of the annual report were ordered to be printed. Mr. Amory was appointed to procure an index to the medical and surgical records. An Annual Committee was constituted to purchase books for distribution under the Warren Fund.

On Feb. 16, the Farm School, having an ultimate interest in the bequest of the late John Parker, on breach of condition by this Corporation, were informed of the number of free beds in the Hospital at his decease. Feb. 25, the subject of the expediency of purchasing the Joy Farm was referred to Messrs. Storrow, Dexter, and the Treasurer; who reported that the price asked, fifty thousand dollars, rendered it inexpedient to purchase. On March 2, the Visiting Committee were directed to inquire into the number and condition of the beds at the Hospital. March 30,

Miss Taylor's wages were ordered to be paid in full during the period of her sickness. Hon. Edward Everett offered to the Hospital his statue of Apollo; and the Trustees presented to him " their grateful acknowledgments for his beautiful gift, valuable as a memorial, that, amidst his arduous public duties in a foreign country, Mr. Everett feels an undiminished interest in the charitable institutions of his native land." On May 4, a bequest of one hundred dollars from the late William Russell was transmitted, and gratefully accepted by the Trustees. The money was invested in silver spoons for the Asylum. A communication from Dr. Warren on the means of preventing erysipelas was received, and referred to Messrs. Dexter and Storrow. June 15, Mr. Joseph Burnett was requested to supply the Hospital with medicines for one year, pursuant to a report of Messrs. Rogers and Amory, recommending this arrangement. June 29, Messrs. Hooper and J. A. Lowell were appointed a Finance Committee to advise the Treasurer as to investments.

On July 11, a legacy of one hundred dollars from the late John Brown, Esq., was received and suitably acknowledged. Mr. Brown was one of the unfortunate victims lost in the burning of the "Lexington." Aug. 3, a communication from Drs. Warren and Bigelow, as to a Lying-in department, was referred to

Messrs. Rogers, Amory, and F. C. Lowell. Aug. 17, John S. Flint was elected House Physician; Alfred Lambert, House Surgeon; Francis A. Holman, Apothecary. Mr. Tappan had resigned in May. Sept. 14, the Building Committee and Mr. Dexter were instructed to finish the two new wings. Sept. 28, Dr. Bowditch resigned his office of Assistant Physician; and, on Oct. 10, Dr. Samuel Parkman was elected as his successor; and the thanks of the Trustees were presented to Dr. Bowditch for "the fidelity, ability, and zeal" with which he had discharged his duties. Messrs. Amory, Andrews, Bowditch, Hooper, and Rogers were appointed a Committee to consider what changes are rendered necessary in the discipline and organization of the Hospital, in consequence of its increased size. Mr. Goodwin's illness was announced, and the Visiting Committee were authorized to confer with Mr. Goodwin as to procuring the services of a temporary Superintendent. Nov. 2, Mr. Francis A. Holman was engaged accordingly.

A letter from Mr. Goodwin, resigning his office of Superintendent of the Hospital, and a letter from Mrs. Goodwin, accompanying it, were read; and it was voted that said resignation be accepted, and that the Chairman and Mr. Andrews be a Committee to express to Mr. and Mrs. Goodwin the feelings of respect and sympathy with which the Board part with them, and to tender to them, on behalf of the Trustees, their heartfelt sympathy in their present trials. Mr. Goodwin's salary was ordered to be paid to the end of six months after the close of the present quarter.

The Treasurer and Mr. John A. Lowell were appointed a Committee to receive the legacy of the late Daniel Waldo. The Committee on the subject of a Lying-in Hospital reported unfavorably, and their report was unanimously accepted. Nov. 16, the extract from Mr. Waldo's will, which gives the munificent sum of forty thousand dollars as a fund, the income of which is applicable generally to the benevolent objects of the institution, was laid before the Board; and the Chairman and Mr. Edwards were appointed a Committee to make a suitable expression of the thanks of the Trustees.

This Committee were also requested to obtain, if possible, portraits of Mr. Waldo and Mr. Munson for this institution. The portraits of these two donors were procured accordingly, and are now in the Trustees' room at the Hospital, by the side of the earlier benefactors of the institution, the example of whose liberality they had so nobly imitated. Nov. 16, a grant of three hundred dollars was made to Dr. John Fox for his services during Dr. Bell's visit to

Europe. Richard Girdler, of Marblehead, was elected Superintendent in place of Mr. Goodwin, with a salary of one thousand dollars.

A special meeting was held Nov. 26; and the death of Mr. Goodwin, the late Superintendent, being announced, it was " voted that, the Trustees having on a recent occasion expressed to Mr. Goodwin the high sense entertained by them of his official integrity and fidelity, would now respectfully assure Mrs. Goodwin of their sympathy for her and her children, who by this event have lost one so deservedly dear to them. Voted that this Board will be happy to unite in a public tribute of respect for the deceased, by attending the funeral services." And copies of these votes were communicated to the family of the deceased.

Mr. Goodwin was a person of cultivation and refinement, of great private worth, and of the most mild and amiable disposition; somewhat wanting, perhaps, in that energy which had characterized his predecessor, Mr. Gurney. Mrs. Goodwin, like her husband, had always taken a deep interest in the patients, and endeavored by all the means in her power to promote their comfort and welfare.

About a week before Mr. Goodwin's death, I called to see him. He was seated in an arm-chair, in the Trustees' room. It was one of the most charming days of the "Indian summer." The south-west wind, cooled by its passage over the water, was admitted freely through the open windows of the apartment. Pleasure carriages and loaded vehicles, in a ceaseless procession, were seen moving rapidly or slowly along the street. and across the bridge to which it led. The river was studded with sail-boats and other vessels. The distant hum of voices, as it arose upon the ear, was drowned by the merry laugh of children just released from the neighboring school. Around us were all the varied activities of a great city, its full tide of business and of happiness. In that quiet room sat an old and a dying man, consciously looking, almost for the last time, and with a pensive interest, upon a scene in which he was never more to be an actor. He reached out his hand, and said, " I was thinking of how little importance man is to his fellow-man; how slight an interruption to the great round of affairs results from the death of even the highest among us. It is wisely ordered, that only a little circle of those nearest to us will be, and that but for a short time, conscious of our departure. Yet," added he, " to the individual himself, how vast and mysterious the change! How inconceivable that a spectacle like this will with me so soon give place to the darkness and silence of the grave!"

SALARY VOTED TO THE TREASURER.

On Nov. 30, a letter from Thomas Oliver Walker, asking the Board to release their right to the family-tomb of the late Thomas Oliver, was referred to Messrs. Bowditch and Edwards. The office of Treasurer, the duties of which had always hitherto been performed gratuitously, had now become very onerous; and it was voted that there should be attached to it henceforth a salary of five hundred dollars. One hundred dollars was granted to Mr. Holman for his services as Superintendent during the illness of Mr. Goodwin. A free bed for life was placed at the disposal of John Tappan, Esq., who was one of the executors of the late Daniel Waldo. Dec. 14, the Committee on Mr. Oliver's tomb reported by Mr. Bowditch, "that said tomb is held by this Corporation, not as their property, but in trust as the burial-place of Mr. Oliver and his family." Mr. J. A. Lowell was requested to advise the Treasurer as to investment of the Waldo Fund. Messrs. Storrow and Amory were appointed to prepare the annual report. This report, like its immediate predecessor, is quite brief, occupying but four pages, and forming, with the accompanying documents, a pamphlet of twenty-five pages. It states the present property of the institution, exclusive of grounds and buildings, at $238,369.91; mentions "the receipt of $40,000, the munificent bequest of the late Daniel Waldo;" also the extra dividend from the Life Insurance Company. It then proceeds : —

"Colonel John M. Goodwin, who for many years past had filled the office of Superintendent of the Hospital, died in November last, after a short and severe illness. The Trustees take this occasion to bear testimony to the fidelity and devotion to the interests of the Hospital which he manifested throughout the period of his connection with it. During his illness, his place was temporarily supplied by Dr. Holman, the House Apothecary; and it has since been permanently filled by the appointment of Captain Richard Girdler, who entered upon his duties on the first day of December last. By this appointment, the Trustees, to some of whom he has long been known, believe that they have secured the services of a gentleman perfectly qualified by his zeal and ability to promote the welfare of the institution."

The weekly expense of each patient was five dollars and fifty-two cents. At the Asylum, at close of the year, were seventy-eight males, seventy-three females. Dr. Bell's report, which is twelve pages in length, is, as usual, clear, interesting, and satisfactory. Dec. 25, twenty-two males and twenty-seven females were in the Hospital.

On Dec. 28, a communication that windows had been opened over the Belknap Estate was referred to Mr. Bowditch and the Treasurer. The Committee appointed Oct. 10 reported a new draft of the rules and regulations, which was ordered to be printed; and, by a subsequent vote, the number of copies was fixed at two thousand. Jan. 16, 1846, an application of the widow of the late George Hallet, to purchase a free bed for life, was referred to the Standing Committee on Free Beds, with full power. At the annual meeting, Jan. 28, 1846, the proposed alterations in the by-laws, received by the Trustees, were adopted. Theodore Lyman was elected Vice-President in place of Jonathan Phillips, and J. Thomas Stevenson, Esq., a Trustee in place of Mr. Storrow, who severally declined. Mr. William W. Stone was subsequently elected by the Board of Visitors a Trustee in place of Henry Edwards. Votes of thanks were adopted by the Corporation, acknowledging the services of the gentlemen who thus retired. Mr. Phillips was son of our first President and earliest benefactor; and he had served as Trustee for sixteen years. Mr. Edwards had likewise been an active member of the Board for ten years. Among the changes introduced by the new rules and regulations, and rendered necessary by the enlargement of the Hospital, was the increase of the Medical and Surgical Staff.

Feb. 1, there were elected, as a Board of Consultation, Drs. James Jackson, George C. Shattuck, John Jeffries, and Edward Reynolds. *Visiting Physicians,

Jacob Bigelow, Enoch Hale, John B. S. Jackson, Henry I. Bowditch, John D. Fisher, and Oliver W. Holmes; the three last being new appointments. Visiting Surgeons, Drs. John C. Warren, George Hayward, Solomon D. Townsend, and Drs. Henry J. Bigelow, Samuel Parkman, and J. Mason Warren; the three last being also new appointments. Admitting Physician, Dr. William Henry Thayer. The officers of the two departments were severally re-elected. The salary of the Steward of the Asylum was raised to one thousand dollars. A Free-bed Standing Committee was appointed, consisting of Messrs. Rogers and J. A. Lowell: Committee on Warren Fund, Messrs. Rogers and Andrews; on the Book of Donations, Mr. Rogers; on Finance, Messrs. Hooper and J. A. Lowell. The subject of a pending petition for a railroad from Waltham to the westerly part of Boston was referred to Mr. Bowditch, with power to employ counsel to oppose the same; Messrs. Stevenson and J. A. Lowell were appointed to oppose any modification of the charters for life insurance which might jeopardize the interests of this institution;—both which Committees reported a satisfactory result at the next meeting. Two thousand copies of the annual report were ordered to be printed.

On Feb. 22, in answer to a communication of Dr.

John C. Warren, inquiring the views of this Board as to the erection of a Medical College in this vicinity, a vote was passed " that they cannot perceive any advantage to this institution to arise therefrom." March 1, a safe was ordered for the use of the Superintendent at Hospital. March 29, a letter from Dr. Bell, recommending open fireplaces in parts of the Belknap Ward at the Asylum, was referred to the Visiting Committee. May 3, Messrs. Andrews and Dexter were appointed a Committee " to erect a suitable monument to the memory of Jeremiah and Mary Belknap, with full powers." Five hundred dollars was placed at the disposal of Dr. Bell for the relief of poor patients. Mr. Dexter reported that the new wing would be ready for occupancy in the present week; and the subject of inviting the benefactors to visit the Hospital was referred to the Visiting Committee. Such an invitation was accordingly issued, and large numbers availed themselves of it. May 17, Dr. Bell's expenses to Washington, to attend a late meeting of the Superintendents of Insane Institutions, were ordered to be paid. The subject of building a new kitchen, and of ventilating the (old) east wing of the Hospital, was referred to the Building Committee, who reported in favor of both measures; the estimated expense of the kitchen, as reported by Mr. Dexter, being ten thousand dollars.

On June 28, a certain gate erected by the Corporation was declared to be with the sufferance and permission of the devisees of Mr. Joy. John C. Dalton, jun., was elected House Apothecary in the place of Dr. Holman, who had asked to be released from his duties. From July 1 to July 31, there were seven deaths at the Hospital, though there had been but nine during the whole preceding quarter. On Aug. 12, Dr. Charles Bertody was chosen House Physician, and Dr. Charles F. Heywood, House Surgeon, for the year ensuing. Aug. 30, the wings of the dwelling-house at the Asylum were ordered to be raised one story; Mr. Dexter, Dr. Bell, and Mr. Tyler being a Committee, with full powers. Oct. 16, books were ordered to be kept as a record of all out-door patients. Oct. 21, an annual extra grant of five hundred dollars was ordered henceforth to be made to Dr. Bell, in addition to his regular salary; he having filled his office for " ten years to the high satisfaction of the Trustees, and benefit of the institution." Nov. 22, this act of the Board was acknowledged in a letter from Dr. Bell, so gratifying to the Board that it was ordered to be copied in their records. The Superintendent of the Hospital was authorized to purchase a chair on wheels for the use of the patients. Dec. 6, a copy of the will of the late John Redman, making this institution his residuary devisee (after certain trusts which will last during the life-time of a son of a feeble intellect), was laid before the Board; and this munificent bequest of what will prove to be at least one hundred thousand dollars was most gratefully accepted. In view of his son's situation, he had intended to leave all his property to the city on certain trusts. He consulted the late Hon. John R. Adan, who satisfied him that the practical effect of such a devise would merely be a very slight reduction of taxes of the citizens, for which no one would thank him. The whole property thus bequeathed to us results from the increased value of the various parcels of real estate in Boston, judiciously selected by Mr. Redman, and purchased as from time to time he found an opportunity. On the back of his will is an enumeration of these estates, the first cost of each, the amount of mortgage, and their present estimated value. It is a document which gives striking evidence of the testator's sagacity and good judgment.*

* This memorandum on Mr. Redman's will was as follows: —

	Cost.	Value.	Difference.
Chamber-street Estate	$16,000	$17,000	$1,000
31, Washington Street	22,000	30,000	8,000
Milk Street	50,000	60,000	10,000
Chauncy Place	19,000	20,000	1,000
Washington and Summer Streets †	60,000	80,000	20,000
Wheeler Estate, Washington Street	10,000	15,000	5,000
Melodeon	45,000	78,000	33,000
Essex and Washington Streets	22,000	33,000	11,000
Bacon Lot, Washington Street	36,000	45,000	9,000
Utica Street	25,000	30,000	5,000
Temple Street	4,500	4,500	
Flats by South Bridge	9,500	15,000	5,500
South Boston	2,200	3,000	800
Roxbury	4,400	4,600	200
Cambridgeport	1,000	1,500	500
Snodon Lot, Roxbury	2,100	2,100	
	$328,700	$438,700	$110,000

† This estate was sold for $94,548.66, making a further gain of $14,548.66.

Messrs. Stevenson and Stone were appointed to prepare the annual report.

This report occupies five pages, and with the accompanying documents forms a pamphlet of twenty-five pages. It states the income of the year, at $24,415.52, and the expenses at $24,318.91; weekly expenses of each patient at Hospital, $6.43; twenty-two out-door patients treated during the year; the new west wing finished and occupied since July last; the erection of the new separate kitchen. It tenders the thanks of the Trustees to the annual subscribers for free beds; mentions that information had been received that Mr. John Redman had made this institution his residuary legatee; and states that " the condition of the M‘Lean Asylum justifies its reputation." Its expenses during the year have been $32,892; its receipts, about $1,300 more than that sum. Mr. Girdler's report occupies four pages, containing various interesting analyses and abstracts, showing the condition of the department under his care. Dr. Bell's report occupies nine pages. It contains a table of admissions and results for the last ten years. It closes as follows: " I cannot deprive myself of the pleasure of again expressing my acknowledgments for the uniformly intelligent and harmonious mode in which I have been supported by all those so many years associated with me in these labors."

Dec. 20, " a letter from Dr. William T. G. Morton offering to the Hospital the right to use his discovery for the alleviation of pain in surgical operations was read; and it was voted that the offer of Dr. Morton be accepted, and that the Secretary be directed to return the thanks of the institution to Dr. Morton in behalf of this Board." The report of Mr. Rogers on the subject of a Lying-in Hospital was taken from the files, and loaned to Dr. Homans for the use of the Trustees of the Lying-in Hospital. It was an extremely interesting and able document. Dec. 31, in Hospital twenty-four males, forty-three females: total, sixty-seven. Jan. 20, 1847, a communication from the State Mutual Life Insurance Company, as to their liability to pay part of their profits to the Hospital, was referred to Messrs. Stevenson and Bowditch.

At the annual meeting of the Corporation, Jan. 27, 1847, the same officers were re-elected; the Board of Visitors subsequently choosing J. Wiley Edmands, Esq., Trustee in place of William W. Stone, who declined a re-election, and was thanked for his services. Feb. 14, there was not a single change in any of the officers chosen or committees appointed in the preceding year. Two thousand copies were ordered of the annual report. Feb. 28, one of Oberhausser's microscopes was ordered to be purchased for use of

Admitting Physician, at the cost of fifty dollars. A grant of fifty dollars was made to Dr. Thayer, the Admitting Physician, in addition to his salary for the past year. March 14, the Board suggest that the exception in the rules as to the admission of patients, allowing the Physicians and Surgeons to send them, applies only to cases of emergency, where a delay of a few hours would be attended with serious consequences. This vote was subsequently rescinded, June 2. April 26, twenty-five dollars was voted towards buying a wooden leg for Ann Kerr, a patient in the Hospital. April 21, five hundred dollars was appropriated towards aiding the poorer patients at the Asylum. May 9, Messrs. Dexter and Rogers were appointed a Committee respecting a new fence round the Hospital-grounds, with directions to ascertain the probable cost, &c.

On May 23, a case of a post-mortem examination, alleged to have been made contrary to the wishes of friends, was discussed; and directions were given to the officer who had performed the same. June 2, a special meeting was held, attended by Drs Warren and Bigelow; and the Physicians and Surgeons were authorized to make regulations as to the treatment of out-door patients, and the dispensing of medicines to them. June 27, the new east wing being completed, the contributors and the pub-

SUPERINTENDENT'S SALARY INCREASED.

lic were invited to visit it. The Committee on the Monument to Jeremiah and Mary Belknap reported, that, after consultation with the family of the deceased, they had erected an appropriate monument. Plans and estimates of a new fence were submitted by the Committee on that subject. Nothing, however, has yet been done: the old and unsightly fence still stands. A neighbor once said to me: "Your institution always reminds me of a fine, likely-looking man disfigured by a rusty coat and a 'shocking bad hat.'" The Visiting Committee's record of July 2, 1847, as made up by Messrs. Stevenson and Bowditch, has the following entry: "One of our patients having been discovered to have the itch, Dr. Holmes was directed to discharge her as soon as it can be done with safety to her, and was instructed never to permit any similar admission." On July 16, the entry is made: "The new east wing is now open for the reception of patients." Aug. 10, Dr. Ralph K. Jones and John G. Sewall were elected House Physicians; Thomas Andrews, jun., and John C. Dalton, jun., House Surgeons; John E. Hathaway, Apothecary, whose salary is to be (if he is re-elected) $250 for the first year, $300 for the second year, $350 for the third year. Oct. 3, the salary of the Superintendent, in consequence of his increased duties, and the highly acceptable manner in which they were performed, was increased, in July 1, to fifteen hundred dollars. On Oct. 15, the free beds were now fixed at eighty.

Nov. 7, the Visiting Committee reported against the word " free " being added to the tickets over the beds of the patients, to distinguish *free* from *pay* patients. On Nov. 21, a communication from Dr. Henry I. Bowditch, as to the formation of a Medical Library at the Hospital, was referred to Messrs. Rogers and Amory, who subsequently recommended an appropriation of two hundred and fifty dollars for that purpose. The devisees of Mr. Joy desiring to sell their farm, and with a view of testing the title, the Hospital agreed to buy, and a case was made for the Supreme Judicial Court. Dec. 5, a communication was received from the executors of the late William Oliver; and the Board expressed their gratitude for his liberal bequest. Messrs. Bowditch and Edmands were appointed a Committee to prepare the annual report. Dec. 31, in Hospital, thirty-seven males, seventy-seven females: Americans, fifty-one; foreigners, sixty-three. Jan. 14, 1848, Dr. Thayer presented the first volume of his Index to the Medical Records, and was thanked for " the very satisfactory manner in which it was executed." Jan. 19, a writ served on the Corporation in favor of William Sohier was referred to Mr. Bowditch, with full powers. This was the amicable suit to try the title of the Joy Estate. Dr.

Thayer to be paid one hundred and twenty-five dollars per volume for these records.

SUMMARY. — No similar previous period of the history of the Hospital was in all respects more brilliant and successful than that which had now closed. The capacity of the Hospital had been doubled by the erection of two new wings and the new kitchen. The Belknap Estate in Washington Street had been rebuilt. The noble public subscription of $62,550; the ten thousand dollars' donation of Mr. Appleton; the bequests of Messrs. Waldo and Munson of forty thousand and twenty thousand dollars; and the bequests of John Parker, William Oliver, and John Redman, which, being subject to life-interests, have not yet been received, but which will eventually be ten thousand, fifty thousand, and one hundred thousand dollars respectively; with several other smaller but gratifying donations, — distinguish this period of five years from all its predecessors. The death of one faithful officer (Mr. Goodwin) had led to the appointment of the present highly acceptable incumbent. A fitting tribute of respect had been paid to the memory of Jeremiah and Mary Belknap. But, above all, the close of this period was signalized by the ether discovery. The importance of this discovery induced the Committee for preparing the annual report at this time to give it their especial consideration, and decides me now to devote a separate chapter to that part of their report. This report is the longest ever published (fifty-four pages), making, with the documents attached, a pamphlet of seventy-two pages. It alludes in the following terms to several of the most recent donations. Of John Redman's bequest it says: " As the legacy of a Boston mechanic, this will ever be a truly memorable instance of munificence; while its amount entitles the donor to be ranked among the very first benefactors of this institution." After mentioning the suitable acknowledgment of Mr. Oliver's bounty, the report proceeds: " With no less gratitude have the Trustees acknowledged another legacy of an especially interesting character received within this period. Miss Sarah Clough (for many years a valued and confidential domestic in the family of Joseph W. Revere, Esq., of this city) bequeathed to this institution the residue of her property, the little savings of her own personal labors. The amount which has been paid to the Treasurer, pursuant to this bequest, is $599.84. There never has been a donation, whatever its magnitude, more honorable either to the donor or to the institution. These new evidences of sympathy and approval cannot fail to stimulate us all to continued and renewed exertions in the discharge of the public trusts confided to us." The report states the whole invested property of the Hospital at $168,092.88; cost of Hospital, $249,572.38; and of the Asylum, $246,850.98. It gives *timely notice* that in A.D. 1916 the Province House will revert to the institution. It states that the current expenses of the Hospital required $20,710.25 to be paid from the general funds. It describes the present condition of the Hospital as follows: —

"The condition of the Hospital in Boston was never, at any former period, more entirely satisfactory. The extensive improvements which were projected a few years since, and which the munificence of the public alone rendered practicable, are now entirely completed. Two new wings have been erected, of which the one last finished was opened for the reception of patients during the past summer. In these wings are four wards, each about fifty feet square. Upon entering one of these apartments, the visitor sees a floor beautifully polished, walls and ceilings of great simplicity and elegance, and twenty neat iron bedsteads arranged around at regular intervals, with their clean coverings and curtains. The ventilation is excellent, and the air in these wards is generally as pure as could be desired. The old wings have also been entirely remodelled, chiefly for the purpose of introducing the same satisfactory system of ventilation. An entirely distinct brick building, of large size, has been erected, designed for all the domestic operations of cooking, washing, ironing, &c.; and containing excellent cellars, store-rooms, &c. The most exact and particular housekeeper may well look with admiration upon the various details of the very perfect arrangements of this building. It is connected with the main edifice by a covered passage-way; and, by means of dumb-waiters, articles sent from the kitchen are speedily distributed throughout the different wards. A new entrance has been made into the Hospital-yard, and a new avenue laid out. Nothing is wanting, except a brick wall or iron railing to enclose the grounds. To this object, as being one of mere ornament, the Trustees have not felt justified in applying the funds of the institution. There is, however, reason to believe, that, at no very distant day, the present unsightly fence may give place to one of a more durable material and elegant design.

"These improvements enable us to accommodate one hundred and forty-one, or, if need be, one hundred and fifty patients, instead of sixty; or, in other words, have nearly trebled our means of usefulness. They have been executed under the superintendence of George M. Dexter, Esq., one of the Trustees, upon whose taste and skill as an architect they reflect the highest credit. The expense attending these measures has been very great, — much greater than was at first estimated. This, indeed, is partly owing to the fact that so much more has been done than was originally contemplated by the Trustees; the whole institution having been, as it were, renovated. The total cost has been $103,276, besides $20,000 called for, but not yet paid, — making $123,276, and being double the whole amount of the public subscription of 1844. Fortunately it has not been found necessary to sell any of the permanently invested stocks of the institution; there having been received from the Massachusetts Hospital Life Insurance Company, since these improvements were undertaken, three annual dividends of $9,000 each, and one extra dividend of $24,000, making in all no less a sum than $51,000. The result, however, has been the reduction of those funds, the income of which was important to meet the increased current expenses of the institution, which will henceforth involve the support of twice our former number of free beds. The receipts during the past year from individual subscriptions ($3,100) and from funds, the income of which is specially appropriated to this object (viz. the donation of Hon. David Sears, and the legacies of the Messrs. Phillips and Belknap, and of the late Misses Tucker and Brimmer), were sufficient only for the maintenance of forty-one free beds. To this increase of the number of free beds, the Trustees feel pledged by their circular, issued in 1844, asking for subscriptions. Any annual deficiency which might otherwise occur will, however, we trust, be obviated by the aid of an increased number of annual contributors. We doubt, indeed, if it is possible for any one to do more good in a year with the sum of a hundred dollars, than by devoting it to the maintenance of a free bed in the Hospital.

"That this enlargement of our buildings had become necessary, seems proved by the fact, that, of the eighty free beds, all except *three* were actually occupied on the first of January, 1848; and it should be remembered, that *two* are, as far as possible, always reserved for cases of sudden accident; such cases, by a fundamental rule of the institution, being admissible without any previous permit.

"A large amount of relief is administered to out-door patients. This class has, however, of course diminished since the opening of the new wings; many of them being doubtless now admitted as inmates. This increase of our establishment has rendered it necessary to double the former number of physicians and surgeons; the present number being twelve. The labors and responsibility of Capt. Girdler, the Superintendent, have also been greatly increased. For this reason, and because his duties have always been performed in a manner so uniformly acceptable to all connected with the institution, the Trustees recently voted to enlarge his salary by an annual grant of five hundred dollars. The neatness, taste, vigilance, and kindness of Mrs. Girdler have caused the Trustees to entertain an equally high sense of the value of her services as Matron. There has, indeed, been a general disposition manifested on the part of all the resident officers, attendants, and nurses, to treat the patients with that attention, tenderness, and consideration which is their due. Any charge of failure or omission in this respect would be sure to receive from this Board the most prompt notice and the strictest investigation.

"To Dr. William H. Thayer, our Admitting Physician, the Trustees are indebted for a folio volume, just completed, which forms a most valuable index to the hundred and twenty-six volumes of *medical* reports of cases in the Hospital. It contains, classified under the head of each separate disease (260 in number), all the cases which have been treated from 1821 to 1845, with the result of the treatment, and a reference to the book and page where the details of each case may be found. We trust that he will proceed to render equally accessible the records of the *surgical* department of the Hospital.

"A small sum has been appropriated for the formation of a Medical Library, to consist of books of reference, for the use of the Physicians and Surgeons; and an annual appropriation will probably be continued for this object."

Among the documents annexed is a table, showing the results of the admissions at the Hospital from its establishment in 1821; being the first table of the sort ever prepared for that department, and containing slight errors and discrepancies, which do not affect its general results. These errors consist in the Superintendent's having omitted from the list of discharges all patients *not treated*, though they were in the list of patients *received*. This alone made an error of twenty-seven in one year. The series of numbers remaining at the end of each year was also made erroneous by each number being placed one year out of the way. I was at the time unable to ascertain or correct these mistakes; and therefore, in preparing this report as Chairman of the Committee, I appended to the table in question a note that it had " a few slight inaccuracies." It is believed, however, that the table prepared at the end of this history is strictly accurate in all particulars, as framed from the official reports of each year; and that its results may be depended on with entire confidence. Mr. Girdler's and Dr. Bell's reports occupy four and five pages respectively. The report closes with the following notice of this department of the institution: —

" There have been under treatment, during the year, three hundred and forty-three inmates, of whom eighty-seven have recovered, and thirty-three have died. The number remaining, Dec. 31, 1847, was one hundred and seventy-three. The whole number received from the opening of the Asylum, Oct. 6, A. D. 1818, to this time, is 2,864.

"The M'Lean Asylum has continued, during the past year, to be conducted upon those salutary principles which the experience of later times, in respect to treatment of the insane, has introduced into this department of medical science.

"The day of physical restraints and coercion has passed away for ever. Kindness, amusements, opportunities of exercise, and agreeable employments, are now our chief remedial agents. The item of 'diversions' has its definite place in all our quarterly accounts of expenditures. The natural beauties of our situation, with its extensive prospects, — our garden, with its terraces and its pond, — the bowling alleys, the billiard room, the dancing hall, the sewing circle, — have solaced and done much to restore many an inmate of our institution. As a pleasing manifestation of the desire felt by its officers to afford innocent gratification to those under their charge, we may mention, that (a reservoir having been constructed near the summer-house, and pipes laid from it) the garden has this year received the additional ornament of a marble basin, tenanted with gold and silver fish, and having a small but graceful jet rising from its midst. The Trustees have also been, as usual, much gratified by promoting the same objects, as they had opportunity, during their weekly visits. Any trifling attentions, which we have been enabled to pay upon such occasions, have always been agreeably received and kindly acknowledged.

"The Board are aware that three railroads already pass very near to the enclosed grounds of the Asylum. Still another has been applied for at the present session of the Legislature. A Committee has been appointed to prevent, if possible, by a most earnest remonstrance, a measure so prejudicial to the welfare of this department of our institution.

SICKNESS AND DEATH OF PATIENTS.

"The past season has been remarkable for the prevalence of dysentery throughout this vicinity, and it will long be remembered with peculiar sadness by those connected with the Asylum. Between July 26 and Sept. 20, no less than seventy decided cases occurred among the patients, whose whole number did not, within that period, exceed one hundred and seventy: twelve of these cases terminated fatally. Of those who died, there were several who had been with us for a long series of years, whose recovery was hopeless. Others, on the contrary, had been with us but a short time, and might, after a brief interval, have carried back joy and happiness to the circles of family and friendship. More than one death we can recall, which must have inspired in those to whom the patients were dear, feelings of the most severe grief and disappointment. There were, besides, ten cases of this disease among the household at the M'Lean Asylum during the same period. That, of those attacked, so large a proportion recovered, cannot fail to excite surprise and gratitude. We doubt not that the result may, in no inconsiderable degree, be attributed to the unremitting efforts of the officers and attendants, whose zeal, patience, and self-denial are most fully acknowledged in the report of the Physician and Superintendent. Mr. Tyler, our Steward, was prostrated by this disease; and his recovery was so slow, that, for some time, the Trustees were apprehensive lest he should find his strength insufficient for a continuance of those duties which he has so long and so ably performed. He has the best wishes of the Board for his speedy and entire restoration to health and strength.

"While oppressed by unusual official cares and anxieties, Dr. Bell, our Physician and Superintendent, was called to experience the bitterness of repeated domestic bereavements. His second child,* a daughter of ten years of age, of a bright and sunny disposition, with rare moral and intellectual endowments, — and another, an interesting boy,† of five years of age, — within a few short weeks, fell victims, the one to this epidemic, the other to consumption. To the afflicted parents we present the assurance of the profound and respectful sympathy of the Trustees. Now that the loved ones of earth have been taken, may these mourners the better see Heaven's love! May their grief be soothed by the gentle ministry of time, — by the hallowed memories of the past, the high duties of the present, and the sacred hopes of the future!"

* Mary Frances died Aug. 22.   † Henry James died Oct. 3.

CHAPTER IX.

1847–1849.

THE ETHER DISCOVERY, AND CONTROVERSY BETWEEN DRS. MORTON AND JACKSON. — LIST OF MORE THAN TWO DOZEN PAMPHLETS. — EXTRACTS FROM A FEW OF THEM. — HOSPITAL REPORT. — VINDICATION OF SAME. — DR. SMILIE'S ADDRESS. — CONGRESS REPORT. — THE CASKET AND RIBBON. — AWARD OF THE FRENCH ACADEMY. — EXTENT TO WHICH ETHER IS USED AT THE HOSPITAL.

THE patience of the public has been long since thoroughly wearied out by the ether controversy. More than two dozen pamphlets have appeared on the subject, which, collected together (as they have been in the Boston Library), fill three respectably-sized octavo volumes.* I have no intention to renew

---

* The following is a list of these pamphlets in the order of publication : —

1. Insensibility during Surgical Operations, produced by Inhalation. By H. J. Bigelow, M.D. Boston Medical and Surgical Journal, Nov. 18, 1846.

2. The Inhalation of an Ethereal Vapor to prevent Sensibility to Pain during Surgical Operations. By J. F. Flagg, M.D. Boston Medical and Surgical Journal, Dec. 2, 1846.

3. Inhalation of Ethereal Vapor for the Prevention of Pain in Surgical Operations. By John C. Warren, M.D., &c. &c. Boston Medical and Surgical Journal, Dec. 9, 1846.

4. Insensibility during Surgical Operations, produced by Inhalation. By H. J. Bigelow, M.D. (in reply to Dr. J. F. Flagg). Boston Medical and Surgical Journal, Dec. 9, 1846.

5. Inhalation of Ether. By J. Mason Warren, M.D. Boston Medical and Surgical Journal, March 24, 1847.

this controversy. I shall merely make such extracts from five of these pamphlets as I think appropri-

6. Circular, by W. T. G. Morton. pp. 88. Boston, March, 1847.

7. History of the Discovery of the Application of Nitrous Oxide Gas, Ether, and other Vapors, to Surgical Operations. By Horace Wells. pp. 26. Hartford, March, 1847.

8. Some Account of the First Use of Sulphuric Ether by Inhalation in Surgical Practice. By George Hayward, M.D. pp. 8. Boston, April, 1847.

9. Discovery by Charles T. Jackson, M.D. of the Applicability of Sulphuric Ether in Surgical Operations. By Martin Gay, M.D. pp. 48. Boston, June, 1847.

10. A Review of Dr. M. Gay's Statement of Dr. C. T. Jackson's Claims to the Discovery, &c. &c. By J. B. S. Jackson, M.D. Boston Medical and Surgical Journal, June 30, 1847.

11. Some Account of the Letheon ; or, Who is the Discoverer ? By Edward Warren. pp. 88. Boston, August, 1847.

12. Mémoire sur la Découverte du Nouvel Emploi de l'Ether Sulfurique par W. T. G. Morton, de Boston, Etats Unis ; suivi des Pièces Justificatives. pp. 60. Paris, 1847.

13. Report of the Board of Trustees of the Massachusetts General Hospital, presented to the Corporation at their Annual Meeting, Jan. 26, 1848.

14. Account of a New Anæsthetic Agent as a Substitute for Sulphuric Ether in Surgery and Midwifery. By J. Y. Simpson, M.D., F. R. S. E., &c. pp. 24. Reprinted, New York, January, 1848.

15. Reprint of the Report of the Trustees of Massachusetts General Hospital, with a History of the Ether Discovery, and Dr. Morton's Memoir to the French Academy. Edited by R. H. Dana, jun. pp. 48. Boston, March, 1848.

16. Rapport des Administrateurs de l'Hôpital Général de Massachusetts, suivi de l'Histoire de la Découverte de l'Ether, &c. &c. R. H. Dana, jun., éditeur. pp. 144. Cambridge, 1848.

17. A Defence of Dr. Charles T. Jackson's Claims to the Discovery of Etherization ; containing Testimony disproving the Claims set up in Favor of Mr. W. T. G. Morton in the Report of the Trustees of the Massachusetts Hospital, and in No. 201 of Littell's Living Age. By Joseph L. and Henry C. Lord. pp. 37. Boston, June, 1848.

18. The Ether Controversy : Vindication of the Hospital Report of 1848. By N. I. Bowditch. pp. 32. Boston, July, 1848.

19. Reports of the First Exhibition of the Worcester County Mechanics' Association at Worcester, September, 1848. pp. 74.

ate to the present publication, viz. "The Hospital Report," and its "Vindication;" "Dr. Smilie's Address;" "The Congressional Report;" and an article in "The American Journal of Dental Surgery," since separately printed under the title of "The Casket and the Ribbon," which is the latest of the series, and reviews the Congressional Report and the Minority Report, presented by two members of the same Committee.

20. Ether and Chloroform; their Discovery and Physiological Effects, &c. By H. J. Bigelow, M.D. pp. 45. Boston, November, 1848.

21. Memorial addressed to the Trustees of the Massachusetts General Hospital, in Behalf of C. T. Jackson, M.D., by his Attorneys, J. L. and H. C. Lord. pp. 27. Boston, December, 1848.

22. Report of the Select Committee of the Congress of the United States, to whom was referred the Memorial of William T. G. Morton, asking Compensation from Congress for the Discovery of the Pain-subduing Property of Sulphuric Ether. pp. 46. Washington, D.C., Feb. 23, 1849.

23. Minority Report of the same Committee. pp. 99. Washington, D.C., Feb. 23, 1849.

24. Rapport du Comité du Sénat et de la Chambre des Représentants des États Unis d'Amérique, auquel on référa le Mémoire de William T. G. Morton, demandant une Compensation, &c. &c. pp. 35. Le 23 Février, 1849.

25. The Casket and the Ribbon; or, the Honors of Ether. pp. 26. Baltimore, 1849.

The Volumes of the Boston Medical and Surgical Journal from August, 1846, to August, 1849, inclusive, contain communications on "Letheon." To these I add —

26. An Address delivered before the Castleton Medical College, on the History of the Original Application of Anæsthetic Agents, May 17, 1848. By E. R. Smilie, M.D.

I. THE HOSPITAL REPORT OF JANUARY, 1848.

This Report was republished in Hays's "Medical Journal." It also reappears (in connection with an article of R. H. Dana, jun.) in Littell's "Living Age." Dr. Morton caused it to be translated into French, and laid before the Academy of Sciences at Paris. After stating the donations, &c., which had been made to the institution, this Report proceeds as follows:—

It is hoped, that, with these various "means and appliances" at command, the institution has hitherto accomplished, and will ever continue to accomplish, the designs of its founders and benefactors. In one striking instance it certainly has not been found wanting. The past year has tested the unspeakable importance of the recent discovery of the properties of *sulphuric ether;* no less than one hundred and thirty-two operations, many of them of much severity, having been already performed with entire success on patients who had been rendered insensible through its benign influence. By overcoming all muscular and nervous resistance, it has extended the domain of surgery; making operations possible which could not have been performed, and which would not have been attempted, without its aid; and, by the removal of the fear of pain, it has greatly increased the actual number of operations. It has already become an established remedy throughout all the chief cities of Europe, and its benefits have reached even the distant natives of Singapore and of Canton.

With just pride, therefore, the Trustees would now record the fact, that within the walls of this building were witnessed the first painless capital operations that were ever performed. The world at large, indeed, is in no small degree indebted to the Medical and Surgical Officers of this institution. But for their immediate appreciation of the importance of this discovery, and their considerate, but, at the same time, zealous and prompt co-operation with Dr. Morton, in availing themselves of its use, its application might have been restricted to the comparatively unimportant operations of the dentist. Who can say what might have been the result, had his overtures been received with excessive caution? An answer may perhaps be found in the fact, that it is only within a few weeks, *if at all*, that the use of sulphuric ether has been introduced into our sister institution in Pennsylvania. This appears by "the Annual Report on Surgery, read before the College of Physicians, Nov. 2, 1847, by Isaac Parish, M. D.," where it is said : "*At the Pennsylvania Hospital in this city, it has not been tried at all;* being considered by the judicious surgeons of that institution as a remedy of doubtful safety, or, at least, as not sufficiently established to warrant them in its employment." And yet, in the same report, we find the following sentence : "But, when we extend our vision to foreign countries, and call to mind that during the past nine months it has been adopted in most of the large hospitals of Great Britain, in the vast hospitals of Paris, and for the last six months in the numerous institutions of like character in Germany, including the immense hospitals at Vienna and Berlin, we can form some idea of the extent to which it has been carried, and of the firm hold which this great American discovery has taken of the mind of the scientific world."

The first operators who applied it were Drs. John C.

Warren and George Hayward, Surgeons of this Hospital. The enthusiasm of one of their colleagues, who had been especially earnest in urging the performance of these operations, led him to become the first champion of ether in this country, by a publication of much merit, and also to transmit the earliest account of the discovery to England, where it was at once hailed with rapturous exultation. And another, a favorite alike of Science and the Muses, has thus vividly described its beneficent effects: "The knife is searching for disease, — the pulleys are dragging back dislocated limbs, — nature herself is working out the primal curse, which doomed the tenderest of her creatures to the sharpest of her trials; but the fierce extremity of suffering has been steeped in the waters of forgetfulness, and the deepest furrow in the knotted brow of agony has been smoothed for ever." Even the grave and dispassionate Dr. Warren himself (in a yet unpublished work, which he kindly communicated to the Committee, and which embodies the matured results of his own experience upon this subject) indulges in equally graphic language: "Who could have imagined, that drawing the knife over the delicate skin of the face might produce a sensation of unmixed delight! — that the turning and twisting of instruments in the most sensitive bladder might be accompanied by a beautiful dream!"

Professor Simpson, of Edinburgh, has discovered that a new agent (chloroform) possesses the same powers as sulphuric ether, and, as he thinks, many and great advantages over it. The universal law of intellect is progress. But, though others may erect the superstructure, the corner-stone of the building will preserve an imperishable record of its founder. The name of Fulton will never be forgotten. Yet how vast is the difference between the first humble steamboat that slowly toiled up the Hudson, and those majestic structures which now defy the storms of the Atlantic!

As philanthropists, we may well rejoice that we have had any agency, however slight, in conferring on poor, suffering humanity, so precious a gift. Unrestrained and free as God's own sunshine, it has gone forth to cheer and gladden the earth. It will awaken the gratitude of the present and of all coming generations. The student who, from distant lands or in distant ages, may visit this spot, will view it with increased interest, as he remembers that here was first demonstrated one of the most glorious truths of science.

Pursuant to an informal suggestion of the Board, who regard this discovery as the most important event which has occurred in the history of this institution, the Committee proceed to make a more extended investigation, in respect to its origin, than would otherwise have been thought necessary.

A recent publication by Dr. George Hayward, entitled "Some Account of the First Use of Sulphuric Ether by Inhalation in Surgical Practice," gives a clear and simple history of this discovery, and of all its attending circumstances, *as connected with the Hospital*. It is interesting to trace the earlier successive steps by which the grand result was at last obtained. These are, to a considerable extent, recapitulated in the British and Foreign Review of April last. It is there stated, that, as early as 1779, "we find many experiments on men and animals on the inspiration of different kinds of airs." — "Dr. Beddoes, in his work on Factitious Airs, published at Bristol in 1795-6," "gives several communications from Dr. Pearson on the inhalation of ether," also "a letter from one of Dr. Thornton's patients, in which the patient himself gives an account of the inhalation of ether, by Dr. Thornton's advice, and its effects in a case of pectoral catarrh. He says, 'It gave almost immediate relief both to the oppression and pain in the chest. On a second trial, he says he inhaled two tea-spoonfuls of ether, which, he adds, 'gave immediate relief as before, *and I very soon after fell asleep*, and had a good night's rest.'" — "Another curious case is given by Dr. Thornton, in which inhalation was prescribed for the relief of a very *painful inflammatory affection of the mamma*, and with very beneficial effect." The Reviewer says, "At this time and subsequently, Dr. Thornton was in the common habit of administering the vapor of ether to his patients." — "In all these trials, no one had distinctly in view the removal or abolition of pain, though this was attained, indirectly, in Dr. Thornton's case. But Sir Humphrey Davy, who it is well known first began his chemical career by assisting Dr. Beddoes," "seems not only to have contemplated such a result by means of medicamentous inhalation, but to have actually put it to the test of experiment on himself. The medium of his experiment, however, was not ether, but the nitrous oxide. Sir Humphrey tells us, that on two occasions the inhalation of the nitrous oxide removed headache. He also tried its effect *in removing intense physical pain*, while he was cutting a wisdom-tooth." — "He says: '*As nitrous oxide, in its extensive operation, appears capable of destroying physical pain, it may probably be used with advantage during surgical operations in which no great effusion of blood takes place.*'" — "In the article 'Ether,' in the Dict. des Sc. Med., vol. xiii., published in 1815, we find the author, Nysten, speaking of the inhalation of *ether* as familiarly known, and as employed for the relief of some pulmonary diseases, and also for *mitigating the pain of colic*." To an eminent medical friend the Committee are indebted for the fact, that in Pereira's Materia Medica, published in London in 1839, it is expressly stated that "*the vapor of ether is inhaled* in spasmodic asthma, chronic catarrh, and dyspnœa, hooping-cough, and *to relieve the effects caused by the accidental inhalation of chlorine gas.*" Dr. Charles T. Jackson, of this city (as we learn from a pamphlet published in 1847, under his own sanction and authority, entitled, "Discovery by Charles T. Jackson, M.D., of the Applicability of Sulphuric Ether in Surgical Operations; by Martin Gay, M.D."), has distinctly admitted that he "was early impressed with the remarks of Davy * concerning the remedial agency of gaseous matters." † As a learned chemist, he was also doubtless familiar with the publication last referred to. Accordingly, two or three years after its appearance, or in the winter of 1841–2, "he inhaled sulphuric ether, to obtain relief from the very unpleasant sensations caused by an accidental inhalation of chlorine gas." In other words, having accidentally inhaled chlorine gas, he resorted to the prescribed remedy. "He at first breathed the ether without producing unconsciousness, but derived from it some relief. Afterwards, still suffering from the chlorine, he continued the experiment to such an extent as to produce complete general insensibility." Subsequently, under precisely the same circumstances, he also prescribed it to one of his students. He had, as he states, on one previous occasion, also about A.D. 1841, inhaled it with safety to the extent of producing "a peculiar sleep or unconsciousness."— "*Before his observations, a state of complete insensibility from this*

---

* Dr. Jackson, in a letter published with Dr. Gay's pamphlet, says: "My interest in the respiration of gases was first excited by Sir H. Davy's experiments; and, since I became acquainted with them, the subject has always seemed to me to deserve further investigation."

† Daily Advertiser of March 1, 1847.

cause was considered by the best authorities as one of greater or less danger; and it had been known to produce fatal results. Young persons had breathed this vapor to the extent of producing unconsciousness, and in some cases without injury."

Dr. Jackson, then, had not discovered any new power or property of ether. *It was known that it could produce insensibility;* and that *that insensibility*, though sometimes fatal, *was sometimes unattended with injury.* It was also known as a specific against the noxious effects of chlorine gas. He had merely tested these known propositions, and found them true in his own person. By so doing he had formed, as he states, a strong opinion, that pure, rectified, sulphuric ether could be inhaled with safety. But its efficacy for the prevention of pain he had, thus far, only verified by actual experiment in the case specified in the text-books, viz. *where chlorine gas had been previously inhaled.* This experiment is stated in Dr. Gay's pamphlet with great particularity, *as if it had been one before unknown.* The motives which led to it, and the philosophical inferences deduced by Dr. Jackson, are set forth with much minuteness. It seems, indeed, to be relied on as the very foundation of Dr. Jackson's claim, as the discoverer of the safety and efficacy of sulphuric ether. *It still obviously remained to be proved,* that it could be safely and effectually inhaled for the prevention of pain under other circumstances.* To establish this point, Dr. Jackson never attempted an experiment on man or animal. It is true that "he communicated to several persons (and, among others, to Mr. Bemis, an eminent dentist, in 1842) his observations and conclusions respecting the pre-

---

* Dr. Gay says himself, "It still remained to be ascertained whether this unconsciousness was so perfect, that, during its continuance, no pain would be produced by wounding instruments." — Pamphlet, p. 10.

vention of pain in surgical operations;" and, in February, 1846, he informed a student in his laboratory (Mr. Joseph Peabody), who wished to have two teeth extracted, " that insensibility would be produced by the inhalation of sulphuric ether-vapor. He advised him to breathe it, and to submit to the operation while in the sleep induced thereby." But what effect did his advice have on Mr. Peabody? " He at last gave up the experiment, because his father, a scientific man, feared irritation of the lungs might ensue, — *because the best authorities on the subject were arrayed against the opinion of Dr. Jackson,* — and because he was unwilling to incur any risk for so slight an operation." And such was really the general state of public opinion among men of science down to that time.* *The discovery was yet to be made by one who was willing to try the experiment, notwithstanding the best authorities on the subject were against it.*

Further, it does not appear, that, from 1841–2 to 1846, Dr. Jackson suggested its use, except for the slighter and instantaneous operations of the dentist. Familiar, as he confesses himself to have been, with the views of Sir H. Davy, who had so long before suggested the use of the nitrous oxide in operations attended *with little effusion of blood*, it was very natural that Dr. Jackson's thoughts should have been exclusively turned to the use of sulphuric ether in the class of minor operations which had been thus specified by so distinguished a philosopher. It would seem, indeed, clear that he had not the remotest conception of its universal applicability and importance. Such, indeed, is the only satisfactory explanation of the fact, that, during an interval of nearly five years, he never once tested his discovery, or

---

* See Mr. Metcalf's letter to the Committee, p. 228.

caused it to be tested, by a single experiment. Upon this point, indeed, the advocate of Dr. Jackson says: " It was more than a quarter of a century after Jenner first heard the milkmaid express her belief in the protective influence of cow-pox, that he vaccinated his first patient;" but, he adds, "*during which period he was much engaged in the investigation of the subject.*" But ether seems to have received only a casual and incidental attention from Dr. Jackson. To make the cases at all parallel, it must be shown, that Jenner, after vaccinating his first patient, waited five years before vaccinating another, *with a like apparent unconsciousness of the importance of his discovery.* Indeed, these two discoveries are of so totally opposite a character, that they suggest a striking contrast, instead of a parallel. In the one case, the truth could be ascertained only by repeated experiments and patient investigation. It had to fight its way against the inveterate prejudices of the world. In the other case, it is fully and for ever demonstrated by the first successful capital operation; and it is at once hailed, as it were, with delight by all mankind.

Within this period, Dr. Horace Wells, of Hartford, used the nitrous oxide while engaged in extracting teeth. His claim, *as a discoverer* in this matter, must yield entirely to that of Sir H. Davy, who, after actual experiments, had, as it were, distinctly suggested the use of this very agent for this object so many years before. There are, doubtless, reasons founded in the nature of this agent, which have prevented these suggestions of Davy, in regard to it, from having been long since realized. And, whatever may have been the result of Dr. Wells's experiments elsewhere, it is certain that his public performance of them in Boston in 1844 was an entire failure. It is also stated by Dr. Wells, that, as early as November, 1844, "a surgical operation was performed at Dr Marcy's office under the influence of *sulphuric ether;*" and he adds, " The doctor then advised me by all means to continue the use of the nitrous oxide." And it seems that the result of this one experiment was such, that, pursuant to this advice, he abandoned the idea of the further use of ether. His claim, therefore, to the discovery in question appears in this view also to be equally unfounded. We cannot but believe, that it has been without due consideration that his claim has received the official sanction of his native State of Connecticut. Indeed, a published letter from Dr. Wells to Dr. Morton seems necessarily to exclude the idea, that he himself claimed to have made any such prior discovery.* All must, however, accord to him the honor of having been an earnest and persevering seeker after truth in this very path of inquiry; and his labors and experiments may, we think, fairly be considered as having had some indirect influence, though not themselves attended with direct success.

Dr. William T. G. Morton, of this city, must now be mentioned. He had been a student of Dr. Jackson's, and formerly a partner of Dr. Wells. He, therefore, occasionally availed himself of the advice of the former; and he was aware of, and (upon the public occasion in Boston before referred to) had taken part in, the experiments of the latter

---

* The letter referred to is as follows : —

" Hartford, Conn., Oct. 20, 1846.

" Dr. Morton, — Dear Sir, Your letter, dated yesterday, is just received; and I hasten to answer it, for fear you will adopt a method in disposing of your rights which will defeat your object. Before you make any arrangements whatever, I wish to see you. I think I will be in Boston the first of next week, probably Monday night. *If the operation of administering the gas is not attended with too much trouble, and will produce the effect you state, it will undoubtedly be a fortune to you, provided it is rightly managed.*

" Yours in haste, H. WELLS."

in the use of nitrous oxide. It does not appear that Dr. Wells had ever mentioned in Boston his one experiment with sulphuric ether. There is evidence, entirely satisfactory, that Dr. Morton's attention had been for some time engaged upon the subject; that he had purchased and experimented upon sulphuric ether; that, as early as July, 1846, a highly intelligent chemist of this city had a conversation with him upon its medicinal qualities; * and that, at this very time, he

---

* Mr. Theodore Metcalf, in a note to Dr. Morton, dated Dec. 20, 1847, says: "I can only state that I remember to have met you at Mr. Burnett's store early in the summer of 1846, and to have had a conversation with you in regard to the medicinal qualities of *sulphuric ether*, a quantity of which you were then purchasing. I cannot, as you desire, give the precise date, but know it to have been previous to July 6, as I left Boston on that day for a tour, from which I have but a few weeks returned." Mr. Metcalf also, subsequently, sent the following letter, before referred to in p. 225:—

"Boston, Jan. 26, 1848.

"Sir,— In answer to your inquiry respecting the nature of my interview with Mr. Morton, I can only add to my note of Dec. 20, that the conversation was commenced by some inquiry on his part, concerning the nature and effects of sulphuric ether, a vial of which he then held in his hand.

"In answer to his several questions, I gave him such information as he could have obtained from any intelligent apothecary at that time, and also related to him some personal experience as to its use as a substitute for the nitrous oxide; adding the then generally received opinion, that its excessive inhalation would produce dangerous, if not fatal consequences. Some reference was made — but whether by Mr. Morton or myself, I cannot remember — to the unsuccessful experiments of his former partner, Mr. Wells, with the nitrous oxide. It was one of those casual conversations which quickly pass from the mind; and it was for the first time recalled to my memory, upon seeing, months after, in a French journal, an account of the anæsthetic effects of ether, the discovery of which was ascribed by the writer to a Boston dentist.

"I am, sir, very respectfully, your obedient servant,
"N. I. Bowditch, Esq." "THEODORE METCALF.

Mr. Metcalf is the well-known predecessor of Mr. Burnett, and, as an apothecary, has long possessed, in the highest degree, the confidence and respect of the medical profession; and there is no one in the community

made an arrangement in business, the express object of which was to relieve himself from the immediate duties of his profession, in order to devote himself to something which would make an entire revolution in dentistry. But we do not think it at all material to go into the minute details of this evidence. Skilful in his particular department, he makes no pretensions to general science. Seeking for this discovery, — accquainted with this very agent, — he calls upon Dr.

whose personal character would give higher authority to any statement of facts distinctly and positively made. *It is therefore certain, that Dr. Morton, months before his interview with Dr. Jackson, purchased sulphuric ether* at the very shop where Dr. Jackson at last advised him to buy some more (pure and rectified), with which the successful experiment was made. And it may be remarked, that the details of the conversation, given by Mr. Metcalf, seem conclusively to show with what intent Dr. Morton was then making his purchase.

The Committee may claim the entire credit of obtaining this most important testimony. Mr. Metcalf, having been absent in Europe, had never been applied to by Dr. Morton, who called upon him only at the express suggestion of the Committee. Besides its direct bearing in the case, it confirms the statement of Dr. Hayden, who had previously testified to the purchase of a small quantity of sulphuric ether at Mr. Burnett's; and not only so, but it seems to prove that Dr. Hayden could not have any motive for misrepresenting the contents of the demijohn, since the point at issue was Dr. Morton's *entire ignorance* of sulphuric ether, not his *greater or less knowledge* of that agent. Dr. Gay, from the omission in the published affidavits of Dr. Morton to state the kind of ether used in his experiments, infers his total ignorance of *sulphuric ether*, down to Sept. 30, 1846. Indeed, Dr. Jackson stated to one of the Committee, that, when Dr. Morton had his interview with him on Sept. 30, 1846, he (Dr. Morton) had never seen sulphuric ether — did not even know it by sight — was wholly ignorant about its nature and qualities — and got from him, for the first time, the idea of using it. To the suggestion that this ignorance was feigned, he replied that he knew it to be real; and remarked, " The Committee may consider it as a *certain fact* in the case. It can be proved beyond all reasonable doubt whatever." The Committee, being aware of Mr. Metcalf's statement, suggested that an unimpeachable witness had stated, that, three months before that interview, Dr. Morton had bought sulphuric ether, and conversed with him respecting its medicinal qualities. Dr. Jackson replied

Jackson; wishing, without betraying his own motives and objects, to obtain all the information which Dr. Jackson's extensive researches and experience might enable him to furnish. Dr. Jackson, at this interview, voluntarily gives him the strongest assurances of the expediency and safety of using pure rectified sulphuric ether; informs him where he can get some of a good quality;* and advises him, as he had more than once advised others, to try the experiment.† Unlike others, Dr. Morton determines to do so. He does

that it could not be,—that it must be an entire mistake, &c. The Committee learned, two days afterwards, from Mr. Metcalf, that he had himself previously informed Dr. Jackson of the fact, that, *before he went to Europe*, he had seen Dr. Morton buying sulphuric ether, and conversed with him about its qualities. He had not, indeed, stated to Dr. Jackson the precise time when this interview took place; but the Committee think that this circumstance affords evidence that Dr. Jackson's conclusions in this case have been formed without a careful and deliberate consideration of the facts, even *when brought directly within his notice.*

* Viz. at Mr. Burnett's shop, where Dr. Morton had himself purchased sulphuric ether three months before.

† In a memorial dated July 31, 1847, transmitted by Dr. Morton to the French Academy, and, as he informs the Committee, subsequently presented by Arago to that body, we find, accordingly, the following paragraph: "I am ready to acknowledge my indebtedness to men and to books for all my information upon this subject. I have got here a little, and there a little. I learned from Dr. Jackson, in 1844, the effect of ether directly applied to a sensitive tooth, and proved by experiment that it would gradually render the nerve insensible. I learned from Dr. Jackson, also in 1844, the effect of ether when inhaled by students at college, which was corroborated by Spear's account, and by what I read. I knew of Dr. Wells's attempt to apply nitrous oxide gas for destroying pain under surgical operations. I had great motive to destroy or alleviate pain under my operations, and endeavored to produce such a result by means of inhaling ether; inferring that, if it would render a nerve insensible when directly applied, it might, when inhaled, destroy or greatly alleviate sensibility to pain generally. Had the ether that I tried on the 5th of August been pure, I should have made the demonstration then. I further acknowledge, that I was subsequently indebted to Dr. Jackson for valuable information as to the kinds and preparations of ether, and for the recommendation of the highly rectified,

not yield to any doubt, from the opposite array of authorities. He is willing to take the risk. Accordingly, on Sept. 30, 1846, — after having, as he states, first inhaled it himself, — he finds a patient who consents to permit him to use it, and *extracts a tooth without pain.* It was, of course, at first still uncertain whether the insensibility so satisfactorily obtained during this brief operation would continue through a more prolonged one. Dr. Morton, on the next day, calls on Dr. Jackson, and informs him of his success; and the latter states that he advised Dr. Morton to get the surgeons of the Hospital to permit its use.* He does not himself, however, see any of these officers. He is not him-

from Burnett's, as the most safe and efficient. But my obligation to him hath this extent, no further."

In this memorial, we find also the following paragraph : "I went to Dr. Jackson, therefore, to procure a gas bag, also with the intention of ascertaining something more accurately as to the different preparations of ether, if I should find I could do so without setting him upon the same track of experiment with myself. I am aware, that by this admission I may show myself not to have been possessed by the most disinterested spirit of philosophic enthusiasm, clear of all regard for personal rights or benefits; but it is enough for me to say, that I felt I had made sacrifices and run risks for this object; that I believed myself to be close upon it, yet where another, with better opportunities for experimenting, availing himself of my hints and labors, might take the prize from my grasp."

The Committee deem it a very important consideration, in respect to this interview, that the information in question was elicited by the visit of Dr. Morton to Dr. Jackson for a specific purpose, viz. to obtain the means of persuading a patient to submit to an operation, under the idea that it would be unattended with pain; and that it was not disclosed in an interview sought by Dr. Jackson to make trial of it for *his* satisfaction, or to accomplish *his* purposes.

* Dr. G. G. Hayden, however, in his affidavit, states that, "on the evening of the 30th of September, after the first experiment had been made with success, Dr. Morton spoke about going to the Hospital, and using the ether there, and thus bringing out the new discovery;" while a witness of Dr. Jackson's testifies, that "Dr. Morton strongly objected at first to going to the Hospital." He certainly showed no such reluctance *at last.*

self present at any of the early operations.* He fears that Dr. Morton may recklessly do some great mischief. He refuses to give him a written certificate of the safety of the application of ether. He openly and strongly expresses his regret that he had ever communicated to Dr. Morton any information upon the subject.† Certainly, then, with respect to all these subsequent experiments, Dr. Jackson is free from the least responsibility; and this alike, whether he doubted the safety of the application of ether, or only, as it would seem, the competency of Dr. Morton to administer it safely. In either case, the risk was wholly confined to Dr. Morton and the surgeons of this Hospital.‡ Dr. Morton thus follows up his first success; and the great truth is at last made manifest, for which so many a prayer had been breathed in vain ever since man had lived and suffered. *It is demonstrated that ether may be applied with safety, so as to produce insensibility during all surgical operations.*

---

* Dr. Jackson was absent from the city when the third operation was performed at the Hospital, and remained absent twelve days; but, besides this expected absence, he had assigned another reason for declining to assist at that operation.

† More than one witness distinctly remembers, that the expression, "I don't care what he does with it, if he does not drag my name in with it," and others of similar import, were used by Dr. Jackson in relation to Dr. Morton's early experiments in confirmation and establishment of this discovery. And one of Dr. Jackson's own witnesses, George O. Barnes, in an affidavit published in Dr. Gay's pamphlet, says expressly : "In fact, he (Dr. Jackson) was sorry that he had communicated his discovery to Morton, and that he had employed him to make those early experiments with the ether. He spoke strongly upon those points."

‡ These were then, as now, Drs. John C. Warren, George Hayward, Solomon D. Townsend, Henry J. Bigelow, Samuel Parkman, and J. Mason Warren. Dr. Gay argues that Dr. Morton *did* not, and from his ignorance *could* not, run any risk in following the directions originally given by Dr. Jackson. That argument is certainly inapplicable to these subsequent experiments.

Upon the whole, then, it seems clear that to Dr. Morton the world is indebted for this discovery; and that, but for Dr. Jackson's scientific knowledge and sound advice, Dr. Morton would not have made it at that precise time, and might have failed to do so at any time. The one, having a strong conviction of the safety of the agent, has the credit of giving the best possible advice : the other, by nature determined and fearless, makes the first actual application. Between the discoverer and his adviser, there will henceforth ever be an indissoluble, however reluctant, copartnership. In accordance with these general views are the published statements of two of our own officers. One of them, Dr. Hayward, says : "It is understood, that Dr. C. T. Jackson, well known by his great attainments in geology and chemistry, first suggested the use of ether; but to Dr. Morton, I think, must be awarded the credit of being the first who demonstrated, by actual experiment on the human subject, the existence of this wonderful property." The other, Dr. Jacob Bigelow, President of the American Academy of Arts and Sciences, in an article published in the Medical and Surgical Journal of July 7, 1847, says : "In the case of Dr. Jackson, if he did make the discovery in 1842, as asserted, or even later, he stands accountable for the mass of human misery which he has permitted his fellow-creatures to undergo, from the time when he made his discovery to the time when Dr. Morton made his. In charity, we prefer to believe, that, up to the latter period, he had no definite notion of the real power of ether in surgery, having seen no case of its application in that science. The first made partial experiments, and recommended, but did not make, decisive ones. The last took the risk and labor necessary to demonstrate or disprove its efficacy, and, above all, the safety of the process, which, until his time, had been believed to be dangerous to life, on various good authorities, from Dr. Christison to Mr. Peabody.

In view alike of the simplicity of the agent employed, the magnitude of the results attained, and the near approaches so repeatedly made to this discovery, how applicable are the lines of Milton, to which a friend has called the attention of the Committee!

> "The invention all admired, and each how he
> To be the inventor missed, so easy it seemed
> Once found, which yet unfound most would have thought
> Impossible."

It is matter of regret that a noble discovery in science should have been attended with discussions and controversy, involving much bitterness, and, as it seems to us, disingenuousness. Dr. Morton distinctly admits, that his original application to Dr. Jackson was made with a studied concealment of his true object, and an assumed ignorance of the whole subject (as it would seem, even to the extent of asking if ether were a gas). The motive of this concealment is explained to have been a fear lest he should otherwise lose the honor of any eventual discovery which he might make. The consequences to Dr. Morton have been, however, that many, relying on the unimpeachable testimony of those present at that interview, have been induced to withhold from him all credit whatever, except that of "a nurse who administers a new and bold prescription of a physician,"* and to re-

---

* This illustration, used by Dr. Gay, seems to the Committee entirely inapplicable. A nurse who refuses to administer even a new and bold prescription may be justly denounced by the attending physician; whereas Dr. Morton was not a student under Dr. Jackson's orders, and obliged to administer his remedies to one of *his* (Dr. Jackson's) patients. He was a free agent, who, after receiving the prescription, voluntarily went and sought out a patient who was willing to submit to it.

gard him, throughout this discovery, in the false light of a mere agent of Dr. Jackson. This culpable step has seemed to increase the merit of Dr. Jackson's advice, by rendering it unsolicited information, instead of a mere answer to a direct inquiry. It has itself furnished the only colorable ground for depriving Dr. Morton of the honor of the discovery. Thus fitly has the majesty of truth vindicated itself! On the other hand, . . . in a communication in the Boston Daily Advertiser of March 1st, Dr. Jackson says he "*was desirous of testing it* (the ether) *in a capital operation*, and that *Dr. J. C. Warren politely consented to have the trial made;* and its results proved entirely satisfactory, an amputation having been performed under the influence of ethereal vapor, without giving any pain to the patient." Whereas we have two distinct published statements of Dr. Warren, one in reply to a letter of Nov. 30, 1846, in which occurs the following sentence: "Two or three days after these occurrences (*i.e. the first two operations at the Hospital*), on meeting with Dr. Charles T. Jackson, distinguished for his philosophical spirit of inquiry, as well as for his geological and chemical science, this gentleman informed me that he first suggested to Dr. Morton the inspiration of ether, as a means of preventing the pain of operations on the teeth. He did not claim the invention of the apparatus, or its practical application. For these we are indebted to Dr. Morton." The other statement is as follows: "Boston, Jan. 6, 1847. I hereby declare and certify, to the best of my knowledge and recollection, that I never heard of the use of sulphuric ether by inhalation, as a means of preventing the pains of surgical operations, until it was suggested by *Dr. W. T. G. Morton*, in the latter part of October, 1846." If it be said that neither of the first two operations was a capital one, we have the authority of Dr. Hayward, who performed the second operation,* for saying that it was the removal of a very large tumor from the arm, — that it occupied seven minutes, — that, as it involved the painful process of cutting through the skin to a great extent, it was as entirely satisfactory as an amputation would have been, — the patient being free from all sense of pain. One present at the operation exhibited to the Committee a sketch of the arm and the tumor upon it, taken at the time, which clearly showed how formidable an operation it must have been, though not perhaps what would be professionally called a *severe* one. Dr. Warren says expressly in his yet unpublished work, "The patient exhibited no sign of physical or intellectual suffering." *And yet it was not until after this operation, that Dr. Warren or Dr. Hayward had received an intimation that Dr. Jackson had any thing to do with the discovery, either from himself or any one else.* The third operation was a capital one, and it was entirely successful. Alice Mohan, a young woman of twenty years of age (who had long been a patient in our institution, and who is doubtless well remembered by all this Board, to whose kind consideration her character and conduct, no less than her misfortunes, so well entitled her), was to submit to amputation above the knee. But if Dr. Jackson's statement is to be understood as applying only to this case, we still find that every part of the statement is entirely irreconcilable with the facts. This operation was performed, not by Dr. Warren, but by Dr. Hayward. And not only was Dr. Hayward still entirely ignorant of Dr. Jackson's participation in this discovery; but the dialogue which actually had taken place

---

* The first operation, the removal of a tumor from the neck, was performed by Dr. Warren, who says that it was a case of imperfect etherization. It was performed Oct. 16, 1846. The second operation took place Oct. 17, and the third on Nov. 6.

between Dr. Warren and Dr. Jackson, in relation to it, was to this effect. Dr. Warren, on being informed by Dr. Jackson that he first suggested to Dr. Morton the use of sulphuric ether, *requested Dr. Jackson to come to the Hospital, and administer it* during this operation, which was to take place the next Saturday. *Dr. Jackson declined doing so*, for two reasons: one, that he was going out of town; the other, that he could not do so consistently with his arrangements with Dr. Morton. Dr. Warren has not given to the Committee any information respecting this conversation; but that such was the substance of the dialogue is capable of judicial proof from other evidence which has been laid before the Committee. So that, if Dr. Jackson at any time requested of Dr. Warren to have the ether administered during a capital operation at the Hospital, it must have been after this conversation, in which he declined to administer it, and after it had been successfully applied by another without his assistance.

This withholding of all credit from Dr. Morton has but caused Dr. Jackson's own claims to be the more strictly scrutinized. Had he been willing to admit that the discovery was a joint one, the world would probably have allowed to him, as a truly scientific man, the largest share of the honors resulting from it. The exclusive claims of Dr. Jackson seem to rest wholly upon the hypothesis, that Dr. Morton was, from first to last, his mere agent, — an idea evidently repudiated by Dr. Morton, when he first went to Dr. Warren, *without even naming Dr. Jackson;* and most openly and unequivocally disavowed by Dr. Jackson himself, during the whole series of Dr. Morton's experiments. The Committee think that Dr. Jackson's own early acts have, indeed, for ever rendered inadmissible these exclusive claims. He at first agreed to receive from Dr. Morton the sum of five hundred dollars, as a compensation for his services. Is it, for one moment, conceivable that the true discoverer would have thus bartered away his birthright for a mess of pottage? And when subsequently, at the suggestion of the Solicitor of Patents, a personal intimate friend of Dr. Jackson, Dr. Morton consented to permit Dr. Jackson's name to be associated with his own in the patent, — he having agreed, instead of the five hundred dollars, to receive one tenth part only of the profits, — we ask again, Is it conceivable that the sole discoverer would have thus associated another with himself, taking even an oath that they were joint discoverers, and, at the same time, have consented to receive only a pittance of what was wholly his own? No! We consider that Dr. Jackson is estopped for ever from such a claim, and that not upon technical grounds, but by the whole equity of the case. We will not, however, further pursue this ungracious part of our subject.

It is further matter of regret that a patent should have been taken out for such a discovery. As well might Dr. Franklin have claimed one for the exclusive use of the electric fluid. A patent in this case, indeed, would seem to be a peculiarly odious monopoly, — a speculation based upon human suffering, — like an exclusive right to sell breadstuffs to a famishing community. It is due, however, to Dr. Morton to state that he tendered the free use of the discovery to this institution, and requested from Dr. John C. Warren a list of all similar institutions in the country, that he might extend its benefits to them.* He, in like manner, tendered the free use of it to the army and navy of the United States. His design was, as he alleges, to charge

---

* He certainly made the offer, without any previous request from this Board; though a witness of Dr. Jackson's states that it was made at his suggestion, and with a reluctant acquiescence on the part of Dr. Morton.

to practitioners a moderate annual sum, which, he thought, would be paid cheerfully, and without inconvenience, by their respective patients.* Dr. Jackson's name would not have been associated in the patent, but at the instigation of R. H. Eddy, Esq., the solicitor, who has publicly avowed that he acted under a mistaken apprehension of facts, and who now awards to Dr. Morton the sole honor of the discovery, which at the time he supposed might fairly be regarded as a joint one. Mr. Eddy's intelligence and truthfulness, and his sincere friendship for Dr. Jackson, are well known in this community. But we must state our conviction, that it was a sad mistake to have resorted to any exclusive legal right in the present instance. This has become the deliberate opinion of the profession and of the public. One of the patentees, Dr. Jackson, after applying to be admitted to a larger share of the profits, ultimately renounced all claims to any benefit from this source; and the patent has also become unavailable to Dr. Morton.† We cannot, how-

* In his licenses was inserted a clause, that such payments were to cease, if the United States, or the State where the practitioner lived, should purchase the right to use the discovery.

† The two gentlemen who acted as legal advisers of Dr. Jackson addressed a letter to Messrs. R. H. Eddy and W. T. G. Morton, dated Boston, January 28, 1847, containing the two following sentences: "Under the present circumstances of the case, we think the least that, in justice to yourselves and Dr. Jackson, you can offer is 25 per cent of the profits arising from the invention, both at home and abroad, in settlement of his claim upon you." . . . .
"It is our wish to settle the matter amicably, if possible. We hope you will see, by our suggestions, that we wish only to have a fair distribution of the profits of a discovery made among those who cannot, if they disagree, effectually sustain the patent; and which, if sustained, *promises to give to all parties large sums of money for their united co-operation.*" Dr. Gay, however, says that Dr. Jackson "deemed it a sort of impropriety to procure letters patent for the practical application of scientific discoveries. He himself never would have procured one merely for his own pecuniary benefit, in a case so important to the interests of humanity."

In the memorial before referred to, as presented by Dr. Morton to the

ever, but wish that it had been originally taken out rather from the hope of securing to themselves the honor than the profits of the discovery. And yet a national benefit of such magnitude is well entitled to a national reward. It may be true that Dr. Jackson does not need or now wish such reward; but it is a mortifying fact that Dr. Morton's pecuniary affairs have become embarrassed, in consequence of the interruption of his regular business, resulting from his efforts and experiments in establishing this great truth, and that his health has also seriously suffered from the same cause, so that he can devote only a small part of each day to his professional labors. He has become poor in a cause which has made the world his debtor. The Committee are, in this connection, authorized to state, that a memorial was prepared by the physicians and surgeons of this institution, to be forwarded to Congress at its present session, and had been already signed by eleven of them (all except Dr. J. B. S. Jackson), when further proceedings were stopped by a remonstrance from Dr. C. T. Jackson. This memorial, as embodying the views of these officers, is placed at the disposal of your Committee; and we cannot better close this discussion than by subjoining the following copy of the document referred to: —

" *To the Senate and House of Representatives of the United States of America, in Congress assembled.*

"The undersigned, Physicians and Surgeons of the Massachusetts General Hospital, beg leave to represent, —

"That, in the year 1846, a discovery was made in the city of Boston, by which the human body is rendered insensible to pain, during surgical

French Academy, the closing sentence is as follows: "But, as the use has become general and almost necessary, I have long since abandoned the sale of rights (under the patent), and the public use the ether freely; and, I believe, I am the only person in the world to whom this discovery has so far been a pecuniary loss."

operations, and during other serious and violent affections, by means of the vapor of ether inhaled into the lungs.

"That a patent for this discovery was taken out by two citizens of Boston, by whom the first satisfactory experiments on the prevention of pain by this means had been made; and the first capital operations, conducted under the influence of this agent, were performed in the Massachusetts General Hospital by the surgeons of that institution.

"That the success of this method of preventing pain has been abundantly and completely established by a hundred and fifteen operations performed in said Hospital during the last year, and by a still greater number out of it in the city of Boston.

"And, in all cases within the knowledge of the undersigned, it has greatly mitigated, or wholly prevented, the pain, when skilfully administered, and in no case has any fatal or disastrous consequence followed its use within their observation; and although inconveniences and temporary disturbances of the nervous system have sometimes followed its application, yet these are exceptions to a general rule, and are not more common than those which result from the employment of other powerful medicinal agents, and are incomparably less distressing than the evils they are employed to obviate.

"The undersigned have reason to believe, that, since the introduction of this process, some thousands of persons have inhaled ether, in Boston and its vicinity, with impunity and benefit; that its value is already recognized, and its employment introduced into most parts of Europe; that the use of the process ought to be, and by judicious arrangements probably will be, extended into all parts of the United States; and that no discovery in medical science, during the present century, has relieved as much suffering, and conferred so great a benefit on humanity, as the discovery of the power and application of ether.

"The undersigned are aware, that the power of ether to produce insensibility, and even death when improperly used, was known in Europe many years ago. They are also aware that other aeriform bodies have been experimented on, and the vapor of ether itself unsuccessfully tried, by other individuals, in surgical operations; but they are satisfied, that the safety of the process, and the effectual mode of applying it, were first made known in Boston in 1846.

"Understanding that the use of this important discovery is now restricted by letters patent granted from the office of the Secretary of State, and believing that it is the policy of wise governments to diffuse among their constituents the blessings of such discoveries as tend to alleviate human suffering, and, at the same time, to reward those who have conferred such benefits upon the world, — the undersigned respectfully pray, that such sums as shall be thought adequate may be paid by the government of the United States to those persons who shall be found, on investigation, to merit compensation for the benefit conferred on the public by this discovery, and on condition of the relinquishment by them of any patent right they may hold restricting its use.

(Signed) " JOHN C. WARREN. | H. I. BOWDITCH.
JACOB BIGELOW. | O. W. HOLMES.
GEO. HAYWARD. | J. MASON WARREN.
ENOCH HALE. | SAMUEL PARKMAN.
S. D. TOWNSEND. | HENRY J. BIGELOW.
JOHN D. FISHER.

" *Boston, Nov.* 20, 1847."

As a general summary of facts and views, the Committee report, that in their judgment the following propositions are satisfactorily established : —

Down to Sept. 30, 1846, Dr. Jackson had discovered nothing that had not been known and in print in London for some years. It was known that ether would produce insensibility ; that such insensibility, though sometimes fatal, was sometimes safe ; and that one of the properties of ether was its power to obviate the ill effects of an inhalation of chlorine gas. The discovery of the safety and efficacy of the inhalation of ether in surgical operations had not yet been made ; the only experiments which Dr. Jackson had tried, or caused to be tried, being those already prescribed by the text-books. Dr. Jackson had for some time entertained a strong impression that it could be used with safety and effect during the operations of the dentist, — a conjecture which a hundred other persons may have made without discovering the fact ; and incidentally, on more than one occasion, he had advised its use for that class of operations, but had been unable to persuade any one to use it, not even persons of science and intelligence, who were most familiar with all that Dr. Jackson knew or thought upon this subject.

Prior to this time, Dr. Wells had used the nitrous oxide for this object, as recommended many years before by Sir H. Davy. His experiments performed in Boston were, however, unsuccessful. He also claims to have performed one experiment with sulphuric ether, which, from the circumstances, must also necessarily be inferred to have been unsuccessful. And there is positive evidence that the most eminent physicians of Boston never heard of the latter experiment till after Dr. Morton's discovery.

Dr. Morton had for some time been engaged in searching for a safe agent for promoting insensibility during dental operations. He knew of, and had upon one occasion taken part in, the nitrous-oxide experiments of Dr. Wells.

As early as July, 1846, he purchased sulphuric ether, and proceeded to experiment upon it. On Sept. 30, 1846, he has an interview with Dr. Jackson, and receives his decided advice to use pure rectified sulphuric ether during a dental operation, accompanied with the strongest assurances of its safety, and with the information where it could be obtained. Dr. Morton, unlike others who had received this advice, and notwithstanding he knew the prevailing belief of the dangerous and sometimes fatal character of this agent,* forthwith acted upon it. That he proceeded to inhale it himself, rests, indeed, on his own assertion. The Committee have no doubt of its truth. He certainly administered it to a patient. *By so doing, he made this discovery.*† On

---

* See Mr. Metcalf's letter, p. 228.

† Indeed, it seems to be distinctly admitted by the advocate of *Dr. Jackson*, that *he* had made no discovery in this case prior to Sept. 30, 1846. Dr. Gay says expressly, in commenting upon Dr. Wells's claims : " Although so much time (two and a half years) has elapsed since Mr. Wells's experiments,

learning this result, Dr. Jackson very naturally suggested to Dr. Morton that he had better get the ether tried by the surgeons of the Hospital, which a witness of Dr. Morton's, however, alleges that he had previously determined to do.

he presents no evidence of its adoption into general surgical practice, even in that flourishing city. *It required little more than the same number of months to diffuse the knowledge and application of Dr. Jackson's discovery throughout the civilized world."*

In fact, the specification accompanying the patent, and signed both by Dr. Jackson and Dr. Morton, and bearing date Oct. 27, 1846, is most distinct in the same admission. We subjoin the following extracts, in proof of this position, and also of the fact that Dr. Jackson did not regard *sulphuric ether* as the *sole* agent which might be used to produce insensibility to pain : —

"It is well known to chemists, that, when alcohol is submitted to distillation with certain acids, peculiar compounds, termed *ethers*, are formed; each of which is usually distinguished by the name of the acid employed in its preparation. It has also been known that the *vapors of some, if not all*, of these chemical distillations, *particularly those of sulphuric ether*, when breathed or introduced into the lungs of an animal, have produced a peculiar effect on its nervous system, one which has been supposed to be analogous to what is usually termed intoxication."

"It has never (to our knowledge) been known, *until our discovery*, that the inhalation of such vapors, *particularly those of sulphuric ether*, would produce insensibility to pain, or such a state of quiet nervous action as to render a person or animal incapable, to a great extent, if not entirely, of experiencing pain while under the action of the knife, or other instrument of operation of a surgeon, calculated to produce pain."

"*This is our discovery,*" &c.

"From the experiments we have made, *we are led to prefer the vapors of sulphuric ether to those of muriatic or other kinds of ether;* but any such may be employed *which will properly produce the state of insensibility, without any injurious consequences to the patient.*"

The testimony of Dr. Keep and of Mr. Barnes, as to Dr. Morton's not being aware of the importance of the admission of atmospheric air, having been commented upon by the Committee, it is proper here to add the fact, that in this very specification occurs the following sentence in the description of the apparatus to be employed : "*Let there be a hole made through the side of the vessel for the admission of atmospheric air,*" &c. And the original apparatus first used at the Hospital by Dr. Morton is, as the Committee are informed, expressly constructed so as to admit atmospheric air. Besides,

But all the subsequent steps were taken by Dr. Morton himself, without the slightest sympathy or co-operation on the part of Dr. Jackson, who, from alleged fear of his recklessness, withheld from him all countenance and encouragement. In view of these facts, the Committee are of opinion, that the *exclusive* claims advanced by Dr. Jackson,* though now very extensively recognized in foreign countries, are unfounded, being unwarranted alike by his acts and by his omissions; and that they involve great injustice towards Dr. Morton; — that their names will be for ever jointly, though not equally, associated in this discovery; Dr. Jackson being entitled to the credit of having rendered readily available the existing knowledge upon the subject of ether, which Dr. Morton was really, though not avowedly, seeking to obtain; and Dr. Morton having first demonstrated its safety and efficacy in the prevention of pain during surgical operations; — and that Dr. Morton, by consenting to permit Dr. Jackson's name to be united with his in the patent, with the right to receive *one-tenth* part of its profits, has shown himself disposed, fairly and honorably, to recognize the amount of his indebtedness to Dr. Jackson's advice.

had no atmospheric air been admitted, his patients would probably have been killed, discredit thrown upon the process, and the discovery perhaps postponed for ages.

It may also be remarked, that, in view of this disclaimer, by Dr. Jackson, of any discovery prior to Sept. 30, 1846, it seems difficult to explain an expression which is quoted by Mr. Warren, in his pamphlet, as extracted from Dr Jackson's letter to M. Elie de Beaumont, originally published in "Galignani's Messenger," Jan. 25, 1847; namely: "I have *latterly* turned this discovery to use, by inducing a dentist of this city to administer the vapor of ether to persons whose teeth he was going to extract."

* That such claims are really advanced by Dr. Jackson is well known. He said indeed to one of the Committee, "I allow of no partnership in this matter. If your report takes from me such a proportion of the sole credit of this discovery *as amounts even to the paring of a finger-nail*, I shall entirely object to it."

The essential conclusions in the case may be thus concisely stated: —

1st, *Dr. Jackson does not appear at any time to have made any discovery, in regard to ether, which was not in print in Great Britain some years before.*

2d, *Dr. Morton, in* 1846, *discovered the facts before unknown, that ether would prevent the pain of surgical operations; and that it might be given in sufficient quantity to effect this purpose, without danger to life. He first established these facts by numerous operations on teeth, and afterwards induced the surgeons of the Hospital to demonstrate its general applicability and importance in capital operations.*

3d, *Dr. Jackson appears to have had the belief, that a power in ether to prevent pain in dental operations would be discovered. He advised various persons to attempt the discovery. But neither they nor he took any measures to that end; and the world remained in entire ignorance of both the power and safety of ether, until Dr. Morton made his experiments.*

4th, *The whole agency of Dr. Jackson in the matter appears to consist only in his having made certain suggestions, which led or aided Dr. Morton to make the discovery, — a discovery which had for some time been the object of his labors and researches.**

The Committee are well aware, that any investigation and opinion which shall have the sanction of this Board, — em-

---

* The results otherwise arrived at by the Committee have received the highest confirmation from Professor Simpson, the discoverer of chloroform, who has transmitted to Dr. Morton a copy of his pamphlet entitled "Account of a New Anæsthetic Agent, as a Substitute for Sulphuric Ether in Surgery and Midwifery," with the following note written upon one of its blank pages: —

"My dear Sir, — I have much pleasure in offering, for your kind acceptance, the accompanying pamphlet. Since it was published, we have had

anating, as all must admit, from those who ought to know most of the circumstances of this discovery, — will be entitled to great weight. That investigation has been conducted by the Committee under a solemn sense of responsibility to the public, to posterity, and to the cause of truth and justice. Personal feelings have been laid aside. When this inquiry was instituted, neither of the Committee had ever seen Dr. Morton; and both of them, on the other hand, were in friendly relations with Dr. Jackson. There had always existed between them and him feelings of mutual respect and regard. No friend of Dr. Jackson would willingly remove a merited laurel from the brows of one whose scientific attainments, upright intentions, and amiable character, all are happy to acknowledge. The Committee, indeed, believe that he is honestly self-deceived in this matter.

We submit our Report upon this subject to the Board, in the assurance that it will receive their deliberate examination,

various other operations performed here, equally successful. I have a note from Mr. Liston, telling me also of its perfect success in London. Its rapidity and depth are amazing.

" In the Monthly Journal of Medical Science for September, I have a long article on etherization, vindicating your claims over those of Jackson.

" Of course the great thought is that of producing insensibility; and for that the world is, I think, indebted to you.

" I read a paper lately to our Society, showing that it was recommended by Pliny, &c. in old times.

" With very great esteem for you, allow me to subscribe myself,
" Yours very faithfully, "J. Y. SIMPSON.
" Edinburgh, 19th November, 1847."

Accordingly, in a note published with the article referred to, is the following sentence: " Within the last few days, I have seen a pamphlet, dated Boston, May 30, 1847, in which it is stated, that, for three months previously, all apparatus had been laid aside, and the sponge alone used for etherization, by Dr. Morton, of that city, — the gentleman to whom, I believe, the profession and mankind are really and truly indebted for first reducing into practice the production of insensibility by ether-inhalation, with the object of annihilating pain in surgical operations."

and that its conclusions will be adopted, if at all, under a like solemn sense of responsibility.*

* A few remarks upon the manner in which this inquiry has been pursued may not perhaps be inappropriate.

The Committee considered, that, as Dr. Morton alone assisted in the early experiments at the Hospital, they were not strictly called upon to mention Dr. Jackson; but, inasmuch as Dr. Gay's pamphlet had been for some time before the world, and also Mr. Warren's reply, it seemed that the whole subject had been submitted by the parties to the tribunal of the public, and that the public would reasonably expect from this institution such a narrative of the facts as might be prepared from these *and from other sources more especially within our reach.* Both these pamphlets were therefore very carefully examined and compared; twenty-two individuals, most conversant with the subject, consulted; and the report substantially prepared. The Committee then deemed it advisable to address a note to Dr. Jackson, informing him that Dr. Gay's pamphlet had been considered by them as containing a full statement of his claims; that if, however, he had any additional facts to communicate, the Committee would be happy to receive them. The result was two personal interviews, besides one of three hours' duration (by express appointment) with Dr. Gay in behalf of Dr. Jackson. Dr. Gay offered to prove certain facts, having no connection with or relation to this discovery, which the Committee declined hearing. He also said he had other evidence of a strictly confidential character, which was also declined. He then proceeded to comment upon the testimony contained in Mr. Warren's pamphlet. All his arguments and objections upon this point have been fairly stated by the Committee from memoranda taken at the time; and the deliberate views of the Committee, in relation to these objections, have been also stated. The Committee, at this interview, wished to know the worst that could be suggested as to the credibility of these witnesses. Few remarks were therefore made to Dr. Gay as to the sufficiency of his objections; but they were noted as subjects for future investigation. The Committee may have said, "Well, putting this deposition aside for this ground, what is your objection to the next deposition?" But it was, on the other hand, distinctly suggested to Dr. Gay, that two of these witnesses were very favorably spoken of, and that the testimony of Whitman, whose character even Dr. Gay admitted to have been above suspicion, was obviously confirmatory of matters stated by the two witnesses referred to; and that even Whitman's testimony alone was sufficient to prove that Dr. Morton was striving to realize the idea of this discovery, and was therefore irreconcilable with Dr. Jackson's *exclusive* claims.

The Committee mentioned to Dr. Jackson, that they had obtained some

HOSPITAL REPORT.   249

[Appended to this Report was the following letter from Mr. Wightman : —]

" N. I. Bowditch, Esq.   " Boston, Feb. 10, 1848.

" Dear Sir, — In answer to your note of yesterday, desiring any information I might be able to communicate with regard to Dr. Morton's application of ether, I am happy to render the following statement for the use of the Trustees of the Hospital, which, if it will aid their investigations, is entirely at their service.

new testimony in favor of Dr. Morton (meaning the letters of Mr. Metcalf and of Dr. Dana) ; but, believing that the testimony in these letters was of a nature not to be rebutted, the Committee did not feel called upon to state the fact that either of these two gentlemen had been consulted. The Committee felt themselves perfectly free, like every one else, to form and to express an opinion upon a matter of universal interest and importance, and which indeed seemed to fall naturally within their peculiar province, *even though they had not the previous permission of Dr. Jackson.* Their report had been unanimously accepted by the Trustees, and presented to and unanimously accepted by the Corporation. While it was in process of publication, a note was received from Dr. Gay, alleging that he supposed his objections to the testimony in Mr. Warren's pamphlet were recognized by the Committee as well founded, and protesting against the course pursued by the Trustees of the Massachusetts General Hospital in giving " any countenance to the attempt of Mr. Morton to rob Dr. Jackson of his sacred right to his own discovery." Dr. Gay, in his note, significantly adds, that " Dr. Jackson has always, excepting in one unguarded moment, declined submitting his claims to any tribunal, either to be agreed upon by the parties, *or self-constituted and forced upon him.*" He alleges that Dr. Jackson has much new evidence, that the investigation of the Committee must necessarily have been partial, &c. This note of Dr. Gay was laid before the Trustees, at a meeting held Feb. 6 ; but they deemed no action necessary thereupon. The Committee claim no judicial powers or functions. Dr. Jackson is perfectly free to continue in his present determination of never submitting his exclusive claims to any human tribunal, or he may hereafter submit them to one which he shall regard as more competent or impartial. If, by any new evidence, he can establish these claims, he is still at liberty so to do. The Committee can only state, that they have endeavored to prosecute their inquiries in a fair, cautious, and thorough manner, and that they feel the utmost confidence in the soundness of the conclusions at which they have arrived ; and, conscious that no proceeding or neglect on their part has justified the remarks of Dr. Gay, they here take leave of this subject *for ever.*

"My acquaintance with Dr. Morton commenced in the summer of 1846, when he applied to me for some information upon increasing the security of artificial teeth by atmospheric pressure. A short time afterwards (I think within a few weeks), he called again, and, in reply to me, stated that he had abandoned his views on atmospheric pressure, which he found were erroneous, *and was then engaged upon something of much greater importance in his profession. He then wished me to show him some bags of India-rubber cloth, made for retaining gas, and inquired whether it would do to put sulphuric ether into them.* My answer was, that ether was used to *soften* rubber, and might dissolve it so as to make the bag leak. He then asked me if an oiled silk bag would retain it. I told him that the silk was covered with a preparation of linseed oil, which I had no doubt would be acted upon by the ether; but, as I could give him no *certain* information respecting the effect, *I advised him to call upon Dr. Charles T. Jackson*, who was well versed in these matters, and could give him the necessary information. He then observed that Dr. Jackson was a friend of his; that he had boarded in his family; had been a student with him; and that he did not think of it before, but would call upon him.

"A few days after this interview, Dr. Morton came to me for some chemical glasses, and appeared inclined to keep from me the purpose for which he wished them; but, in the course of the conversation, I had no question in my mind but they were for experiments with ether. The article he then took not answering his purpose, he visited my rooms a number of times during the week; and, after trying various articles, he informed me that what he wished to have was something which would allow ether to be inhaled from it, to produce insensibility to pain in his dental operations. I inquired of him whether this would not injure the lungs. He replied that he had tried it himself, and administered it without experiencing any ill effects, and that Dr. Jackson said that it was not injurious.

"After suggesting various forms for an inhaler, we decided upon a tubulated globe-receiver, into which he proposed to put a piece of sponge, to be kept saturated with ether, and have the opening through which the retort usually enters placed over the mouth, and the air admitted through the *tubulure*, or hole for the stopper. I advised him to try this, and, if it answered the purpose, to have an appropriate vessel made. He then left me, and I did not see him again, until one afternoon he called upon me in great haste, and begged me to assist him to prepare an apparatus with which he could administer the ether to a patient at the Hospital the next day, as Dr. Warren had consented to use it in an operation. He appeared much excited; and although, from a pressure of other engagements, it was very inconvenient for me, yet I consented to arrange a temporary apparatus under these circumstances. This apparatus was composed of a quart tubulated globe-receiver, having a cork fitted into it instead of a glass stopper, through which cork a pipette or dropping tube was inserted to supply the ether as it was evaporated. *I then cut several large grooves around the cork to admit the air freely into the globe to mix with the vapor,* and delivered it to Dr. Morton.

" From this time I have had but one interview with Dr. Morton, and I regret that I am unable to furnish specific dates for these transactions; but, from the variety of articles tried and returned by Dr. Morton, and the trifling value of those taken by him at different times, I made no charges to him in my books. I am therefore indebted to other circumstances for the date of these occurrences, one of which is that I returned to Boston from the country with my family on the 28th Sept. 1846; a fact which appears from an actual entry in my books. In the cars I met Dr. Morton; and, from my recollection of the circumstances at that time, I am satisfied that the conversation about the effect of sulphuric ether upon the gas bags was previous to that time. My attention was called to the date and circumstances of this interview in the winter of 1846-7, and I then satisfied myself upon the matter.

" On the appearance of the article signed ' E. W.' in the Daily Advertiser of March 5, 1847, in which some allusion was made to me, Dr. Jackson and Mr. Peabody called upon me in reference to my knowledge of the dates of Dr. Morton's interviews with me. I explained the matter to them at that time; and although we differed in opinion as to the date of Dr. Morton's *first* application to me, yet I am happy to state that Dr. Jackson has since admitted to me, that my view of the dates of the transactions was substantially correct, adding that he could substantiate his discovery as far back as 1842. — Yours respectfully,

" JOSEPH M. WIGHTMAN."

The Committee make the following remarks on this letter : — The date of Mr. Wightman's coming to Boston is fixed beyond all doubt. The circumstances connected with this occasion have been verbally stated to the Committee, and are of a nature, rendering, in their judgment, a mistake impossible. This letter, then, proves that, prior to

Sept. 28, 1846, *or more than two days before his interview with Dr. Jackson, Dr. Morton called on Mr. Wightman, alluded to some intended discovery of great importance, and inquired about bags, suitable for holding sulphuric ether. And it would seem probable, that it was owing only to a casual suggestion then made, that Dr. Jackson, rather than some other learned chemist, was subsequently consulted by Dr. Morton.*

The letter also proves, that Dr. Jackson had heard *from Mr. Wightman* (as well as from Mr. Metcalf, see p. 228) facts which it seems difficult to reconcile with his (Dr. Jackson's) conviction, expressed so strongly to the Committee, *that Dr. Morton was wholly ignorant of sulphuric ether*, down to the interview with him. Dr. Jackson, and his friend Mr. Peabody, seem, indeed, to have been aware of the important bearing of Mr. Wightman's testimony on this point. Therefore in March, 1847, they endeavored strenuously, but in vain, to satisfy him that he was mistaken as to the date of his first interview with Dr. Morton, about the gas bags. *It would seem that Dr. Jackson had not yet resorted to the hypothesis, that he had made his discovery in 1842; since that, of course, rendered all these transactions with Dr. Morton of no consequence.* Accordingly, in his later interview with Mr. Wightman, Dr. Jackson said, in effect, " You may be about right in your dates; *but it is immaterial to me,* as I can substantiate my discovery as far back as 1842." *Unfortunately, Dr. Jackson,* in the specification accompanying the patent, *had, under oath, disavowed any discovery prior to that which he made jointly with Dr. Morton;* and the Committee have proved, that what Dr. Jackson knew about ether in 1842 had been published by Pereira in 1839.

II. VINDICATION OF THE HOSPITAL REPORT.

BY N. I. BOWDITCH.

In the month of April last, a card of Dr. Charles T. Jackson appeared in various newspapers of the city of Boston, cautioning "the friends of science and humanity" against a combination of interested persons, and proposing to expose the falsehoods in the Report of the Trustees of the Massachusetts General Hospital, presented to the Corporation, Jan. 26, 1848. "A Defence of Dr. Jackson's Claims to the Discovery of Etherization," by his attorneys the Messrs. Lord, was published a few weeks afterwards. Prepared with this deliberation, and heralded with this solemnity, it doubtless presents all the important points upon which Dr. Jackson relies. The notice which the writers take of me is somewhat personal. The other Trustees of the Hospital are declared not to be "held responsible for the truth of my statements, the legitimacy of my inferences, or the justness of my conclusions." Without recognizing any such exclusive responsibility, I am perfectly ready to meet its consequences. Having engaged in this investigation only from the wish that truth and justice might prevail, I am induced by the same motive to ask the attention of the public to a brief vindication of the Hospital Report. I feel it unnecessary, before this community, to defend either my motives or my conduct from the charges made or insinuated by the Messrs. Lord.

It will be remembered, that the Hospital Report alleges that Dr. Morton, previous to his interview with Dr. Jackson (Sept. 30, 1846), had bought sulphuric ether, and conversed about its qualities, especially its effects when inhaled, as a substitute for nitrous oxide, for the prevention of pain in dental operations, &c.: in other words, that Dr. Morton was seeking for *this* discovery by means of *this* agent, and did *not* get the first idea of using it from Dr. Jackson. These positions are, it is believed, fully established by the statements of Mr. Metcalf and Mr. Wightman. The Messrs. Lord are obviously aware, that it is absolutely necessary for them to do away with those statements. This they attempt, in the case of Mr. Metcalf, by declaring that they *understand* that he (Mr. Metcalf) will not be willing to swear that it was *sulphuric* ether which he saw Dr. Morton buying, — that he merely thinks the vial was so labelled, — that he probably would not swear that Dr. Morton did really purchase said vial of ether, &c. Now, will it be believed, that the Messrs. Lord have never asked a question of Mr. Metcalf upon the subject; and that, on the contrary, Dr. Jackson himself knew from Mr. Metcalf's own lips, that he was entirely certain it was sulphuric ether? What is this, on the part either of Dr. Jackson or his attorneys, but an absolute perversion of truth? I subjoin a note of Mr. Metcalf upon this subject: —

"Boston, June 4, 1848.

"Dear Sir, — The writers of the reply to the Report of the Trustees of Massachusetts Hospital have never been informed by me, that I was not ready to swear that the vial in Mr. Morton's possession, early in the summer of 1846, contained *sulphuric* ether. Neither can I believe, that they have been so informed by Dr. Jackson; for, *on the evening of the day after the date of my letter to you*, I called at Dr. Jackson's office, and informed him of its purport. He expressed surprise that I was able to fix a purchase of sulphuric ether by Mr. Morton of so early a date, and asked if I was sure that it was *sulphuric*, and not chloric, ether in the vial. *I told him that I knew it to be sulphuric ether*, because, while conversing with Mr. Morton, I had uncorked the vial, and smelt it.*

* Besides the interview here described, Mr. Metcalf previously spoke to

"That the vial contained *sulphuric* ether, — that I made the above statement to Dr. Jackson, — and that Mr. Morton purchased the ether, as I have stated in my note published in the Hospital Report, *I am ready to swear.* Yours respectfully,

"THEODORE METCALF.

" N. I. Bowditch, Esq."

Now as to Mr. Wightman's letter. The "Defence" speaks of its vagueness and uncertainty, and suggests many ingenious and elaborate theories to prove that Dr. Morton's interview with Mr. Wightman was *after*, not *before*, his interview with Dr. Jackson. Whatever uncertainty, however, there may be as to the exact time when Mr. Wightman first became acquainted with Dr. Morton, the date of the particular interview with him, which is important in this case, is fixed so securely that it is hardly possible for any thing to be more definitely established by human testimony. Mr. Wightman came to Boston with his family, Sept. 28, 1846, or *two* days before the interview between Dr. Jackson and Dr. Morton. This date is fixed by an actual entry in his books, and subsequent entries of articles sold Sept. 29, &c. When coming to Boston in the cars, he met Dr. Morton. I have obtained from Mr. Wightman a supplementary note, stating the circumstances which then occurred. These are of such a nature as to make it impossible for him to be mistaken in the fact that it was before this time Dr. Morton had consulted him about bags of India-rubber cloth for holding sulphuric ether, and on which previous occasion he had advised Dr. Morton to call on Dr. Charles T. Jackson, for the purpose of obtaining more definite and certain information as to sulphuric ether

Dr. Jackson of the fact, that, *before he went to Europe*, he had seen Dr. Morton buying sulphuric ether, &c. — a fact commented upon in the Hospital Report.

than he himself could give him. The following is Mr. Wightman's note: —

"N. I. Bowditch, Esq.   "Boston, June 15, 1848.

"Dear Sir, — In reply to your note asking for a written account of the circumstances which I mentioned to you verbally, as alluded to in my letter of Feb. 10, I would state as follows: —

"It appears by my books of account and entries of cash made on those days, that on Aug. 1, 1846, I went to Dover with my family, and that on Sept. 28, 1846, I returned with my family to Boston; there being also in my account-books, for the month of September, separate subsequent entries under dates of Sept. 29 and 30. I distinctly recollect, that, on several different occasions within that period, I met and conversed with Dr. Morton in the cars; and these must have been separated by intervals of at least one week, as I only went to Dover on Saturdays, returning on Monday mornings. We went up together in the five-o'clock trains, and I always returned in the first train; and it was only by reason of my taking a later train, when I brought my family back to Boston, that I met Dr. Morton. On this occasion, Sept. 28, 1846, he had a bouquet in his hand. I was sitting by his side. He asked me if the lady near me was Mrs. Wightman: I replied, 'Yes.' He said, 'Will she accept these flowers?' I assented, and thereupon introduced him to my wife. She asked me in a low voice who Dr. Morton was. I told her he was a dentist, who was making experiments about extracting teeth without pain. Mrs. Wightman recollects distinctly, that in conversation I observed to her, 'Dr. Morton thinks that I do not know what he means to use for this purpose; but I do.' From all the circumstances in the case, I have not the least doubt in my mind that the agent he intended to use for that purpose was *sulphuric* ether. This I infer from his inquiries as to the effect of sulphuric ether in dissolving India-rubber bags, &c., as alluded to in my former letter. From that time I have never met Dr. Morton in the cars.

"There is one other circumstance, affording internal evidence, that makes me entirely certain that Dr. Morton really called upon Dr. Jackson pursuant to my suggestion. It is this: Dr. Morton and I had talked of mesmerism, and he asked me if I believed in it. I told him no; that much of its effects was probably nervous, and much the result of imagination. *I* then proceeded to relate to him *myself* the very anecdote which it is proved, both by Barnes and M'Intyre, that he (Morton) related to Dr. Jackson, viz. that of a criminal upon whom certain French surgeons tried the experiment of merely pricking his arm while he was blindfolded, and letting warm water trickle down from his arm into a bowl; the result being, as I informed Dr. Morton, that his pulse became more and more feeble; and when the surgeons thought that the experiment had been carried as far as was safe, the bandage was removed, when, to their great surprise and alarm, they found that they could not revive him, and he actually died from the effect of imagination.

"Yours respectfully,

"JOSEPH M. WIGHTMAN."

Further, the "Defence" admits, that Mr. Wightman and Dr. Morton had an interview, and *within a very few days*, either *before* or *after* the interview with Jackson. Now, throwing out of the case all circumstances by which Mr. Wightman is enabled to fix the date to be *before* the interview with Jackson, what is the other evidence in the case? On the one supposition, all is very natural. Dr. Morton calls on Mr. Wightman, and asks about India-rubber bags for holding sulphuric ether. *He tells him to call on Dr. Jackson* for more definite information. Dr. Morton calls accordingly. At this interview we find him "having in his hand an *India-rubber bag* belonging to Dr. Jackson;" and a conversation commences. *The subject of nitrous oxide is introduced.* At a former interview with Mr. Metcalf, this same subject had led to a conversation about using sulphuric ether for inhalation, instead of nitrous oxide; and the same result follows on this occasion.

On the hypothesis that the interview with Mr. Wightman was after that with Jackson, two obvious questions arise. If Dr. Morton had already received such definite and particular instructions from Dr. Jackson as to the use of ether, and how to apply it, and had actually performed his first experiments, why should he call on Mr. Wightman at all, and ask about India-rubber bags, and whether ether would dissolve them? Why not take Dr. Jackson's opinion on this point; and, when Mr. Wightman tells him to go to Dr. Jackson for definite information, what possible motive could he have had for not replying, "I have been to see him a very few days ago, and he has told me all about sulphuric ether"? No, this internal evidence, of itself, would be enough to settle the question of priority as to these interviews.

It is, then, a fact for ever established, that Dr. Morton's conversations with Mr. Metcalf and Mr. Wightman were *before* his visit to Dr. Jackson. Of course it follows, that when, at this interview, he asked if ether were a gas, and said, "What queer-smelling stuff!"* he was designedly concealing what he knew. And what motive could he have had for such concealment, except that subsequently assigned by himself, viz. that he was seeking for this discovery, and was fearful that, if he made any direct inquiries of him, Dr. Jackson would claim it as his own?*

Now, suppose that all four of Dr. Morton's witnesses, Spear, Leavitt, Hayden, and Whitman, are perjured; that no demijohn of ether was purchased; that no experiments were tried from the contents of such demijohn; still these two statements of Mr. Metcalf and Mr. Wightman prove, as I conceive, beyond a possibility of doubt, that Dr. Morton was seeking for this discovery before Sept. 30, 1846; and that he was *not* indebted to Dr. Jackson for the first idea of using sulphuric ether, as claimed by Dr. Jackson and his friends. Mr. Wightman, indeed, as he expressly states, feels certain that it was only in consequence of his casual

---

* It has been stated in the Hospital Report, that the facts proved by Mr. Metcalf make it certain that the degree of ignorance expressed by Dr. Morton, in his interview with Dr. Jackson, was assumed. Yet the "Defence" says upon this point, "We have to depend on Mr. Morton's word alone."

suggestion that Dr. Jackson was consulted at all in the case. The facts proved by these two statements utterly overthrow Dr. Jackson's exclusive pretensions.* The concurrent testimony of the other four witnesses is merely cumulative. It may be wholly rejected, without affecting one of the conclusions arrived at in the Hospital Report. Three of these witnesses are living, and can take such steps as they consider necessary for the vindication of their characters; but the late Francis Whitman, one of these witnesses, is spoken of by many who knew him well, in high terms, as a man of truth and honor. Even Dr. Gay, then not pretending to doubt the existence of the demijohn, said to me that Whitman was *too honest* to allow that it contained sulphuric ether, and therefore in his deposition states it contained chloric ether. That such a man would lend himself to this base conspiracy to injure Dr. Jackson, I, for one, entirely disbelieve; and yet, if his testimony is to be credited, it establishes a secret purchase of some sort of ether. The "Defence" itself introduces no evidence to impeach this witness, except the allegation, that all the witnesses, after giving their depositions, began to talk of matters respecting which they had been before silent. I designedly abstain from any comments upon the testimony by which Dr. Jackson endeavors to impeach the credibility of these four witnesses, as I think the whole matter comparatively irrelevant and unimportant. I will, however, make one or two suggestions. Mr. Brewer's affidavit is merely that his firm sold ether of a certain quality, and never such as that in the demijohn. Now, such is the volatile nature of ether, that, if the vial containing it be left open or insecurely closed, its whole spirit will evaporate. A physi-

---

* Indeed, Mr. Metcalf's letter alone is of itself sufficient to do so.

cian of high scientific attainments, and a member of the Academy, informs me that, last year, he ordered a vial of ether at an apothecary's, and, on opening it, perceived that it had no smell of ether, and, calling the apothecary's attention to its worthless character, asked an explanation. The reply was, "I don't understand this. *It was some of Stevens and Brewer's best.*" It was probably at first a good article; and, like it, the contents of the demijohn had deteriorated, from the same or some other cause. This explanation disposes of that one of Dr. Morton's alleged " lies " which is founded on this affidavit. Indeed, some half-dozen of these " lies " relate to this demijohn and its contents.

Some most puerile remarks are made upon the discrepancies in the testimony. Thus Leavitt says, that he was sent to Dr. Gay, but could not find his residence; while another witness swears that Leavitt came back and said Dr. Gay was not in. Do not the Messrs. Lord, as " counsellors-at-law," know that these slight discrepancies are really satisfactory as proving a want of concert among the witnesses? Similar discrepancies are actually adduced by commentators as evidence of the genuineness even of the Gospels.

Again, there has always been a system of concealment and secrecy on the part of Dr. Morton, manifest throughout all the testimony, and expressly recognized in the Report. This very ether is sworn to have been bought in the name of a fictitious purchaser, as if to be sent into the country. Whitman's testimony also seems to imply, that this system extended to the demijohn and its contents. Thus he says, "I told Dr. Morton I knew what it was that William had bought, and said it was chloric of ether." This system of concealment explains the fact, that many of those employed in Dr. Morton's office may never have happened to see the demijohn. But one credible witness, who swears positively to its existence, is to be believed, though twenty others equally credible swear that they never saw it. Further, this system of concealment may explain the silence of the four witnesses, prior to the giving of their depositions; since, of course, all injunctions of secrecy would then be removed. It is obvious, that a controversy may be carried on interminably by *ex-parte* affidavits made without any cross-examinations; each set of witnesses impeaching the characters of those on the opposite side, and the public having no means of judging of the degree of credit to be given to either. It may be remarked, that Dr. Morton has always been willing to leave the question to reference, when perjury on either side would be sifted by the cross-examination of intelligent referees. But I repeat, that the vindication of the Hospital Report requires no such prolonged discussions. No one impugns the integrity or doubts the intelligence of Mr. Metcalf or Mr. Wightman. Both are free from the slightest bias or interest; and their statements form the all-sufficient basis upon which rest these positions of the Hospital Report.

The " Defence " contains a mass of testimony to the effect that Dr. Morton habitually admitted that it was Dr. Jackson's discovery, and not his. But it is expressly stated in the " Defence," that Dr. Morton sought to obtain a patent without Dr. Jackson's previous knowledge or permission; thus publicly claiming before all the world, that, in performing the first experiment, he had acted for himself, not as the agent of Dr. Jackson. So, likewise, printed circulars were published in the newspapers, and distributed as handbills, in which Dr. Morton most positively and emphatically claimed this discovery as his own. These are still extant. One of them has been submitted to me. Dr. Morton, of course, always admitted his obligations to Dr. Jackson. I have no doubt, that he did most fully and openly declare, on many occasions, the truth, — namely, that Dr. Jackson told him to try this new agent, and pronounced it to be safe, — that it was by his express advice and sanction that he performed his first experiment of pulling out a tooth. But, whatever may have been his language on these occasions, it cannot alter the facts proved by Mr. Metcalf and Mr. Wightman, namely, that, before he saw Dr. Jackson, he was himself seeking to learn the properties of this agent, for the purpose of realizing this discovery. Dr. Morton had an obvious and very powerful pecuniary motive for thus uniformly declaring and setting forth Dr. Jackson's claims as the discoverer, viz. that of getting the discovery more generally introduced than it could be otherwise. Indeed it is stated expressly in Mr. Eddy's testimony, that he advised Dr. Morton to admit Dr. Jackson as a joint patentee, because he thought "that his association with Dr. Morton would give immediate character to the discovery." After the joint patent was taken out, and when no dispute could therefore be anticipated, and Dr. Morton's object was merely to sell his rights as extensively as possible, he did doubtless put Dr. Jackson prominently forward, and award to him in the fullest terms the credit of having made the immediate scientific suggestion which led him to try the first experiment. It is somewhat amusing to find Dr. Jackson insisting that these verbal declarations of Dr. Morton shall debar him from proving the previous steps which he had taken towards this discovery, and for ever oblige him to admit as true, what certainly is not true, that he got the idea of using sulphuric ether for this purpose, for the first time, from Dr. Jackson; while, on the other hand, the statements of Dr. Jackson, actually written, signed, and *sworn to* (in the specification accompanying the patent), to the effect that the discovery was a joint one, — that no human being ever discovered this power of ether before this joint discovery, &c. — are quietly set aside by him as the mere formal " wording of an official paper."

If the claim to this scientific discovery is to be decided by the application of the technical doctrines of estoppel, those rules certainly ought in fairness to be applied to both parties.

The "Defence" next insists upon Dr. Jackson's having been induced to become a party to the patent " for the single purpose of securing the *credit* of the discovery." This uniform disinterestedness is again alleged. The "Defence" says, "That he did not wish to make any thing out of the public is sufficiently proved by," &c. The reader, however, will remember that the letter of Dr. Jackson's legal advisers, published in the Hospital Report, demanding an increased share of the profits, speaks of the patent as one "*which, if sustained, promises to give to all parties large sums of money for their united co-operation.*" . . .

Again, it is most positively stated in the "Defence," that there is no pretence that Dr. Morton ever made a gratuitous offer of any sort to the army and navy of the United States, as declared in the Report; he having really only offered to *sell* his discovery to the Government. But, in fact, subsequently to the offer to sell to Congress, letters *were* addressed by his agent to those two departments, offering its use forthwith, on account of the existing war with Mexico.

The "Defence" claims for Dr. Jackson the honor of introducing this discovery into the Hospital. It is abundantly proved by the Report, that the first capital operation, and two others preceding it of a less serious character, were performed by surgeons who knew only Dr. Morton; Dr. Jackson's name not having been mentioned to them at all.

Dr. Jackson, however, attempts to connect himself with these first operations by evidence that he told Dr. Morton to call on Dr. Warren. The idea of generalizing and extending the discovery was, of course, perfectly obvious; and (even if we disbelieve the testimony of Dr. Hayden, that Dr. Morton had already decided to go to the Hospital) Dr. Jackson can hardly claim much merely from such a suggestion. The reluctance testified to, as manifested by Dr. Morton to Dr. Jackson with regard to going to the Hospital, I suppose indeed to have been part of his system of concealment. It was a reluctance to go there *as the agent of another.* He was unwilling probably to accede to this suggestion, lest he should be deprived by Dr. Jackson of all credit which might result from taking this step. But what is Dr. Jackson's actual relation to the Hospital in this matter? He sends to the surgeons of this institution an agent whom he avowedly regards as ignorant and reckless. He does not trouble himself to call personally upon any one of these surgeons to give them a word of caution or advice, though all six of them live within five minutes' walk of his house.* For many successive weeks, he does not go once to the Hospital to see these operations, though absent from the city only during a brief period as stated in the Report. And, when at last he concludes to do so, Mr. Burnett sees him at his office, and is informed by him that he is going to take a bag of oxygen to the Hospital, as he thinks Morton will probably kill somebody yet with the ether, before he has done. All this, surely, is a singular mode of manifesting his interest in, and promoting the success of, these Hospital operations. During the same period, Dr. Morton is not the reluctant agent of another. He acts for himself. While, on

---

* A casual interview with Dr. Warren, *after* the two first operations, forms no exception to the truth of this remark.

the one hand, it would be difficult to exaggerate the degree of indifference shown by Dr. Jackson during the whole series of these early experiments, it would, on the other, be equally difficult to do more than justice to the earnest and indefatigable efforts of Dr. Morton. One of the surgeons of the Hospital says that he absolutely haunted them.

Dr. Jackson, upon this state of facts, and in compliance with alleged applications from numerous quarters, concludes to give to the world a true narrative of this great discovery, and of the circumstances attending its introduction. This he does in the form of a paper addressed to the American Academy, and published in the Boston Daily Advertiser, March 1, 1847. He there thinks it best to suppress all mention even of Dr. Morton's name in connection with the Hospital. He deliberately claims all himself. "I was desirous of testing it (the ether) in a capital operation," &c. "Dr. Warren *politely consented* to have the trial made." But mark the result. At the meeting of the Academy on the very next day, Dr. Jackson learns from Dr. Hayward that *he* performed the first capital operation at the Hospital. Dr. Jackson forthwith alters his text, so as to make *Dr. Hayward* "politely consent" to perform that very operation. In other words, Dr. Jackson, by his own showing, did not know till March 2, 1847, who it was that had politely consented, at his desire, to do this important act four months before. Dr. Hayward states, that, when he performed this operation, he had not the slightest suspicion that Dr. Jackson had any thing to do with this discovery. Nor, as it appears, had Dr. Jackson the slightest suspicion that Dr. Hayward had any thing to do with performing the operation. In alleging any polite consent of Dr. Hayward, under these circumstances, Dr. Jackson certainly drew largely on his imagination.

After all, then, Dr. Jackson cannot, it would seem, complain of Dr. Morton's conduct in this instance. If Dr. Morton suppressed Dr. Jackson's name, when, pursuant to his advice, he asked Dr. Warren to perform these operations, Dr. Jackson in return suppressed his in his true and perfect history of their performance. The one, it may be, wrongfully appropriated a suggestion; the other, in return, appropriates its verification.

The fundamental proposition of the Hospital Report is, that "Dr. Jackson does not appear at any time to have made any discovery, in regard to ether, which was not in print in Great Britain some years before." Does the "Defence" adduce any additional evidence on this point? The only new testimony is that of Mr. Blake, who relates a conversation, in the spring of 1842, on the subject of nitrous oxide and sulphuric ether, when Dr. Jackson said, "Are you aware that, when inhaled, it (sulphuric ether) produces complete insensibility?" or words to that effect. Is it gravely pretended, that this question implies any extraordinary knowledge of this agent on the part of Dr. Jackson? Why, twenty-five years before, we find in a London publication ("Journal of Science and Arts," 1818) an article upon the effect produced by the inhalation of the vapor of sulphuric ether; where it is expressly stated, that its effects resemble very much those of nitrous oxide. The best apparatus or mode of inhaling it is exactly described, and the necessity of an admixture of atmospheric air, &c. shown, as in Dr. Jackson's final advice to Dr. Morton; and the result, in one case mentioned, is declared to have been the production of a lethargic state, which was regarded as highly dangerous.

Dr. Jackson and his friends (?) wish the world to believe, that, as early as 1842, he had arrived at the mature and well-considered conclusion, that pure rectified sulphuric ether could be inhaled with safety and effect for preventing pain in all surgical operations. The utmost of the evidence adduced by him to support this proposition is, that he once inhaled this ether to the extent of producing unconsciousness, *when he was not suffering any pain;* and once more to the like extent, when suffering from the effects of chlorine gas, for the relief of which it was the prescribed remedy in the text-books. Now, Davy had suggested that the nitrous oxide, by producing insensibility, might be used for the prevention of pain in surgical operations attended with little effusion of blood; and the writer in 1818 had ascertained, that sulphuric ether produced effects analogous to those of nitrous oxide. These suggestions and facts were before the world. Dr. Jackson, from his own limited experience in the two instances above stated, seems to have formed the opinion, that pure rectified sulphuric ether could be inhaled with safety, to the extent of producing insensibility; — an opinion which he never could persuade any one else to entertain, who knew the opposite authorities on the subject. This opinion he apparently thought of little value. He, in casual conversations, incidentally suggested the use of sulphuric ether for the prevention of pain in dental operations. The only positive, explicit testimony, however, that he actually mentioned this very agent, even for this object, is a case where one of his students was desirous of being mesmerized, with a view to the extraction of two teeth without pain; whereupon Dr. Jackson suggested the use of sulphuric ether instead. There is not a tittle of evidence, that in any case, not even in this last, Dr. Jackson expressed the wish to have the experiment tried for his own satisfaction, or to verify his suggestion. And yet we find, from the " Defence " itself, that Dr. Jackson was all along conscious, that, until such actual experiment was performed, nothing could be published to the world *as a fact*. Knowing this to be so, he yet takes no voluntary, deliberate step whatever *to ascertain whether it be a fact or not*. He does not try, or cause to be tried, a single experiment on man or animal; nor does any one else to whom he makes a suggestion venture to do so; *because ether had been known to produce fatal effects*, and the decided weight of authority was against Dr. Jackson's opinion of its safety.* At last comes Dr. Morton. The subject of inhalation to prevent pain had been long in his mind. He had been a partner of Dr. Wells, and knew of his nitrous-oxide experiments. These, having been attended with but partial and doubtful success, were abandoned by Dr. Wells. The object aimed at by them was of great importance to Dr. Morton in his profession. He buys sulphuric ether. Mr. Metcalf talks with him about its character and properties, about Dr. Wells's unsuccessful experiments with the nitrous oxide, and about the inhalation of ether as a substitute therefor; telling him " the generally received opinion, that its excessive inhalation would produce dangerous, if not fatal, consequences." Dr. Morton then calls on Mr. Wightman, asks

* A recent *jeu-d'esprit*, in the ether controversy, describes the case of a man, who, being told by another that there was honey in the hollow of a tree, subsequently *verified* this suggestion, thus made the discovery himself, and secured the honey. It would have spoiled the joke to have added, that the informant had repeatedly told others of the same honey, all of whom feared that there was a deadly snake concealed in the hollow, and therefore did not like to put their hands into it. This was, indeed, the " generally received opinion " of the whole neighborhood. Truly, under such circumstances, the verifier of the suggestion deserved the honey. And it will be in vain for the informant to cry out, "I saw it first: I won't leave it to anybody to decide which of us shall have it. I have, indeed, sworn that it belongs to us jointly; but it really all belongs to me. You sha'n't have a mouthful of it."

for India-rubber bags made for retaining gas, and inquires "whether it would do to put sulphuric ether into them." Mr. Wightman refers him to Dr. Jackson for more certain and definite information on the subject than he can give.

To a mind thus prepared to receive it, the final impulse was now to be given. The same casual suggestion which he had before made to others, Dr. Jackson at last makes to Dr. Morton, — to one whom he had known for years, whose personal and scientific character he distrusted, and of whom he always spoke most disparagingly, — one to whom, after the very first successful experiments, he refused to give a written certificate of the safety of ether, on the grounds, as the "Defence" alleges, of a conviction of his ignorance, and an unwillingness to figure in his advertisements. This information, be it remembered (as stated in the Report), was elicited by Dr. Morton in an interview *sought by him* for an alleged specific purpose, viz. to obtain the means of persuading a patient to submit to an operation, under the idea *that it would be unattended with pain*. It was not disclosed in an interview sought by Dr. Jackson. Dr. Morton was not asked to make trial of it for Dr. Jackson's satisfaction, or to accomplish his purposes.

Now, is not every act and every omission of Dr. Jackson, from first to last during these five years, utterly inconsistent with a conviction in his own mind that he had made this great discovery? Had his breast been warmed with the faintest consciousness of this great truth, could he have been thus totally and uniformly indifferent? And knowing, as he must have done, the importance of those experiments by which alone it could be verified "*as a fact*," would he at last have suggested their performance, and resigned their exclusive management and control, to one whom he deemed thus ignorant and reckless? Having such a glorious conception, would he thus voluntarily and knowingly have incurred such imminent risk of miscarriage? As well believe that Columbus would have suggested and relinquished to a common sailor the attempt to discover his new world!* Contrast for one moment his conduct during these five years with his proceedings afterwards. The discovery is no sooner promulgated, and its importance recognized, than his ardent, impulsive character, and his thirst for reputation and popular applause, at once display themselves. The discovery is his own — wholly — exclusively — no partnership in it with Dr. Morton. *He* is to have no participation in the credit which it brings — "not even to the extent of the paring of a finger-nail." Through private and through official channels, in conversation and by the press, Dr. Jackson communicates *his* discovery, and claims for himself the gratitude of mankind. With what face, however, can he now appeal either to the friends of science or of humanity, after the folly and the heartlessness involved in this five years' delay? What are *his* claims to gratitude who has proved himself so long utterly insensible to the dictates of nature and the sufferings of the world? In alleging that he made this discovery in 1842, Dr. Jackson seeks, as it seems to me, to vindicate his scientific claims

---

* Dr. Jackson has compared himself, in this matter, to Columbus; and his friends have done so likewise in previous publications. I was not surprised, therefore, to find that the writers of the "Defence" recognize in Dr. Jackson, Columbus; and in Dr. Morton merely the sailor who first shouted "land" from the mast-head. I would suggest, as a truer estimate of their relative positions in regard to this discovery, that Dr. Morton was the energetic commander of a vessel, somewhat deficient, it may be, in nautical science; and Dr. Jackson, a skilful pilot, summoned when the voyage was just at its close, by whose aid the vessel was brought safely into port; where it would, in all probability, have arrived, without that aid.

at the expense alike of his character and his understanding; and this although his entire recent conduct demonstrates, that, if he had made this discovery in 1842, the whole world would have known it forthwith. But no! The supposition is too monstrous. The true explanation is contained in the Hospital Report. Dr. Jackson merely thought that the insensibility produced by sulphuric ether might last while a tooth was extracted, — a conjecture of so little consequence, that he wholly neglected all attempts to verify it, and merely suggested it in a casual manner when his attention was accidentally called to the subject.

And now I have done with this controversy. Whatever be its issue, it will always be to me a source of satisfaction, that, placed in a situation which as I thought devolved upon me the duty of engaging in it, I have, according to my convictions and to my ability, candidly stated and earnestly enforced the claims of truth. I am no "heated advocate of Dr. Morton." I am not even his apologist. It was of him, of his want of frankness, and of the consequences which it had entailed upon him, that the Report says, "Thus fitly has the majesty of truth vindicated itself!" But, whatever may have been his deficiencies or his mistakes, I feel certain that to him the world owes this discovery. Should posterity ever erect a commemorative statue, I believe that it will be inscribed with his name. He has, indeed, already received a slight "testimonial of the gratitude of his fellow-citizens," in a limited subscription, for the purpose of contributing "towards indemnifying him for his services and losses." On the other hand, I have always recognized the value of the suggestions made by Dr. Jackson. There is no evidence, that, until the interview with him, Dr. Morton had ever heard that sulphuric ether, *when pure and rectified*, could be inhaled to the extent of producing insensibility, with more safety than the common ether of the shops. For this opinion, strongly expressed, and the soundness of which was proved by Dr. Morton's subsequent experiments, he was, as I believe, indebted to Dr. Jackson. The Report accordingly speaks of this suggestion as one "which led or aided Dr. Morton to make this discovery," without which " Dr. Morton would not have made it at that precise time, and might have failed to do so at any time." But I regard the *exclusive* pretensions advanced by Dr. Jackson as the most preposterous that any man of science ever laid before an intelligent community; and such, I sincerely believe, will be the final judgment of mankind.

Testimonial to Dr. Morton, referred to above.

The following details may not be without interest in relation to the ether-controversy: —

LETTER TO DR. MORTON.

"Boston, May 12, 1848.

" Dear Sir, — At a meeting of the Board of Trustees of the Massachusetts General Hospital, a few weeks since, it was informally suggested, that a limited subscription of one thousand dollars shall be raised for your benefit, in acknowledgment of your services in the late ether-discovery; no one to be asked to subscribe more than ten dollars. We consented to act as a Committee to receive and apply the proceeds of this subscription. The proposed sum having been obtained, we have now the pleasure of transmitting it to you. We also enclose the subscription-book in a casket which accompanies this note. Among its signatures you will find the names of not a few of those most distinguished among us for worth and intelligence; and it may be remarked, that it is signed by every member of the Board of Trustees.

" You will, we are sure, highly value this *first* testimonial, slight as it is, of the gratitude of your fellow-citizens. That you may hereafter receive an adequate national reward is the sincere wish of your obedient servants,

" SAMUEL FROTHINGHAM.
" To Dr. William T. G. Morton." " THOS. B. CURTIS.

Dr. Morton's Reply.

"Boston, May 15, 1848.

"Gentlemen, — I need hardly say, that your communication of the 12th inst., and the accompanying casket, subscription-book, and donation, have been received by me with gratification of no ordinary degree.

"Apart from the positive value of the gifts, the kind feeling which has led to this manifestation on the part of so many of the first citizens of Boston has affected me in a manner that I am not likely soon to forget. The circumstances in which I have been placed for some time past give them an additional value; and by my children the testimonial will be appreciated hardly less than by myself.

"In recognizing among the names those of each of the Trustees of the Massachusetts General Hospital, I am bound to acknowledge this renewal of my indebtedness to that institution. It was the first to receive, verify, sustain, and promulgate the ether-discovery; and, from the earliest, I have received from its officers, surgeons, physicians, and trustees, nothing but constant courtesy, liberality, and kind consideration.

"Allow me to acknowledge your personal kindness in acting as a Committee for the purposes of subscription, and the tasteful manner in which you have given to it an enduring value and significance.

"You are pleased to speak of my services as deserving a national reward. I am glad to have your concurrence and sympathy in this opinion; and it is not unknown to you, that, if received, it would be to me, not only a reward, but an indemnification and relief.

"Respectfully, your obliged and obedient servant,
"WILLIAM T. G. MORTON.

"To Messrs. Samuel Frothingham and Thomas B. Curtis."

The box accompanying this note had upon it the following inscriptions: — In front, "Testimonial in honor of the Ether Discovery of Sept. 30, 1846." And on the lid, "This box, containing one thousand dollars, is presented to William Thomas Green Morton by the members of the Board of Trustees of the Massachusetts General Hospital, and other citizens of Boston, May 8, 1848." — Under which is a line extracted from the late Hospital Report, viz. "He has become poor in a cause which has made the world his debtor."

The subscription-book has one hundred and fourteen signatures. It is headed as follows, viz. : —

"In view of the benefit received by the public from the late ether-discovery, and with the desire of aiding towards the remuneration of Dr. W. T. G. Morton, of this city, for his services and losses, — we, the subscribers, agree to pay the sum set against our respective names; the same to be applied by Samuel Frothingham and Thomas B. Curtis, Esqrs., as they shall judge best for the benefit of Dr. Morton and his family.

"Boston, April 3, 1848."

III. DR. SMILIE'S ADDRESS.

Dr. Smilie is a man of science and ingenuity. He details his own near approaches to this discovery. But he adds, "'There was a lion in the way,' which served to restrain me at bay, until Mr. Morton proved himself fitted for the encounter. And, although it is urged by his opposers that he lacked knowledge which should have stimulated his discretion, it is now proved upon their own grounds, that valor, supported by ignorance, is, in some instances, the better part of discretion, in conferring benefits upon mankind." This pamphlet awards the whole scientific credit to Dr. Wells, but admits that "the peculiar character of the Massachusetts General Hospital Report has given an almost irresistible strength to the favorable tide of Mr. Morton's claims." It ends with the following paragraph : —

Having, in the foregoing, given a correct history of the rise and progress of the discovery of the power of ether to produce insensibility to pain in surgical operations, in connection with the claims of each person, directly or indirectly interested in bringing it before the public, I will now offer an analysis of their claims, to expose the merit that they are separately entitled to from the character of the aid rendered. In the first place, a question is raised or a suggestion made, whether the nitrous oxide might not be used for the production of insensibility to pain during surgical operations? But, notwithstanding the high character of its source, emanating as it did from Sir Humphrey Davy, it remained a recorded suggestion through the many editions of his works, for the lapse of nearly half a century, and had been read and re-read by persons of almost every grade of talent in every department of study, from the student to the professor, — long trained in the preparation of its basis for the purpose of experiment. Still it passed through an ordeal so varied, without ever being subjected to a single test in that direction; while the mesmerizer was affording daily stimulus for its trial, by the record of his painless operations upon persons under the influence of his reputed science. But it passed the gauntlet of minds engaged in the various combinations of investigation exercised in different directions, without meeting an organization adapted for its development, by making it the subject of trial, until it fortunately met the eye of Horace Wells, a person possessing qualities of mind of an order required for its development, although deficient in the stamina derived from early education, which led, from the disappointment of cherished and just expectations, to his sadly premature death. From that suggestion, and his acquaintance with Mr. Morton and Dr. Jackson, and the aid derived from them in gaining him an introduction at the Hospital, may be traced the studied, motive influence, which directly aided in making the latter the accidental suggester of ether as a substitute for the agent applied in Mr. Wells's experiments. The former was the adventurer, who with negative merit demonstrated its power, and placed it under the guarantee of high authority in the hands of the profession. And if there is to be an award of merit, we cannot consistently bestow it upon Sir Humphrey Davy, who, with the evidence which led him to make the suggestion, neglected to test it by actual experiment. Neither can we attach merit to the course adopted by W. T. G. Morton, the accidental instrument in developing the resources of ether, as he acted in his application to Dr. Jackson according to the instructions of Mr. Wells, for the express purpose of obtaining the agent employed in his experiments; and least of all to Dr. Jackson, who, to avoid the trouble attendant upon its preparation, in the press of more urgent duties, gave qualified advice for the use of ether from the known similarity of effect producing exhilaration, — which he directly specified at the time, with the probable danger incurred by its use. But merit is naturally directed to Horace Wells, who tested an untried suggestion of long standing, from his knowledge of the composition of its basis and harmless effect, and proved its applicability, which directly laid the foundation for the discovery of a more ready and certain agent, derived through the fortunate instruments of chance.

IV. CONGRESSIONAL REPORT.

THIRTIETH CONGRESS, SECOND SESSION. — REPORT, No. 114. — HOUSE OF REPRESENTATIVES.

WILLIAM T. G. MORTON. — SULPHURIC ETHER.

Feb. 23, 1849, laid upon the table, and ordered to be printed.

Dr. Edwards, from the Select Committee, to whom the subject was referred, made the following Report : —

The Select Committee, to whom was referred the memorial of William T. G. Morton, asking compensation from Congress for the discovery of the anæsthetic or pain-subduing property of sulphuric ether, report, — That the following memorial was presented to the House on Jan. 19, 1849, and was on the next day referred to the Committee : —

" *To the Honorable the Senate and House of Representatives of the United States of America in Congress assembled:*

" Your petitioner, William T. G. Morton, respectfully represents, that he is a dentist in the city of Boston; that in the year 1846, and for several years previously thereto, he was in the prosperous and lucrative practice of his profession in that city; his actual annual receipts from his business, as his accounts will show, being between nine and ten thousand dollars.

" That his occupation obliging him to see frequent instances of physical suffering, he was, as many others had been, induced to consider whether there might not be some means of alleviating such sufferings, and rendering operations less painful to those obliged to submit to them.

" That, in pursuance of this object, he examined such known and approved treatises on materia medica as he could obtain, and consulted with the most learned persons to whom he could get access, but found the scientific knowledge on this subject wholly vague and unsatisfactory; that, nevertheless, he continued the investigation, and, gathering all the information he could, was led, step by step, after many examinations and experiments, to the belief that sulphuric ether, properly administered, might produce partial if not total insensibility; that, desirous to verify his belief by actual experiment on the human system, and finding the idea prevalent among the scientific that any application which would be productive of such effects would be injurious to health, if not fatal to life, he made the experiment upon himself, and, after an unconsciousness of several minutes, awoke with no injury to health; that, thus confirmed in his views, he proceeded, against much opposition and amidst many obstacles, until at last, in the presence of the most eminent surgeons and physicians of a public institution, and on a public occasion, he was enabled to manifest the truth of his conception, and exhibited a patient submitting to an amputation of a leg, without the slightest sentiment of pain, or the least injury to general health in consequence of the application which produced this insensibility.

"Your petitioner would further state, that, interested in the investigations which resulted in this discovery, he devoted himself exclusively to them, to the neglect of his ordinary and regular business, in consequence of which his practice became almost entirely lost to him; that his experiments and the various arrangements and preparations which the calls upon him from all parts of the country, as well as from foreign countries, obliged him to make, and which a belief in the validity of his patent induced him to suppose would not be unrequited, were very expensive, and involved him deeply in debt; that the patents which he obtained, though legally valid, were in fact wholly valueless in a pecuniary sense; and that he finds himself now, after all his outlays, exertions, and endeavors, with his practice greatly abridged, his reputation injured by the efforts of those who opposed with great warmth the introduction of his discovery; his health impaired by mental anxiety and over-exertion; himself reduced to poverty, embarrassment, and pecuniary distress; and probably the only being living who has been a sufferer from a discovery which enables the world to rejoice in an exemption from many sufferings.

"Your petitioner states only facts which are well and widely known. He therefore respectfully prays your honorable body, that — considering the nature of the discovery; the benefit which it confers, and must continue to confer so long as nature lasts, upon humanity; the price at which your petitioner effected it, in the serious injury to his business; the detriment to his health; the entire absence of any remuneration from the privileges under his patent, and that it is of direct benefit to the government, by its use in the army and navy — you should grant him such relief as might seem to you sufficient to restore him at least to that position in which he was before he made known to the world a discovery which enables man to undergo, without the sense of pain, the severest physical trials to which human nature is subject.

"And your petitioner will ever pray, &c.

"WM. T. G. MORTON."

The day on which the above memorial was presented to the Committee, the Chairman addressed the following letter to Dr. Charles T. Jackson, of Boston, knowing that a controversy had long existed between him and the memorialist in relation to the discovery claimed : —

"House of Representatives, Jan. 20, 1849.

"Sir, — I write to inform you that a memorial of Wm. T. G. Morton was presented to the House of Representatives, and referred to a Committee on the patenting of compound medicines, of which I am Chairman. The memorialist claims the discovery and practical application of sulphuric ether in producing anæsthesia, and asks remuneration from Congress. I have long known of a controversy as to this discovery, and am aware that you claim this as yours. I shall with pleasure receive any communications on this subject.

"Your obedient servant,

"T. O. EDWARDS, Chairman, &c.

"Dr. Charles T. Jackson."

The following reply was received : —

"Boston, Jan. 23, 1849.

"Dear Sir, — I have the honor of acknowledging the receipt of your favor of 20th instant, in relation to the claims set up by Wm. T. G. Morton to the discovery of etherization, and most heartily thank you for this prompt and friendly intelligence, and shall very speedily send a remonstrance from the physicians and citizens generally of Boston. You will very much oblige me by waiting a few days before bringing up the subject; for we are taken by surprise in this matter, the movements of Morton and his friends having been concealed and unknown to us. The moment I heard that Morton had gone to Washington with some scheme of gaining notice from Government, I wrote you a letter, having learned that you were interested in the protection of our profession from quackery, and that as a physician you would be likely to interest yourself in this subject. I was very glad to learn by your letter that you were Chairman of the Committee before whom the question of the discovery of etherization would come. I am satisfied that ample proof will be laid before you, showing that Morton was in no sense the discoverer of etherization.

"I will visit you in person before long, and then shall be able to explain every thing that may not be perfectly clear.

"Were it not that my urgent duties as United States geologist required all my time, I should rejoice in being able to lay my case before Congress; knowing that there is much more facility in arriving at the truth, when both sides are examined, where there is not so much local feeling as exists in the vicinity of our Hospital.

"I shall deem it necessary, for the cause of truth, science, and for the credit of our profession, to lay my case fairly before you; and you shall soon have all the documents we can furnish. I now send you Dr. Gay's statement, which please accept.

"With the highest regard, I have the honor to be, your obedient servant,
"CHARLES T. JACKSON, 31 Somerset Street, Boston.
"Hon. Thomas O. Edwards."

"Professor Silliman, Professor Hare, Professor Gibson, and all our men of science who have examined the evidence, decide in my favor.
"C. T. J."

The following remonstrance was presented to the House, and referred to the Committee: —

"*To the Senate and House of Representatives of the United States in Congress assembled:*

"The undersigned begs leave to represent, that, whereas a memorial has been presented to the Congress of the United States by William Thomas Green Morton, of the city of Boston, in the State of Massachusetts, representing that, in the year of our Lord one thousand eight hundred and forty-six, he, the said Morton, made, in the city of Boston aforesaid, a discovery by which the human body is rendered insensible to pain during surgical operations, and during other serious and violent affections, by means of the vapor of sulphuric ether inhaled into the lungs, — praying also for a national remuneration or reward for making the said discovery, and for its practical application; and whereas the said discovery was made by the undersigned, without the knowledge of the said Morton, and without the co-operation or assistance of any person whomsoever, and was communicated by the undersigned to various persons, from the spring and autumn of eighteen hundred and forty-two to the thirtieth day of September, eighteen hundred and forty-six inclusive, and on the said thirtieth day of September was also communicated by the undersigned to the said Morton, — he, the said Morton, being, previous to the said communication of the discovery to him, wholly ignorant of the anæsthetic properties and effects of sulphuric ether aforesaid; and whereas the undersigned did also, on the thirtieth day of September, eighteen hundred and forty-six, devise and commit to the said Morton the performance of an experiment for the verification of the said discovery, so far as the extracting of teeth is concerned; and whereas the said Morton, acting in strict conformity with the instructions and upon the exclusive and expressly-assumed responsibility of the undersigned, did, to the extent of a painless extraction of a tooth, successfully verify the said discovery; and whereas the undersigned did, shortly afterwards, cause the discovery to be further verified by the surgeons of the Massachusetts General Hospital, in the first painless capital operation ever performed under the influence of the ether-vapor; and whereas the signature of the undersigned to certain letters-patent, taken out in the joint names of the undersigned and of the said Morton, declaring the discovery to be their joint invention, was obtained through the representation of Robert H. Eddy, Esq., of said Boston, the solicitor by whom the said letters-patent were procured, and copartner with the said Morton in the profits thereof, that the undersigned ' might lose all his credit as a discoverer,' if he did not consent to become a party to the said letters-patent; and whereas the undersigned, after being instructed by eminent legal counsel that the said Morton had not rendered himself in any sense a joint discoverer, by reason of the painless extraction of a tooth as aforesaid, and that he had not thereby acquired any right either to an exclusive patent or to participation with the undersigned in any patent upon the said discovery, did publicly repudiate all connection with the said letters-patent, and did refuse any part of the proceeds arising from the sale of licenses under the same; and did, as he originally intended, give the discovery freely to the world, to the full extent of his interest; evidence of all which is herewith submitted. The undersigned does, therefore, earnestly remonstrate against the memorial of the said

Morton, and prays that his petition may not be granted; and that there may not be, on the part of the Congress of the United States, any recognition whatever of his claims to the said discovery.

"CHARLES T. JACKSON.
"Washington, D.C., Jan. 29, 1849."

Dr. Jackson and Dr. Morton each appeared before the Committee on several occasions; and Mr. J. L. Lord, attorney for Dr. Jackson, presented the testimony in his favor. Various pamphlets and numerous letters, together with numerous conflicting and irrelevant affidavits, were referred to us; and, after an examination of more than a month, and a patient and careful weighing of all the facts as presented, we report that, —

On the 12th day of November, 1846, a patent was issued by the Department of State to Dr. William T. G. Morton, for a new and useful improvement in surgical operations, which consists in rendering the patient insensible to pain, by the inhalation of the vapor of sulphuric ether.

The interest of Dr. Jackson in the patent was previously assigned to Dr. Morton, who now brings it before Congress with his memorial, and offers to surrender it. He asks from Congress some consideration for the valuable boon which he claims to have conferred upon his country and the world, and remuneration for his own personal sacrifices in making the discovery. And he avers that he himself is the sole discoverer, aided only by the current knowledge of the day, which he derived from books, and from conversation with Dr. Jackson and other scientific men. Dr. Jackson, on his part, denies that Dr. Morton is the author of the discovery; but claims the whole merit as his own, and avers that in the experiments made and operations performed by Dr. Morton, testing the truth and value of the discovery, and bringing it before the world, Dr. Morton acted as agent, and that all was done by his special directions, and on his personal and professional responsibility. The contending parties have presented to the public their respective statements, and have adduced much evidence in their support; all of which your Committee have felt it their duty carefully to examine and consider.

The specifications which accompany the patent show what the contending parties admit to have been known on the subject prior to alleged discovery, and also what they claim as exclusively their own contribution to the existing mass of human knowledge. It is sufficient to refer to the following clause in the specification: "It has been known that the vapors of some, if not of all these chemical distillations, particularly those of sulphuric ether, when breathed or introduced into the lungs of an animal, have produced a peculiar effect upon its nervous system, one which has been supposed to be analogous to what is usually termed intoxication. It has never, to our knowledge, been known until our discovery, that the inhalation of such vapors (particularly those of sulphuric ether) would produce insensibility to pain, or such a state of quiet of nervous action as to render a person or animal incapable, to a great extent, if not entirely, of experiencing pain, while under the action of the knife or other instrument of operation of a surgeon, calculated to produce pain. This is our discovery."

In addition to this, the vapor of ether, for the last half-century, has been known as a nepenthe both in Europe and America, and has been inhaled for the relief of inflammations, spasms, and the effect produced by the inhalation of chlorine gas. Sir Humphrey Davy long ago suggested that the inhalation of a gas (the nitrous oxide) might be used to prevent pain in surgical operations; and the inhalation of it was publicly tried in a dental operation, but without success, by Dr. Horace Wells, in Boston, in 1844, in the presence of many persons, and Dr. Morton aided in the experiment.

In July, 1847, after the right to the discovery had become a matter of contest, Dr. Morton drew up a narrative, in the form of a memorial to the Academy of Sciences at Paris, which was, in the autumn of the same year, presented by M. Arago, in which he gives a detailed statement of what he claims as his discovery and the steps by which he arrived at its consummation. In this he states, that, in the summer of 1844, he was a student of Dr. Jackson and a boarder in his family. He details a conversation, in which Dr. Jackson explained the well-known effects of sulphuric ether on the nervous system, when taken by inhalation, and adds that Dr. Jackson, in the same conversation, said that he had sometimes used ether as a local application to relieve pain in the teeth, and recommended it to him for that purpose, and afterwards sent him a vial of highly rectified chloric ether, which he subsequently used.

This conversation with Dr. Jackson; the effect produced by the use of ether, directly applied to the teeth, in deadening pain; the experiment of Dr. Horace Wells, in the following winter, with nitrous oxide, in which he assisted; and his subsequent reading, which now took a decided turn, directed his mind to the subject, and led to further experiments. He gives the necessities of the profession as the cause which urged him on in the path of discovery. He details several attempts in the summer of 1846, none of which were entirely successful, to produce insensibility to pain by the inhalation of ether; and various efforts to provide some apparatus from which it might be conveniently inhaled. At last, on the 30th of September, he again called on Dr. Jackson for the purpose of obtaining further information as to the preparation and use of the ether, and, at the same time, studious to conceal the object which he had in view, lest Dr. Jackson should turn his thoughts in the same direction, and anticipate him in the discovery. He states a conversation with Dr. Jackson on that day, opened on his part in a manner most likely to cover his real purpose, and, at the same time, elicit the information desired He says his declared purpose was to get a refractory patient in his power, so that he could operate; and that he said nothing about performing the operation without pain. He first proposed to act on the imagination of the patient, merely by administering atmospheric air from a gas bag. This Dr. Jackson condemned; spoke of Dr. Wells and his nitrous oxide with derision, on which Dr. Morton asked him why he could not use the sulphuric ether. This Dr. Jackson at once approved; spoke of the stupefying effects of the sulphuric ether, and of the students taking it at Cambridge, and said that the patient would be dull and stupefied, so that the operator could do what he pleased with him and he would not be able to help himself; and, after some conversation about the preparation of ether, and directions as to the shop at which the best could be had, Dr. Jackson gave him a flask, with a glass tube, with which to administer it; and they parted. Dr. Morton states that he procured the ether, went to his office, locked himself up, and tried its effects on himself; and afterwards, on the same day, extracted a tooth without *pain*, or even *consciousness*, from a patient whom he had put under its influence. And that, in order to bring out the discovery, he applied to surgeons of the Hospital to suffer it to be tried in some surgical operations, which they consented to do.

Dr. Jackson denies the truth of this statement, thus far, in all its material parts. He denies that Dr. Morton, prior to their interview on the 30th of September, 1846, had any knowledge of sulphuric ether, or its effects on the nervous system; — that he was, prior to that time, in pursuit of any discovery to prevent pain in dental operations, or that he had made any experiments whatever tending to that object; and he avers that the operation of the 30th September was performed by Dr. Morton as his *agent*, by his direction, and on his sole responsibility; — that, in other words, he was the actor and Dr. Morton his instrument; and that such also was the case in the application to the surgeons of the Hospital, and the successful experiments there tried in sundry operations. On these questions much evidence is adduced, and on their determination rests the whole merit of the discovery.

To prove, amongst other matters, that Dr. Morton had no knowledge of sulphuric ether prior to September 30th, Dr. Jackson takes the testimony of two persons, — George O. Barnes and James M'Intyre, — who were his students in chemistry, and present at the interview. Barnes details a conversation about the use of atmospheric air to operate upon the imagination of the patient, which Dr. Jackson condemned; says that nitrous oxide was named, but not sulphuric ether, when Dr. Jackson said, " Now, Morton, I can tell you something that will produce a real effect. Go to Burnett the apothecary, and get some very strong sulphuric ether, — the stronger the better; *spatter* it on your handkerchief; put it to your patient's mouth; take care that it be well inhaled; and, in a minute or two, perfect insensibility will be produced." " Sulphuric ether," said Morton, " what is that? *Is it a gas?* "

It will be remarked, that the witness here professes to speak with perfect accuracy, giving this part of the conversation in its order in the form of a dialogue; but, if he be entirely correct, it involves a singular absurdity. Dr. Jackson directs that the ether shall be administered by *spattering* it on a handkerchief; on which Dr. Morton asks him, " Is it gas?" as if gas could be spattered on a handkerchief, and then administered to a patient. It is possible, however, that the very language put in the mouths of the interlocutors was, in fact, used; but, if so, Dr. Morton could not have asked the question, "*Is it gas?*" in *ignorance*, for the fact that it was a liquid was explained to him in the very directions of its use; but it must have been to disguise his knowledge, and with it his purpose.

The statement of James M'Intyre, the other witness, is less positive, and more consistent with probability. After stating the conversation about the atmospheric air and the nitrous oxide, he says: —

"As Morton was going away, Dr. Jackson told him that he could tell him something that would make the patient insensible, and then he could do what he had a mind to with him; Morton asked what it was; Dr. Jackson then told him to go to Burnett's, and get some pure sulphuric ether, and *pour* it on a handkerchief, and let her inhale it. Morton asked what sulphuric ether was; what kind of looking stuff it was. I stayed in the front room, while Morton and Dr. Jackson went to look at the ether. From Morton's questions about the ether, I am satisfied he knew nothing about its properties or nature."

There is no inherent difficulty in this statement, and that Mr. Barnes is incorrect is rendered the more probable from another consideration. If, after Dr. Jackson had directed Morton to go to a drug-store and get sulphuric ether, and administer it by *sprinkling* or *pouring* it on a handkerchief, Morton had asked if it was *gas*, how could the absurdity have escaped the observation of the students in chemistry? Would the two young men have failed to make it a subject of ridicule, in conversation with each other, so that it would have been impressed on the memory of both? But the witnesses concur in this, that, at the time of that conversation, Dr. Morton had, or pretended to have, no knowledge of sulphuric ether, or its effects upon the nervous system.

This does not militate against the general effect of the statement of Dr. Morton. He went, as he says, to Dr. Jackson to obtain from him certain information, but at the same time anxious to conceal from him the object of his pursuit, being fearful lest Dr. Jackson might anticipate him in bringing the discovery to perfection. We deal with this matter as a question of fact, not of words, and do not decide whether Dr. Morton might consistently, with the obligations which trust imposes, use artificial means to conceal a mental conception which he did not wish to divulge. We believe, however, where a person has a right to his secret, and is under no obligations to disclose it, a direct denial of that which was fact for the purpose of such concealment has not been visited with strong moral censure. We would instance the case of Walter Scott, who, at the table of George IV., when toasted by his majesty as the author of Waverley, declared that he was *not* the author. But as to the fact of Mr. Morton's knowledge : —

The statement of Theodore Metcalf, a gentleman of undisputed veracity, shows that, as early as July 6, 1846, Dr. Morton talked and thought of sulphuric ether; had been informed of what was then currently known in the scientific world as to its effects on the nervous system; that nitrous oxide was spoken of by him, and the unsuccessful experiment made by Dr. Wells. Dr. Morton had in his possession at this time a vial of sulphuric ether, which Mr. Metcalf smelled and examined; so that, after July 6, 1846, Dr. Morton could not but have known, until he forgot his knowledge, "what kind of stuff" sulphuric ether was, and, generally, something of its application and effects. There is much evidence corroborating that of Mr. Metcalf on this point, which will be considered hereafter. Suffice it to say, that we think Dr. Morton's knowledge to this extent well established; and we think it equally clear, that, in his conversation with Dr. Jackson in the presence of his students, he used artifice to conceal his knowledge. But did Dr. Morton, prior to the 30th of September, 1846, engage in the attempted discovery of some agent to prevent pain in dental operations? And did it occur to him to try the vapor of sulphuric ether as such agent? This is also affirmed on the one side, and denied on the other.

The testimony of Francis Whitman goes to this point. He says: "One day, I think it was previously to July, 1846, Dr. Morton, in speaking of improvements he had made in his profession, and of some one improvement in particular, said if he could only extract them without pain, 'he would make a stir.' I replied I hardly thought it could be done. He said he believed it could, and that he would find out something yet to accomplish his purpose." "Some time in July last, he spoke of having his patients come in at one door, having all their teeth extracted, and without knowing it, and then going into the next room, and having a full set put in." He adds, "that Dr. Morton came into the office one day in great glee, exclaiming that he had found it, and that he could extract teeth without pain."

There is nothing in the case to cast a shade over the testimony of this witness. His statement involves no contradiction or improbability; he speaks of matters which would be likely to make a distinct impression at the time: therefore your Committee could not refuse him credence, even if he were uncorroborated; but this is by no means the case. Dr. Granville G. Hayden testifies that Dr. Morton applied to him about the last of June, 1846, and desired to make some arrangement that would relieve him from the cares of his office, as he had an idea in his head connected with dentistry, which he thought would be one of the greatest things ever known, and that he wished to give all his time to its development. He at first declined to state its nature, but at length told Dr. Hayden it was something he had discovered which would enable him to extract teeth without pain; said that he had already tried its effects upon a dog, and described its operation. He said it was not nitrous oxide, and requested Dr. Hayden to say nothing about the matter. This contract with Dr. Hayden was reduced to writing on the 30th of June, 1846, as appears by the statement of Richard H. Dana, jun., the counsel who drew the instrument; and, at the time he was preparing it, Dr. Morton told him that he was in progress of a discovery, which, if successful, would revolutionize the practice of dentistry.

In the month of August, he told Dr. Hayden that his agent was sulphuric ether, taken by inhalation; said he had inhaled it himself, and tried to get three young men in his office to inhale it. He afterwards spoke of ill success and discouragement in the use of ether, and Dr. Hayden suggested that he should consult a chemist on the subject.

William P. Leavitt and Thomas R. Spear, jun., who were students in the office, testify to the purchase of sulphuric ether for Dr. Morton, in July and August; that he prevailed on them to inhale the ether; and that he offered them a reward, if they would find some one who would consent to have a tooth extracted under its influence; and that, after Dr. Hayden came, Dr. Morton seemed wholly absorbed with his experiments; that he had bottles and India-rubber bags in a small room in his office, in which room he frequently locked himself up.

Joseph M. Wightman, a gentleman of very high character, states that, in the summer of 1846, Dr. Morton applied to him for information upon increasing the security of artificial teeth by atmospheric pressure; a short time after, he stated he had abandoned his views, which he found were erroneous, and was then engaged in something of much greater importance in his profession. " He then wished me to show him bags of India-rubber cloth made for retaining gas, and inquired whether it would do to put sulphuric ether in them." It is very clearly shown that these interviews occurred prior to the conversation with Dr. Jackson, on the 30th of September, 1846; nor is the mass of evidence above referred to weakened in its force, so far as it bears on the points now under consideration, by the opposing testimony. This consists of statements alleged to have been made by Dr. Morton, attributing the discovery to Dr. Jackson; statements that he had never inhaled the ether, and statements on the part of Spear and Leavitt that they inhaled the ether for the first time, after the 30th of September, 1846. Generally, this is a species of evidence little to be relied upon, less in a heated controversy like this in which the community participate, than in ordinary cases; but we will refer to this more especially by and by, when we come to consider the several depositions. But in no wise can evidence like this weigh against a chain of facts and circumstances, proved, as in this case, by the testimony of many disconnected witnesses. There are no contemporaneous facts or declarations stated by the rebutting witnesses on this branch of the case, except by Don P. Wilson, who says he was *in and out* of Morton's office quite frequently during the summer and the month of September, 1846; never saw sulphuric ether there; never heard Morton speak of it, that he can remember; never perceived its odor about the clothes of Morton or otherwise, and thinks it could not have been used in the office without his having perceived its odor. He says, that, during the summer of 1846, he often heard Morton speak of a new discovery which he was about to publish to the world, and which, to use his own words, " would revolutionize the whole practice of dentistry, and secure to him a fortune ; " but he never hesitated to tell me and others, that " it consisted in a new preparation for filling teeth and a new mode of making teeth, and setting them to plate." This was Morton's great hobby during the summer of 1846, and during the month of September, the same year.

And John E. Hunt, whose statement on those subjects is the same with that of Wilson, except that he says he was " connected with the office in the summer of 1846," — how connected he does not say, but that he " entered the office early in the month of November of that year," — and was assistant-dentist. Now, it is sufficiently apparent, that the discovery of which Dr. Morton did not hesitate to speak publicly to these young men " and others," could not be the one which he was at the same time carefully concealing ; and, for the rest, the whole amount of this evidence is, that these persons, who occasionally visited the office of Dr. Morton in the summer of 1846, did not discover what he took especial pains to conceal. The affidavit of William A. Brewer, that the house to which he belonged sold nothing but the best sulphuric ether, is no doubt true, according to the opinion of the witness ; but it is hardly possible for him to know that none of an inferior quality left the shop, even if the best only were purchased or prepared, as it is an article greatly subject to deterioration by time, especially if the vessel containing it be often uncorked or remain open for a length of time, in which case the pure volatile ether flies off in vapor, and the dregs remain. Hence the chemical analysis had of the ether remaining in the demijohn does, in our judgment, fall far short of proving its true quality when purchased at the druggist's.

But, on the whole, the evidence thus far leaves no doubt on the minds of your Committee, that, prior to his interview with Dr. Jackson, on the 30th of September, 1846, Dr. Morton was possessed of the idea that the inhalation of sulphuric ether would render a patient insensible to pain during a dental operation; that his time and attention were for several months previously devoted to the bringing about this result; and that he called on Dr. Jackson that day to obtain information by which he could obviate certain difficulties which he encountered in his experiments, and that he disguised his knowledge and purpose from Dr. Jackson, lest he should penetrate his secret and anticipate his discovery. And as to that interview, of the two witnesses present, one, James M'Intyre, gives an account of the conversation, agreeing in all matters of substance with the account of Dr. Morton, except only that, according to him, Dr. Jackson, and not Dr. Morton, first spoke of the use of ether.

George O. Barnes said that Dr. Jackson, after directing Dr. Morton how to give the ether, said " that the patients, after breathing a dozen breaths, would fall back insensible, and you can do with them as you please *without their knowing any thing about it, or feeling any pain;* so that you can take out their teeth at your leisure." This suggestion as to *insensibility to pain* had become, as was no doubt supposed, the very point in issue. It was a most striking remark, and, if in truth it was made, was most likely to impress both the young men present. Both state the conversation in its immediate context; so that the statement of this impression by one, and its omission by the other, amounts to a discrepancy which greatly weakens the force of the affirmative statements. We have already shown a still more striking discrepancy between these witnesses in the question attributed by Barnes to Morton — "Is it a gas?" — after Mr. Morton had been told to get it at an apothecary's, and *spatter* it on a handkerchief; and we are well satisfied, in this particular as in that, it is more safe to rely on the evidence of M'Intyre.

The evidence, then, amounts to this: Dr. Morton came into Dr. Jackson's office, having in his hand a gas-bag, with which he proposed to operate on the imagination of a refractory patient by administering to her atmospheric air. Dr. Jackson ridiculed the idea. Nitrous oxide was spoken of; Dr. Jackson objected to that, saying to Morton, that, if he attempted to make it, it would become nitric oxide. He then suggested sulphuric ether, and said it would make the patient insensible, and Morton could do what he pleased with her. This conversation, it will be noted, all took place about a refractory patient; the object considered was the mode of bringing a nervous patient to a condition in which she could be operated upon, not in which she would feel no pain from the operation, — Mr. M'Intyre says not one word about pain or its absence in the operation, — but that the operator could do what he pleased with the patient under the influence of sulphuric ether. If this conclusion be correct, the information given by Dr. Jackson to Dr. Morton was no more than the current knowledge of the age, — no more than he would have been told by any scientific man, or than he would have read in books which treat of chemistry and medicine; and, if it differed in any thing from the general opinion of scientific men, it was in a stronger than ordinary assurance that the vapor was not injurious to health. At the same time, it is very clear to your Committee that Dr. Morton relied more implicitly on information which he obtained from Dr. Jackson than from any other source, and that the information was given with the unhesitating confidence arising from a consciousness of high scientific attainments.

This view of the subject awards to Dr. Jackson the merit of greatly aiding, by his advice and instructions, in the discovery. He did not himself produce the result, which was new; or, by his information, carry knowledge in that direction beyond the point it had already reached. He was a safe and reliable guide to its then utmost limit in that direction, — the Calpe and Abyla of scientific research, — but left the sea beyond to be explored by others. Nor is the result changed as to the merit of the discovery, if we take the testimony of Barnes instead of M'Intyre, as to what occurred at this conversation. On that hypothesis Dr. Jackson suggested to Dr. Morton, that his patient, under the influence of the vapor of sulphuric ether, would be insensible to pain during his dental operations; but this was no new idea to Dr. Morton: he had thought and spoken of it long before. He had for months given himself up to its consideration, and he had talked of it to a host of witnesses referred to above; some directly, some in ambiguous phrase; but so, as now, when the facts and their connection and dependence are known, to leave no doubt of the object of his study and pursuit. Then if, on the 30th of September, 1846, Dr. Jackson told him that the vapor of sulphuric ether would render his patients insensible to pain, he gave him no new information; for he was armed with no fact to show it. He gave a speculation of his own, an inference he had drawn from his scientific knowledge; but the idea was already in the mind of Dr. Morton: he had speculated on the same subject, and in the same direction. He had drawn the same inference from the same general knowledge, and he had tried an experiment on his own person, with a view of testing its correctness. It is the case of one man in the pursuit of a discovery, who has his mind fixed upon the object, and the mode of effecting it determined on, who consults with another who confirms and support his previously entertained opinions.

Nor is it, in our opinion, at all material whether Dr. Jackson had or had not been long before impressed with the conviction that this great object could be effected by the same agent, and in the same manner in which it has been brought about. If he made the discovery, he did not give it to the world. The case would have been different if he had communicated the idea to Dr. Morton prior to his researches in the summer of 1846. But this is nowhere claimed by Dr. Jackson or averred by any of his witnesses.

It is, however, contended by Dr. Jackson, that, in the administration of ether to his patient on the 30th September, and in the subsequent exhibition of it in the Hospital, Dr. Morton acted as his agent merely; that he was, in fact, the experimenter as well as the discoverer, and the merit of success or the responsibility of failure rested on him. This position your Committee will now proceed to examine.

This claim is not supported by the evidence which has been thus far considered: indeed, it bears strongly against it, and your Committee can find no contemporary matter touching this point, except a statement of George O. Barnes, not yet commented upon. The witness, after stating Dr. Jackson's efforts to overcome the scruples of Morton, says: " Indeed, Dr. Jackson urged the matter very earnestly and with perfect confidence, taking on himself the whole responsibility." Now, if this be a deduction, an inference from the conversation stated, it is of no value whatever, except to show a certain earnestness in the witness. If it be but a further declaration, it is unsupported by the testimony of M'Intyre; and, in a third important particular, differs from and goes beyond him. But the well-attested conduct of the parties themselves, at the time of the transaction in which this agency is claimed to have been conferred and accepted, what is termed by lawyers the *res gestæ*, shows more clearly than every thing else the true relation which they then bore to each other, and each of them to the subject-matter in controversy.

Dr. Jackson claims that he had long had in his mind a conviction that the vapor of sulphuric ether could be inhaled without danger or injury to the patient, and that, under its influence, surgical operations could be performed without pain. All admit him to be a man of science, fully aware of the mighty value of such a discovery, and not at all indifferent to his own reputation in the scientific world. In this state of things, we cannot conceive it possible that he could have remained inactive for years, waiting till chance should send him some one to bring out his great discovery, instead of proceeding himself by direct experiment. It is not at all disputed, that Dr. Morton went to Dr. Jackson's shop that day uninvited; that *his* wants, and not Dr. Jackson's wishes and purposes, led to the conversation; that there was nothing of an especially confidential nature between them; and that what Dr. Jackson said to him, he said in the usual manner of public conversation, and not like a man who was engaging another to bring out a most important discovery to the world.

But, take Dr. Morton to be just what Dr. Jackson and his two witnesses represent him to have been at the time of that conversation, was he the man whom Dr. Jackson would have trusted to represent him in a matter so deeply involving his character and his fame? Say it is Jackson's discovery, the experiment is his, *he* is responsible for the consequences. If it succeed, he has made the noblest contribution to surgical science which the century has witnessed; if it fail, the consequences might be most disastrous. Whom does he select to carry out this, the most important conception of his life or of the age? Let his two witnesses answer.

According to them, a man profoundly ignorant of the powerful medicinal agent which he was directed to employ, one who did not know what kind of "stuff" sulphuric ether was, and who wished to see it in order thus to test its qualities, is selected by one of the first scientific men of the age to conduct a delicate and dangerous experiment with this same sulphuric ether, on the success of which even more than reputation depended. If Dr. Jackson had dwelt upon the subject, conceived the discovery in his own mind, considered it with a view of making it known to the world and useful to mankind, he knew that much depended on the first public exhibition; and he also knew that it required science, prudence, and skill to render the experiment successful, and prevent its becoming disastrous. Sulphuric ether would produce insensibility to pain; *too little* of it would make the experiment ineffectual, and bring the operator and his nostrum into ridicule; *too much*, or the proper quantity *unskilfully administered*, would produce asphyxia, probably death. Under these circumstances, how can your Committee believe that Dr. Jackson would have trusted such a man, as his witnesses represent Dr. Morton to be, with his first experiment upon his great discovery? Would it not have been inexcusable in him to have done so? Would it not have shown a recklessness of his own fame and the lives of his fellow-men?

Such a conclusion, your Committee are satisfied, cannot be imputed to him with justice. Had Dr. Jackson made the discovery and felt that it was his, could he have failed to be at once aware of its vast importance, and the world-wide reputation it would give him? Would he have trusted it for a moment in the hands of a man less skilful and scientific than himself? — indeed, would he have intrusted it with any one? But would he not have himself seen that it was administered in a proper manner, and under proper conditions to make it safe and effectual? Would he not have stood by, and watched the sinking pulse of his first subject, until insensibility was complete, and have been careful to withdraw it when he saw it was likely to endanger life, and thus done all that science and skill could do to avoid a failure or a catastrophe? But there was nothing of this. Having given the information which he did give in the conversation with Dr. Morton, he turned neither to the right nor left, nor troubled himself further on the subject, until he was advised by Dr. Morton that the experiment had been successful. He expresses no surprise, no emotion : it is an incident of the day, — an occurrence. According to the testimony of Barnes, he advises Dr. Morton to try it in some capital operation in the Hospital; does not say he will try it himself, which he might or ought to have done, if Morton had been his agent. He does not propose to get permission for Dr. Morton so to try it; though he well knew the application by himself, or in his name, would ensure the permission. He advises Dr. Morton to get permission, and try it in the Hospital, and does not propose to be present, and in fact is not present, when the trial is made, though the Hospital was but five minutes' walk from his door. That operation was successfully performed, and another was noticed to take place the next day, about which Dr. Jackson gave himself no concern, and at which he was not present. The Committee feel that his conduct during this time was wholly inconsistent with the fact, that he recognized the discovery as his own, and that these were his experiments.

It is urged as a reason for his absence at the first operation in the Hospital, that Dr. Morton did not inform him at what time it was to take place. As to this, there is no proof that he did or did not inform him; but surely had Dr. Jackson felt the solicitude which the discoverer would naturally feel, he would have informed himself, and his daily associations naturally led him to the knowledge. On the other hand, after the successful operation of the 30th of September, and after Dr. Morton had seen his patient and ascertained that he had suffered no injury from the ether, — elated with his success, he consulted Dr. Hayden as to the mode of bringing out the discovery, and suggested at once that he would introduce it into the Hospital. A few days afterwards, he told Dr. Hayden that Dr. Jackson would not countenance the discovery, and again said he would go to Dr. Warren and endeavor to have it introduced into the Hospital. The fact that Dr. Jackson refused to give Dr. Morton a certificate that ether was harmless in its effects, or might be used with safety, is admitted by Dr. Jackson in his defence by the Messrs. Lord; but they say it proves nothing but Dr. Jackson's "unwillingness to figure in Dr. Morton's advertisements, *and his prudence in refusing to make himself responsible for any thing and every thing Morton, in his ignorance, might do, with an agent liable to the most dangerous abuse.*"

This, if it stood alone, might be satisfactory; but one of the witnesses, Geo. O. Barnes, says, that, on the 30th of September, Dr. Jackson employed Dr. Morton to use this very agent. He assured him it would "*not do the least injury.*" He "urged the matter very earnestly, *expressly taking on himself* all the responsibility;" and it was on the 1st of October, the morning after the *successful* experiment, that Dr. Jackson refused to give a certificate "that ether was harmless in its effects," and yet, on this same day, the witness Barnes says, on being advised by Dr. Morton of the success of the operation, Dr. Jackson said to him: "You must go to Dr. Warren, and get his permission to administer it in the Massachusetts General Hospital, and, if possible, it should be on a capital operation." And he goes on to say that Morton strongly objected at first to going to the Hospital; that everybody would smell the ether, and it would not be kept secret; but that, after learning something to disguise the odor, he agreed to apply to the Hospital.

We have already adverted to the fact, that Dr. Morton, the very evening after the successful operation, suggested to Dr. Hayden that he would go to the Hospital and get permission to try the ether there; that he went next morning to Dr. Jackson, and returned, saying Dr. Jackson would not give his countenance to the discovery; and it is admitted that Dr. Jackson refused him the certificate he wished for, and one of the reasons given is that he did not think him fit to be trusted. Is it, then, probable that he urged him to go to the Hospital, and there bring out his (Dr. Jackson's) great discovery? But James M'Intyre was also present on the 1st of October, when Dr. Morton returned and advised Dr. Jackson of the entire success of the experiment; and he says not a word of Dr. Jackson's proposing to Dr. Morton to try an experiment in the Hospital. Your Committee has already remarked on several other points of difference in the testimony of these two witnesses; and in each case, as in this, they felt themselves constrained by the testimony of other witnesses, and by the inherent character of the evidence, to rely on the accuracy of M'Intyre rather than of Mr. Barnes, where these discrepancies occur.

Another difficulty in sustaining the position assumed by Dr. Jackson forcibly impresses itself upon your Committee. According to this, on the 30th of September, Dr. Jackson entrusted Dr. Morton with his discovery, and not only suffered him, but "earnestly urged" him, to use it, assuring him it was perfectly safe; Dr. Morton tried it on the same evening; his success was complete; he brought to Dr. Jackson the next morning conclusive evidence of all this, and Dr. Jackson refused him a certificate because he would not " make himself responsible for any thing and every thing Morton in his ignorance might do with an agent liable to the most dangerous abuse." While nothing is shown to shake Dr. Jackson's confidence in Dr. Morton since the previous day, or at all to change his opinion of him except the triumphant success of the operation which he reported and proved. On the 16th of October, the first operation was performed in the Hospital, at which, as we have already shown, Dr. Jackson did not attend, and at which his name was not known. The second operation at the Hospital took place on the 17th, Dr. Jackson taking no part in it by his presence or his counsel. Both operations were entirely successful, and both conducted on the part of Dr. Morton to the entire satisfaction of the surgeons of the Hospital. But at this time Dr. Jackson's confidence in Dr. Morton, if he ever did confide in him, is wholly gone. He denies, in the conversation with his neighbor and friend, Caleb Eddy, that under the influence of ether the flesh of a patient can be cut without pain; says Morton " is a reckless man for using it as he has; the chance is he will kill somebody yet;" and, in the interval between the 30th of September and about the 23d of October, he declared that he did not care what Morton did with it or how much Morton advertised, if his own name was not drawn in with it.

It would seem, that, as Dr. Morton acquired eclat by his constant success, as he continually and rapidly rose in the estimation of other scientific men, he as continually and as rapidly sunk in the estimation of Dr. Jackson. The evidence of Francis Whitman and Mr. Caleb Eddy shows, that, prior and up to the 23d October, Dr. Jackson spoke doubtingly of the effect of ether, and condemned its use; and there is no proof whatever, that within that time he lent the slightest countenance to Dr. Morton to sustain the discovery; and all his remarks, except those stated by Dr. T. E. Hitchcock to have been made to him on the 2d and 3d of October, tend to create distrust and destroy confidence both in the operator and the agent used. His favorable mention of it to Dr. Keep occurred *after* the 26th of October, the actual date not fixed, and was accompanied with a strong general charge of ignorance and recklessness against Morton, who was then in the full tide of successful experiment. This state of facts is, in the opinion of your Committee, wholly inconsistent with the assumption that Dr. Jackson was the discoverer; that he had employed Dr. Morton to bring out the discovery, and that the experiments of Morton were tried on the responsibility of Dr. Jackson.

On the 30th of September, the first successful operation took place. On the first of October, Dr. Morton applied to R. H. Eddy, agent for patents, to aid him in procuring a patent for the discovery. Mr. Eddy took the case into consideration, and did not see Dr. Morton again until the 21st. In the mean time Dr. Morton's experiments had been attended with the most flattering success. Two operations had been performed in the Hospital to the entire satisfaction of the faculty, and the discovery had acquired a footing in the medical world; and prior to the 21st, but the precise day is not stated, Dr. Jackson had a conversation with Mr. Eddy, was informed of the application of Dr. Morton for a patent, and claimed that he had some connection with Dr. Morton in making the discovery. He called on Dr. Morton on the

23d; and it was then arranged that Dr. Jackson was to have $500 for the information he had given Dr. Morton, if ten per cent on the proceeds of the patent would produce that amount.

This arrangement between the parties, settled by and between themselves in a private conference, proved by their subsequent conversation with Mr. Eddy, and not now denied, shows conclusively the view that each had of his respective participation in the discovery. It was between them both distinctly a business-transaction, — an affair of dollars and cents, and as clearly Dr. Jackson called and introduced the conversation, — not to assert his rights to the discovery, — not to inquire as to its success, for of this public report had advised him, — not to give any advice or caution as to its further use, but to claim a compensation in money for the advice and information he had given to Morton on the 30th of September; and $500, if ten per cent on the proceeds of the patent would produce it, was agreed upon as the sum to be paid for that information. This conversation and agreement is entirely consistent with the view we have thus far taken of the case; but it is wholly inexplicable on the ground assumed by Dr. Jackson. But the representations and advice of Mr. Eddy, the common friend of the parties, modified their arrangement. He represented to Dr. Morton, that Dr. Jackson, from having given him the information and advice spoken of on the 30th of September, was entitled to participate in the patent as a joint discoverer; that, if he were not joined in the patent, the fact of his giving that information would be used to impeach the patent; and that, if Dr. Jackson were joined as a patentee, his name and his advice and assistance would be useful in bringing out the discovery and giving it celebrity. With these arguments, Dr. Morton was satisfied, and consented that Dr. Jackson should be named as a joint discoverer in the patent. Mr. Eddy also advised with Dr. Jackson, who informed him, that, " by the laws of the Massachusetts Medical Society, he would be prevented from joining with Dr. Morton in taking out a patent, as he would be expelled from the association if he did so. He further stated, that he intended to make a professional charge of $500 for the advice he had given him, and that Dr. Morton had acceded to this; that he did not wish his name coupled with Dr. Morton in any manner; that Dr. Morton might take out a patent if he desired to do so,.and do what he pleased with it." At a subsequent interview prior to the 27th of October, Mr. Eddy urged Dr. Jackson to waive his objections to associating with Dr. Morton, as " I was confident that he was mistaken in his views as to what would be the action of the medical association; that Dr. Morton could not properly take out a patent without him; and that, by joining in the patent, he would of a certainty be obtaining credit as a discoverer; whereas, should he not do so, he might lose all credit, as in the case of the magnetic telegraph, which I understood from Dr. Jackson he had suggested to Professor Morse." The objection as to the Medical Society was removed on consultation with Dr. Gould. Dr. Jackson consented to join in the patent, and it was agreed that he should have ten per cent of the proceeds for his interest in it.

Your Committee do not feel, that on this question of fact the parties ought to be bound by the legal conclusions of their common friend, Mr. Eddy, or by the papers which they executed in pursuance of his legal advice. But they do consider the communications made by them at the time to Mr. Eddy; the mutual agreement of the parties between themselves, as touching the discovery and the facts admitted by them on the consultation, as matter of the utmost importance and significance. A voluntary agreement took place between the parties on that day, of which both must have understood the full force and effect, and to which neither seems to have been, or probably could have been, impelled by advice or counsel. It was that the whole right to use the discovery under the patent should be and was assigned to Dr. Morton, he paying to Dr. Jackson ten per cent on all sales for licenses.

Your Committee cannot here fail to remember the unqualified terms of contempt and reprobation in which Dr. Jackson had during the preceding part of that month, down almost to the very date of this arrangement, spoken of Dr. Morton and his alleged ignorance and recklessness in the use of this agent. They cannot conceive it possible, that, if he felt himself to be the true discoverer, he would, by solemn contract, relinquish all power over his discovery, and place it solely in the hands of a man of whom he thought so illy. Dr. Jackson indignantly repels the idea that it was done for the purpose of gain; and we think it could not be the case, as the pittance reserved to him, if he conceived himself the discoverer, was despicably small. And how could he hope to acquire *fame*, by abandoning the most important discovery of the age; one which, if it were his, and if under the auspices of his reputation, with his skill and science, it were presented to the world, could not fail to place him on the highest scientific and professional eminence? How could he hope to acquire fame, by thus surrendering all control over this discovery, and placing it in the hands of such a man as he had represented, and still represents, Dr. Morton to be?

A careful examination of the above detailed acts and conversations of the parties, down to the 27th of October, about which it would seem to your Committee there could be no doubt, renders it clear almost to a demonstration, that neither Dr. Jackson nor Dr. Morton, nor any of those who had witnessed or aided in the operations, supposed that Dr. Jackson was entitled to the merit of this discovery, or any other merit than that of having communicated important information to Dr. Morton; and, if we trace the conduct of the parties further, this opinion is but confirmed.

On the 7th of November, a capital operation was performed by Dr. Hayward in the Hospital; the patient being under the influence of sulphuric ether administered by Dr. Morton. Dr. Warren, being informed by Dr. Jackson that he suggested the use of sulphuric ether to Dr. Morton, invited him to attend, and administer the ether. He declined for two reasons: one was, that he *was going out of town;* the other, that he could not do so consistently with his arrangements with Dr. Morton: so the first capital operation under the influence of ether was successfully performed, Dr. Jackson not yet thinking fit to attend. But, in a communication published in the Boston Daily Advertiser of March 1st, 1847, he says: " I was desirous of testing the ether in a capital operation, and Dr. Warren politely consented to have the trial made; and its results proved entirely satisfactory, an amputation having been performed under the influence of the ethereal vapor without giving any pain to the patient." It strikes the mind with some surprise that Dr. Jackson should claim this operation as an experiment, made by him at his request, and to satisfy himself of the efficacy of the "ethereal vapor" in a capital operation; when the only connection which he had with the operation was to decline attending it when specially invited. Indeed, so entirely did he omit to inform himself on the subject of this experiment — which he declares to be his — that, in the above communication, he names Dr. Warren as the surgeon who performed the operation, which was in fact performed by Dr. Hayward.

Another surgical operation was performed at the Bromfield House on the 21st of November, the ether again administered by Dr. Morton. Dr. Jackson was then present for the first time on invitation, but merely as a spectator. On the 2d of January, 1847, an operation was performed in the Hospital, when Dr. Jackson attended, and brought with him a bag of oxygen gas to relieve the patient from asphyxia, in case it should supervene. Nothing of the kind occurred, and the gas was not used. This is the first and only act of Dr. Jackson's made known to your Committee which implied that he had any duty to perform in the administration of the ether, or that he rested under any responsibility as to its effects.

The testimony of Don P. Wilson and J. E. Hunt, who were assistants in Dr. Morton's shop for a few months, commencing in November, 1846, is adduced to impeach the evidence of Leavitt, Spear, and Hayden, by *their* alleged declarations, and the title of Dr. Morton to the discovery, by his declarations. This is a species of testimony against which the books on evidence especially put us on our guard. It is a sweeping kind of evidence which covers every thing; and, if the imputed conversation be *private*, or if it be general (as he often said, or always said), it is often difficult to subject the evidence to the ordinary tests of surrounding circumstances and inherent probability, so as to fix its value. There is enough, however, in these depositions to show that they are of but little weight. It is to be remembered, in the first place, that they are in direct contradiction to the testimony of Whitman, Spear, Leavitt, and Hayden; and they contradict by strong implication the testimony of Mr. Metcalf and Mr.

Wightman, the character of all and each of whom is most satisfactorily vouched. The testimony of these two witnesses cannot be true, unless the four first above named entered into a conspiracy to carry a point by perjury; but, as to them, we have examined their evidence — we have tested it by its agreement with surrounding circumstances, and we are satisfied of its truth.

This, of itself, would be enough to dispose of the testimony of Wilson and Hunt; but it is proper to look at the inherent character of their evidence.

Wilson, in the commencement of his deposition, *swears*, by way of recital, that Dr. Charles T. Jackson was the discoverer of the application of ether to produce insensibility to pain in surgical operations; and, among other things, he says, "*Morton first claimed the discovery to be his own*" in February, 1847. To say nothing of the looseness and total want of caution with which the fact of the discovery is stated, — a fact of which Mr. Wilson certainly had no knowledge whatever, — he testifies directly against the recorded fact in the second particular; for Dr. Morton did *claim* the discovery as early as September 30, 1846, and his claim was given to the world the next day in the public prints. *His* claim, and *his* alone, was known to the surgeons of the Hospital during the month of October; and his public circulars, and the numerous answers to them, which he has exhibited to the Committee, show that during all that time, and at all times, he claimed the discovery publicly and to the world as his own. The witness goes on to say: "In the administration of ether, I was guided by and solely relied upon the advice and assurances of Dr. Jackson, received through Morton. *We never dared to follow Morton's own directions*" — and adds that, if they had, the consequences would probably have been fatal, and etherization a failure. And further, that he never knew Morton "*to apply it to a patient in the office.* This was from a most apparent fear and shunning of responsibility."

Now, as to the advice and assurances of Dr. Jackson, alleged to have been received from time to time through Dr. Morton, we have no reason to suppose that any such repeated intercourse and communication took place during that time, and we have no evidence of the actual fact of any such meeting and instructions. On the contrary, there is evidence of unkind feelings existing on Dr. Jackson's part towards Dr. Morton; and, in the opinion of your Committee, the testimony of Dr. Keep *indirectly* contradicts the testimony of Wilson on that point, and *directly* upon each of the other points last named. Dr. Keep's object and the tendency of his evidence is to depreciate Dr. Morton, but for faults the very reverse of those with which he is charged by Wilson, namely, a "*rash recklessness*," instead of "*a most manifest fear of responsibility*," in administering the ether; and he evidently is impressed with the belief, and designs to let it be known, that the success of etherization depended upon his skill and prudence. He says, "*It was his (Morton's) practice during that time to administer the ether*, without any adequate provision for the admission of atmospheric air; *and, whenever operations were performed by other persons in the office* and under his supervision, he directed the application in the same way, in consequence of which many of the operations were unsuccessful, and great distress and suffering were induced." Dr. Keep then states that he made ample provision for the admission of atmospheric air, and advised the assistants to do the same thing; "but they, being influenced by his (Morton's) directions and known wishes, did not at all times follow my advice." Not a word is said by Dr. Keep of any advice or directions coming from Dr. Jackson, which, if it had actually occurred, must have been known to him, and would have formed an important item in the current incidents of the time. The evidence of these two witnesses stands thus. They were in the office of Dr. Morton, during the same " thirty days," — Keep, the superior; Wilson, the assistant. Keep says Dr. Morton was in the habit of administering the ether in a particular manner, and that he was *rash* and *reckless*. Wilson says he never administered it at all, and that he was *timid* and shrank from responsibility. But the surgeons of the Hospital agree with neither one nor the other, but show that he repeatedly administered it in the Hospital *himself*, to their entire satisfaction and with entire success. Wilson says the assistants in the office would not follow the directions of Dr. Morton, but relied upon such as were brought from Dr. Jackson. Keep says nothing about instructions from Dr. Jackson, but that the assistants in the office were influenced by the directions and known wishes of Dr. Morton, so that his salutary advice and remonstrances were often of no avail. Wilson says Dr. Morton explained to him, an assistant in his office, very fully all the particulars of the discovery and patent; but to Dr. Keep, his partner, he extended no such confidence. We leave these two depositions to be viewed in their strong contrast; and as to the testimony of Don P. Wilson, considering its inherent improbability, the suspicious nature of the species of testimony to which it belongs, the manner in which it is contradicted directly and indirectly by the evidence of Dr. Keep; and when we further consider that it is directly opposed to the evidence of Whitman, Spear, Leavitt, and Dr. Hayden, and indirectly to that of Metcalf and Wightman; and that it is also in direct conflict with numerous public printed cards and notices of the day, — we feel that we cannot give it the slightest weight or consideration.

The testimony of John E. Hunt is subject to the same objections with that of Don P. Wilson, and other objections which your Committee will now proceed to notice. In order to bring out a declaration on the part of Spear, that he had never taken the ether, he represents him as taking it one evening, and, in the excitement produced by it, seizing upon a countryman present, and handling him roughly. The apology which Spear makes to the countryman is, "*this was the first time he had ever taken the ether;*" not that it was the first time that ether so affected him, or that the rudeness was committed under the influence of ether, but that it was the first time he had ever taken ether, — a fact which had little to do with the act of rudeness, and was a most irrelevant apology. But the inquiry thereupon made by Hunt is most remarkably inconsequent: he, having heard Spear say that it was the first time he had ever taken ether, asks him if it "ever affected him in the same way before." Now, if he had been pressing Spear with a cross-examination, in order to entrap him in some important admission, the inquiry might perhaps have been made; but it was *then* a matter of no importance whatever whether Spear had breathed the vapor of ether or not, and it becomes in the highest degree improbable that both branches of the conversation, so inconsistent with each other, actually occurred; and as the statement contradicts the testimony of so many respectable witnesses, and is in itself improbable, your Committee do not feel bound to give it credence. Again: in a walk with Spear, Hunt gets from him a full disclosure of the discovery, and a statement that it belonged to Dr. Jackson. According to this, Dr. Morton got the requisite information and instructions from Dr. Jackson; came home; *tried it on a woman, and it worked first-rate;* and he had since then continued to use it under the directions of Dr. Jackson. The evidence shows that Spear well knew that the *experiment* was not tried on a *woman*, but on a *man*, whose certificate was read next day by hundreds in the city of Boston. But the witness evidently took this part of his story from the narrative of Don P. Wilson (whose deposition was taken on the same day) about the refractory female patient named in the conversation with Dr. Jackson on the 30th of September, who was to be cheated with atmospheric air, administered from a gas-bag.

From among the thousands with whom Dr. Morton communicated, touching this discovery, during the winter of 1846 and '47, some six or seven, with whom he had personal controversies, testify to his admissions that he was not the discoverer. They differ as to the degrees of directness and fulness with which he opened the matter to them; but it will be found, as your Committee believe, to be a rule in this case, having no exception, that the more violent the hostility of the individual, the more fiercely he assailed Dr. Morton's patent, the more free Morton became in his communication, and the more fully did he unbosom himself; and his statements always went directly to defeat his own claims, and support the defence of the opponent, to whom he made it. For example, H. S. Payne says " that, in the early part of December, 1846, he commenced applying the vapor of ether to produce insensibility to pain in surgical operations. This was after I had heard of the discovery of the preparation by Charles T. Jackson, of the city of Boston." He then states that Dr. Clarke purchased of Dr. Morton a right, under the patent, for Rensselaer and several adjoining counties, who sold to Dr. Bordell, and Dr. Payne was notified by Dr. Blake, as the agent of Dr. Morton, to abandon the use of ether in his practice. After failing in an attempt at negotiation with Dr. Bordell, he went to Boston, and had an interview with Dr. Morton, who not once only, but repeatedly, declared that Dr. Jackson was the *sole discoverer;* " that all the knowledge he possessed in relation to its properties and application came from Dr. Jackson; and that he never had any idea of applying sulphuric ether, or that sulphuric ether could be applied, for the aforesaid purposes, until Dr. Jackson had suggested it to him, and had given him full instructions." This most frank communication raises at once a difficulty about the patent, which is obviously void if that statement be true; and Dr. Morton attempts to remove it by saying, " that he had been very fortunate in effecting an arrangement with Dr. Jackson before any one else had the opportunity, and that he was the first man to whom Dr. Jackson communicated the discovery." And he adds : " Dr. Morton *again and again* said that he was not in any way the *discoverer of the new application of ether, but that the idea had been first communicated to him by Dr. Jackson, who was its discoverer, and that his (Dr. Morton's) interest in the patent was merely a purchased one; and, moreover, that he was very lucky in anticipating all other persons by first receiving so precious a discovery from the lips of Dr. Jackson.*"

After seeing the fulness and unreserved character of this important conversation, and the apparent earnestness with which Dr. Morton attempts to impress the fact that he had no participation whatever in the discovery; not satisfied with suffering it to escape him inadvertently, or even stating it once, but repeating it "again" and "again," as if he were anxious to impress it, — one could not but be surprised to know that Dr. Payne, before this conversation, had *pirated* this discovery; had set up for himself; bade defiance to Dr. Morton and his assignees; and, on his return home, published a card, in which he by no means denies that Dr. Morton discovered the *thing* which he and his assignees are using, but averring that his (Dr. Payne's) *anodyne vapor*, which in his affidavit he admits to be sulphuric ether, "is not the invention of the great Dr. Morton, but an entirely superior article, and all persons must beware how they infringe on his rights." And the more especially is it surprising when we reflect that this state of facts, which Dr. Morton took such unusual pains to repeat and to impress upon this his most determined opponent, would, if true, render the patent wholly void in his hands, and put his discovery entirely in the power of Dr. Payne, and all others who should see fit to avail themselves of it. There can be no absolute proof that Dr. Morton did not make these statements; but it is clear that it was against his interest to make them; and there is also full proof that they are not true, and that they are in direct opposition to his numerous printed and published statements. They are not true; for, besides the six witnesses who testify directly or indirectly to the discovery in its inception and progress, it distinctly conflicts with the conversation of the parties, and their mutual understanding on the 26th and 27th of October, as testified to by R. H. Eddy. It is in direct conflict with the claim promulgated by Dr. Morton, and received and accredited by the scientific gentlemen in the Medical Hospital, who performed the operations testing the efficacy of the discovery.

Dr. Warren says : —

"Boston, Jan. 6, 1847.

"I hereby declare and certify, to the best of my knowledge and recollection, that I never heard of the use of sulphuric ether by inhalation, as a means of preventing the pains of surgical operations, until it was suggested by *Dr. W. T. G. Morton*, in the latter part of October, 1846."

And alike opposed to all the numerous printed circulars which Mr. Morton and his agents had distributed and were then distributing in every part of the United States. It appears that, prior to this date, Dr. Morton's attention had been called to an opposing claim to the discovery, and to the experiments at the Hospital, and he had taken a decided public stand against them, as witness his circular, published the 20th day of November, 1846, and the note thereto attached : —

"DENTAL OPERATIONS WITHOUT PAIN.

"*Dr. Morton has made a great improvement in dental and surgical operations*, for which letters-patent have been granted by the Government of the United States, and to secure which measures have been taken in foreign nations.

"Having completed the necessary preparations for the purpose, and greatly enlarged his establishment, Dr. Morton respectfully announces to his friends and the public that he is now ready to afford every accommodation to persons requiring dental operations.

"His assistants and apartments are so numerous, and his entire arrangements on so superior a scale, that immediate and the best attention can be given to every case, and in every branch of his profession.

"The success of this improvement has exceeded the most sanguine expectations, not only of himself and patients, but of the very skilful and distinguished surgeons who have performed operations with it at the Massachusetts General Hospital and other places in Boston, or witnessed its use at his office. Rooms, No. 19, Tremont Row.

"Boston, Nov. 20, 1846.

"*⁎* Inasmuch as one or two persons have presumed to advertise my improvement *as their own*, and even issued notices to the effect that the applications of it at the Hospital were made *by them*, and that the certificates of its efficacy and value were given *to them* by the SURGEONS OF THAT INSTITUTION, I feel it my duty to warn the public against such false and unwarrantable statements; and at the same time to caution all persons against making, aiding, or abetting in any infringement of my rights, if they would avoid the trouble and cost of prosecutions and damages at law."

And your Committee do not think it credible that Dr. Morton, resting his claims to the discovery on the grounds which he did, — having a most decided public opinion at home in his favor as the discoverer, — having freshly tasted of the intoxicating draught of fame, and recently, in the public papers and in circulars, asserted his authorship of the discovery and defied his rivals, — they do not think it credible that he should seize the first occasion which offered, in conversation with a most determined opponent, to declare the falsehood of all that he had written, published, and claimed; to disclaim the honor which the world so generally and freely accorded him; confess away all his pecuniary rights under the patent; and even support his surrender, disclaimer, and sacrifice, by a self-debasing assertion which he well knew was false. The improbability is too strong to allow it credit.

But Dr. Payne says, that, in the early part of December, 1846, he commenced his operations with sulphuric ether; and that this was after he had heard of the discovery of Dr. Charles T. Jackson, of Boston. How he heard of the discovery of Dr. Jackson, he does not say; surely not by the information of the scientific men of Boston, for they attributed the discovery to Dr. Morton; not by the public prints, cards, and advertisement, for the name of Dr. Morton alone appeared there; and he says, in conclusion, that *he was very much astonished* in learning, some time after his visit to Boston, that Dr. Morton "asserted any claim whatever" to the discovery; and this after the publication and circulation of the notices, cards, and circulars of Dr. Morton, and after the witness had long been engaged in an embittered contest with Morton and his assignees, and the publication of his (Dr. Payne's) card.

Dr. Allen Clarke — who also testifies to admissions by Dr.

Morton, but much less strongly than Dr. Payne, and whose statement may well be the result of a misunderstanding, made the more decided by hostility to Dr. Morton, and a desire to defeat his patent — was the purchaser of a right, for which he gave his note for $3,350. He at length determined not to pay the note, but to join in contesting the patent; and he expresses the opinion, that, by keeping up the controversy for one year, the patent would be broken down. Dr. Blaisdell says: "Clarke would not pay you; for he could get the use of the letheon for one year, before you could get the license from them, and by that time they could ruin the sale of it there," and he might well have added, and with it the discoverer; a very common fortune to men who render the most important services to their race.

Time, and the reasonable limits of a report, will not allow your Committee to dwell upon the few remaining items of kindred testimony. The weight and strength of them have been considered; and the residue, like them, are composed of alleged statements by Dr. Morton to persons with whom he then had or has since had personal controversies touching his discovery, and they are all in contradiction to the claims which Dr. Morton daily promulgated in print to the world. Those printed papers are, as your Committee conceive, the best evidence of what Dr. Morton all that time claimed, and what he conceded; they are of the time and of the transaction; they do not admit of misstatement, misconstruction, or falsification; they are of unvarying and exact memory; and they speak the language of undoubted truth as to the claims, though not as to the rights, of the author. His claims, contemporaneous with these papers, are what these witnesses attack. His *rights* we have already considered; and, as to the evidence of his *claims*, that which he insisted and said was his, the published papers stand against the testimony of these witnesses, as written or printed evidence against parol. His alleged confessions, made under the most improbable circumstances, are in direct contradiction to his printed circulars, daily and contemporaneously promulgated to the world. If, then, these alleged parol admissions stood against the printed and published papers, without any thing beside to add strength to either, we could not, in our conscience, in weighing the conduct of men by rational probabilities, hesitate to give the decided preponderance to the printed over the parol evidence. But the parol evidence runs counter to all the leading facts in the case heretofore considered and established, in the opinion of your Committee, by the most indubitable proof; while the printed circulars and notices entirely agree with them, and make with them one uniform and consistent whole. The objects of the parties, their claims, their efforts, their purposes, are the same throughout. The deposition of A. Blaisdell is, however, worthy of especial comment. At the time he professes to have had the conversation in which Dr. Morton accords all the merit of the discovery to Dr. Jackson, he was the agent of Dr. Morton, spreading his circulars throughout the land; had taken care to send one of them to each and every surgeon-dentist in New York; and yet now declares that he was especially charged with the information which he takes care to inculcate, that these circulars were all false in the most material point, and that the patent which he is selling is void by reason of that falsehood. He was, at the same time, in habits of almost daily correspondence with Dr. Morton; and the difficulties which he met with occurred while he was absent, and it would most naturally have suggested itself to him to communicate them to Dr. Morton by letter, and in that way get his assent to obviate them by declaring Dr. Jackson the *sole discoverer*. But he does not do so : if he had, his letter and Dr. Morton's answer would have been in writing; and then, if there were truth in the statement of those alleged admissions, there would have been one item of written evidence to support them. But this is wholly wanting. Blaisdell professes to have waited till his return to Boston, and then to have held a private conversation with Dr. Morton, who at once and eagerly admitted away his *whole claim*, both to money and reputation.

It is remarkable that, in more than three months, during all which time these witnesses say Dr. Morton conceded to Dr. Jackson the merit of being the "sole discoverer," and during all which time he was daily writing and almost daily publishing, there is not produced one line written by Dr. Morton, or written to him, countenancing the idea ; nor is there one act of his which looks to such admission. A written admission or an ambiguous paragraph in writing, which could be fairly construed into an admission, or a letter written *to him* during that time, which could be reasonably construed to refer to such admission, would be tenfold the value of all the parol testimony now presented of those admissions. Dr. Morton has shown to the Committee several bound volumes of letters addressed to him upon this subject, all of which recognize him as the discoverer. Viewing these statements in this point of light; comparing them with the printed and published papers, in which Dr. Morton contemporaneously and continually asserted his claims to the discovery ; and finding them opposed, as they are to the well-settled facts of the case already considered, — they weigh, in our opinion, as dust in the balance, and in nowise affect the well-settled facts of the case.

Considering the case presented on its own merits, and independent of any authority whatever, your Committee has come to the same conclusion that was arrived at by the Board of Trustees of the Massachusetts General Hospital, at their annual meeting in January, 1848, and subsequently confirmed in 1849; and they cannot better state the propositions, which they consider established, than by adopting to this extent the language of the report of that institution. It is as follows: "1st, Dr. Jackson does not appear at any time to have made any discovery, in regard to ether, which was not in print in Great Britain some years before. 2d, Dr. Morton, in 1846, discovered the facts, before unknown, that ether would prevent the pain of surgical operations, and that it might be given in sufficient quantity to effect this purpose without danger to life. He first established these facts by numerous operations on teeth, and afterwards induced the surgeons of the Hospital to demonstrate its general applicability and importance in capital operations. 3d, Dr. Jackson appears to have had the belief, that a power in ether to prevent pain in dental operations would be discovered. He advised various persons to attempt the discovery: but neither they nor he took any measures to that end; and the world remained in entire ignorance of both the power and safety of ether, until Dr. Morton made his experiments. 4th, The whole agency of Dr. Jackson in the matter appears to consist only in his having made certain suggestions, which led or aided Dr. Morton to make the discovery,—a discovery which had for some time been the object of his labors and researches."

And although your Committee have deduced their conclusion from the evidence, without resting on opinion or authority, they are greatly strengthened by the concurrence of that highly intelligent and scientific body of men who examined the subject on the spot, while the transaction was yet recent, and who were acquainted with the conduct of the parties during the progress of the discovery, and with the character of the witnesses. This conclusion being reached as to the exact state of fact, your Committee are satisfied thereon that Dr. Morton is entitled to the merit of the discovery. *The great thought was of producing insensibility to pain; and the discovery consisted in that thought, and in verifying it practically by experiment.* For this the world is indebted to Dr. Morton; and even if the same thought in all its distinctness and extent arose also in the mind of Dr. Jackson, at or prior to that time, yet he did not carry it out by experiment, and thus give it to the world; and on that supposition it was the case of an important thought occupying two minds at the same time, one only of whom brought it out by experiment, and is therefore the discoverer. It was clear that the discovery was destined soon to be given to the world. Science had almost reached it; but a single step, and it was compassed; and it happened in this case, as in many others, that the necessities of the profession, a want deeply felt in the daily business of life, rather than scientific induction, at last produced the consummation.

That it is a discovery we cannot doubt; that it is an advance beyond the heretofore known walks of science, we know; and scientific men of all civilized nations, even to the extremities of the earth, acknowledge and proclaim it.

As to the question whether a sum of money shall be appropriated by Congress as a reward for this discovery, your Committee beg leave to refer that subject to the consideration of this House. Numerous cases, however, have occurred, to which your Committee beg leave to refer, in which compensation in money has been made by Congress as a reward for like discoveries of less importance to the country and mankind. . . . . .

This discovery is the long-sought desideratum of surgeons. His sinking heart, when witnessing the writhings and agonies of his patients, has looked to this as a consummation devoutly to be desired. Various narcotics have been employed. Mesmerism, and its kindred neurology, were tendered as this great boon; but they have passed, and with them the expectations of the profession, and the promises of their discoverers. Dr. J. C. Warren, page 3, in his work on Etherization, says, "A new era has opened on the operating surgeon. His visitations on the most delicate parts are performed, not only without the agonizing screams he has been accustomed to hear, but sometimes with a state of perfect insensibility, and occasionally even with the expression of pleasure on the part of the patient. Who could have imagined that drawing a knife over the delicate skin of the face might produce a sensation of unmixed delight? — that the turning and twisting of instruments in the most sensitive bladder might be accompanied by a beautiful dream? — that the contorting of anchylosed joints should co-exist with a celestial vision? If Ambrose Paré and Louis and Dessault and Cheshelden and Hunter and Cooper could see what our eyes daily witness, how would they long to come among us, and perform their exploits once more! And with what fresh vigor does the living surgeon, who is ready to resign the scalpel, grasp it, and wish again to go through his career under the new auspices!"

We quote also from the same: "In order to form a proper estimate of the value of the new practice, we should endeavor to realize the mental condition which precedes a surgical operation. As soon as a patient is condemned to the knife, what terrors does his imagination inflict! How many sleepless nights, and horrible dreams, and sinkings of the heart does he experience! What apprehensions of dangerous bleedings, of wounds of vital parts, and even of sudden death, does he paint to himself! And when to these is added the dread of insupportable pain, what a frightful picture presents itself to the mind! No wonder that many persons are unable to bring themselves to submit; no wonder that some, wrought to desperation, are led to anticipate their sufferings by a voluntary death. Horror of the knife led a gentleman in this city, afflicted with a stone in the bladder, to commit suicide. When the terror of corporeal suffering is taken from this load of apprehension, the patient may indulge a hope which leads him cheerfully to uncertain dangers."

In reply to communications addressed to the Surgeon-General of the Army, and Chief of the Medical Department of the Navy, we learn that chloroform and ether are used in both these departments, and that they constitute in part the supplies for the service, and have been used during the recent war with Mexico. This would, in justice, entitle the memorialist to compensation, as the laws of the United States guaranty to him all benefits in its use by all persons. Had we not already exceeded the usual limits of a report, we would gladly introduce numerous testimonials of the advantageous use of anæsthetic agents in various diseases, besides those subject to surgery. And we deem the subjoined tables, showing its introduction into the hospitals of the United States, will give a general idea of the usefulness of the discovery, and its general applicability to disease. They are taken from the Transactions of the American

Medical Association, assembled in Baltimore in May, 1848. [The tables are here omitted.]

The effects of chloroform and ether are similar; each has its advocates; yet your Committee are assured, that, amongst the hundreds of thousands of cases of various diseases in which ether has been used, no case has terminated fatally, in which any injurious effect could be traced to ether. We cannot assert the same for chloroform. The effects of ether are more readily controlled, and its strength is supposed to be but one-tenth that of chloroform.

As citizens of the United States, we feel we have just cause of pride, that this discovery, the most important in science, had its origin on our shores; and that its general adoption by the European world, numerous admissions of the discovery here and its usefulness, are alike honorable to the recipients of its favors and the discoverer. Professor Simpson, the discoverer of chloroform, in transmitting to Dr. Morton a copy of a pamphlet, entitled "Account of a New Anæsthetic Agent, as a Substitute for Sulphuric Ether in Surgery and Midwifery," writes the following note. [This note is copied into pp. 246, 247.]

We close our communication with an extract from the work on Etherization by Dr. J. C. Warren, a name confessedly among the first in the United States in the department of medicine and surgery : —

"This discovery certainly merits a notice from the American Legislature, since it may take rank perhaps of all the great improvements which adorn the present age of surgery. The establishment of union by the first intention, the safe ligature of the great arteries, the substitution of lithotrity for lithotomy, the rejection of pernicious ointments and plasters in the management of wounds, the constitutional treatment of local diseases, and the free external use of cold water, mark the present as the golden period of surgical science.

"The introduction of ether, enabling us to perform operations and apply remedies without pain, crowns all these improvements.

"While we would pay a willing and liberal tribute to the individual who has been made the instrument of this discovery, we should look higher for its author, and elevate our fervent attributions of praise and thanksgiving to Him who has been pleased, from the rich treasures of his goodness, to confer so wonderful a gift on our generation."

The subjoined resolutions were ordered to be appended to the report.

Dr. Lord offered the following resolutions, which were adopted : —

"*Resolved*, That, the Committee having refused to recommend any remuneration to be given to the contestants of the ether-discovery, the report of the Committee be made in conformity to the above decision.

"*Resolved*, That, believing the report of the chairman does fairly express the opinions of the Committee, and the real views as embodied in the resolutions of Dr. Fries, herewith published, it is hereby adopted as the report of the Committee."

Dr. Fries offered the following resolutions, which were adopted : —

"*Resolved*, That, in the opinion of this Committee, to Dr. C. T. Jackson is due the credit of having suggested to Dr. W. T. G. Morton that pure sulphuric ether might be inhaled with safety, and that the effect of such inhalation is to produce insensibility; but that, in expressing this opinion, the Committee do not wish to convey the idea that Dr. Morton had not previously experimented with this important agent, but refer to the strong proof herewith published, for the evidence that he had thus experimented.

"*Resolved*, That to Dr. W. T. G. Morton is due the credit of having made the first practical application of sulphuric ether as an anæsthetic agent, and demonstrating to the world its power to destroy nervous sensibility to such an extent as to enable surgeons to perform all the various surgical operations upon the human body without pain.'

[And two other resolutions, which relate only to not having kept a journal of proceedings.]

NOTE. — During the preparation of this report, there was forwarded to the Committee the affidavit of Henry C. Lord, one of the counsel for Dr. Jackson, and also the affidavit of George H. Palmer, and one by Dr. Jackson himself, from which it appears that Mr. Lord, the counsel, called upon Thomas R. Spear, — induced Spear to visit him at his chamber, and held a conversation with him; and that his effort in that conversation was to get some admission from Spear, that his testimony, given under oath in the case, was untrue. Lord and Palmer say that he did so admit. The witness Spear, who was afterwards called upon, testifies that he *did not*, and states facts which show an effort to entrap him in a mode not usually practised by the legal profession in the United States. Your Committee give no weight to the alleged statements, considering the manner in which they were procured, even as stated by Mr. Lord himself. There was a like attempt to get a contradictory statement from Leavitt, similar in its character with that made with Spear, but more strongly marked by professional irregularity. These depositions in no respect modified the opinion of your Committee as to the facts given in question, and only present another most striking example of the caution with which testimony of the declarations of parties and witnesses should be received unsupported, and especially when contradicted by written papers.

There was also forwarded to us the deposition of N. C. Keep, which is in the following words : —

"COMMONWEALTH OF MASSACHUSETTS, *Suffolk*, ss.

"I, N. C. Keep, M.D., of Boston, in the County of Suffolk, and Commonwealth of Massachusetts, dental surgeon, being called upon by the Hon. Thomas O. Edwards, Chairman of a Committee at Washington, on patenting compound medicines, to give my testimony in the matter in hearing concerning the claims of Dr. W. T. G. Morton as the discoverer of etherization, depose as follows: —

"I became associated in the business and practice of dentistry with Dr. Morton, on the twenty-eighth day of November, in the year 1846. On the next day, we were about to prepare an advertisement for publication, when Dr. Augustus A. Gould called at our rooms. Being pressed with business, I requested him to write the advertisement; with which request he complied. After he had written it, which he did at his own house, he brought it to me, and we read it together. In it the discovery of etherization, without any suggestion having been made by me to that effect, was ascribed in explicit terms to Dr. Charles T. Jackson. Dr. Gould, pointing with his finger to the words in which this ascription was expressed, said to me, 'That will please Jackson.' I then showed the advertisement to Dr. Morton, and we read it together. He then exclaimed with emphasis, 'That is good; I like that. I'll take it to the printer.' Copies of the advertisement were made under the direction of Dr. Morton, and, as I supposed at the time, without alteration, and published by his order in three evening newspapers. On seeing the advertisement in the 'Evening Traveller' on the evening of the same day, I was greatly surprised to find that the words which ascribed the ether-discovery to Dr. Jackson had been struck out. The next morning I called the attention of Dr. Morton to the fact, and asked him why he struck out those words. He hesitated, and seemed not to know what to say, when I said to him, 'Morton, why do you quarrel with Jackson? You injure yourself, and injure the cause.' His reply was, 'I wouldn't if he would behave himself. The credit of the discovery belongs to Dr. Jackson; Jackson shall have the credit of it; I want to make money out of it.'

"I stated the foregoing facts to my family on the aforesaid evening, and afterwards to other individuals. I have heretofore declined voluntarily testifying to them, but consider that I have no right, upon a call of such a nature as is now made upon me, to withhold this testimony.

"N. C. KEEP."

"Boston, Feb. 8, 1849."

When this deposition was received, the Chairman of your Committee showed it to Dr. Morton, who in a few minutes brought to him a bound book, entitled "Miscellaneous

Notes." On the 91st page was a manuscript in the handwriting of Dr. A. A. Gould, written evidently on the outside sheet of a letter addressed to Dr. A. A. G., and postmarked "Washington City, D.C., July 9," from all which it was most manifest that this was the original draft of the advertisement testified to by Dr. Keep. This paper, contrasted with the evidence of Dr. Keep as the contents of an original draft, fixes in the minds of your Committee the just value of this species of evidence. This paper is as follows: —

"The subscribers, having associated themselves in the business of dental surgery, would respectfully invite their friends to call on them at their rooms, No. 19, Tremont Row. They confidently believe that the increased facilities which their united experience will afford them of performing operations with elegance and despatch, and the additional advantage of having them performed without pain, by the use of the fluid recently invented by Drs. Jackson and *Morton*, will not only meet the wishes of their former patients, but secure to them additional patronage."

V. THE CASKET AND THE RIBBON, OR THE HONORS OF ETHER.

In this review, the writer, after alluding to the importance of the ether-discovery, and the bitterness of the controversy to which it had given rise, proceeds thus: —

That controversy is now substantially ended. The masterly Report of the Committee of Congress, presented by the Hon. Thos. O. Edwards, M.D., — its clear and simple statements of the question at issue, — its searching analysis of the evidence, — its striking illustrations, — its conclusive and logical deductions, have, as we believe, convinced all, except those few partisans of Dr. Jackson who, from personal friendship, professional bias, or the natural reluctance to abandon an early and cherished opinion, still adhere to his cause with unwavering fidelity. Without any parade of learning or scientific research, this document sets forth certain acts of the parties, and then, by the plainest and most cogent arguments, irresistibly leads the reader to infer the motives and views of the actors. Without any severity of language, it quietly sets aside the false pretences which came under its notice. Thus Dr. Jackson claims that he made his discovery in 1842. If, however, he had the least realizing sense of this great truth (it is argued), then he must have known that immortal honor awaited its disclosure. He hears around him the cries of suffering, — he is admitted to be an eager aspirant for fame, — and no one doubts his kindly disposition. But he remains torpid for four years, deaf alike to the call of ambition, and even to the dictates of common humanity. The unavoidable inference is, that he could not have had any strong, clear convictions in the case. We accede, therefore, at once, to the conclusion, that he merely had arrived at an induction or hypothesis on the subject which he thought of little or no value (probably as tending only to a slight improvement in *dental* surgery), and thus entirely omitted to take any step to verify it.

Again, Dr. Jackson claims, that at last Dr. Morton performed his experiments as *his* agent, — being the mere "nurse who administered *his* prescription." This claim likewise is shown to be surrounded by insuperable difficulties. Dr. Jackson, in an interview, *not sought by himself*, makes a mere casual suggestion to Dr. Morton, one whom he represents as grossly ignorant and reckless, to whom he refuses to give a written certificate of the safety of the application, and from whom he thenceforward holds himself wholly aloof. He is not present at the early experiments. He publicly denounces Dr. Morton as likely to kill somebody yet before he is done; expressing, in the strongest manner, his regret that he had ever given him any information on the subject, &c.

Now, the inference of the Committee seems absolutely unavoidable, that Dr. Jackson — knowing, as he must have done, the importance of these first, test experiments; what science, skill, and caution were necessary for their safety and success — could not have selected as his agent such a man as his own witnesses represent Dr. Morton to be; and that, having selected him, he could not thus have conducted himself throughout the series of these experiments.

Indeed, the deliberate claim by Dr. Jackson, that these experiments were *his*, performed by *his* agent, and in *his* behalf, seems to us the act of a man, who, shunning all responsibility during the period of danger and uncertainty, seeks at last to snatch away the prize which had been fairly won by the labors and services of another.

The legal acumen shown by the Committee is remarkable: it would do high honor to the most eminent practitioner. The fact that Dr. Morton's ignorance (as manifested at his interview with Dr. Jackson) was assumed, seems certain, from his having previously learned from Mr. Metcalf the general properties of ether. The Committee, however, discover one circumstance, in confirmation of this position, which had before been wholly unnoticed, viz. that Dr. Jackson directed ether to be *spattered on a handkerchief;* thus really telling *that it was a liquid,* — so that when Dr. Morton, in reply, asked *if it were a gas,* he must have been concealing what he knew.

The comparison of the testimony of Barnes and M'Intyre is also most able and satisfactory. Dr. Keep and Don Pedro Wilson are placed in an interesting contrast — without a word, however, charging either with intentional falsehood; and Dr. Keep's affidavit, that a certain paper contained a certain statement in favor of Dr. Jackson, is amusingly nullified by the production of the paper itself, containing nothing of the sort.

This report is brief, pertinent, searching, decisive, encumbered with no array of documents, and no irrelevant opinions or certificates. It adopts the four propositions contained in the Report of the Trustees of the Massachusetts General Hospital. It closes with a stricture upon the "*professional irregularity*" of which one of the Messrs. Lord, the attorneys of Dr. Jackson, had been guilty.

We repeat, that we consider that this document has brought to an untimely end the claim of Dr. Jackson as the discoverer and first applier of etherization.

A Minority Report was subsequently presented by two members of the Committee of Congress, which is certainly a more plausible statement in Dr. Jackson's behalf than had before appeared. It does not, however, as we conceive, disprove or even weaken the conclusions of the prior Report, from which it dissents. It sets forth what no one has ever denied, — that Dr. Jackson communicated to Dr. Morton *an induction* which he had made, viz. that ether could be used with safety and effect during a dental operation.

The Committee next proceed with a long array of opinions of different individuals as to Dr. Jackson's merit of having made this suggestion. President Everett and other remonstrants (among whom, we regret to learn, are to be found many·of the Boston dentists) give all the credit to Jackson.

After criticising the letters contained in the Minority Report, from Hon. Franklin Dexter, Drs. Walter Channing, Luther V. Bell, J. B. S. Jackson, John D. Fisher, and Mr. Bowen, the editor of the " North American Review," which were all in favor of Dr. Jackson, the writer proceeds: —

A letter from Mr. Prescott, the historian, with more discrimination, awards to him the suggestion; but to Dr. Morton "*a share, and no mean one,*" in the discovery; viz. its verification. A letter from Charles G. Loring, Esq., one of Dr. Jackson's counsel, of course takes the side of his client. It is not an uncommon circumstance for gentlemen of the legal profession to think favorably of their own cases, — to regard their own geese as swans.

Having duly paraded these letters in behalf of Dr. Jackson, the Committee next proceed to introduce others highly complimentary to Dr. Morton; which, however (as they would make it appear), refer merely to his meritorious services "in demonstrating the practical value of the discovery, and in contributing, perhaps (!) more than any other person, towards its introduction into general use." It is certainly evidence of great ingenuity on the part of the Committee, in this manner, to qualify and fritter away the most absolute and unequivocal recognitions of Dr. Morton's claims. Dr. Jackson can never despair, if his friends can find any ground for his pretensions left in such a letter as the following from Dr. John Jeffries, of Boston, to Mr. Speaker Winthrop: —

" Boston, January 10, 1849. Dear Sir, — Mr. Morton, who visits Washington to seek some remuneration from Government for the benefit which he has conferred on the country by the introduction of sulphuric ether, requests me to express to you my opinion; which I do most unreservedly, — that the world is indebted *entirely* to Mr. Morton for the introduction of this agent to produce insensibility to pain, and that it is a physical blessing not second to any that has been conferred upon suffering humanity," &c.

The Committee dispose of similar letters from his Excellency Gov. Briggs and Ex-Gov. Morton, of Massachusetts, and Hon. John P. Bigelow, Mayor of Boston, by suggesting, that, as the writers use general terms, they probably rely more upon information from others than upon any investigation of their own. The whole of these opinions, *pro* and *con*, have nothing to do with the subject. They *change* no *fact*, and they *prove* no *fact* in the case.

After some dozen pages of the Report have been thus occupied, the Committee next proceed to comment upon the character and competency of the Board of Trustees of the Hospital. It is announced as a fact, that there are few or no legal or scientific men among the members of that Board; and they courteously suggest that the Trustees have shown partiality towards Dr. Morton, caused, doubtless, by a *thirst for distinction*, and a wish to identify their institution with the discovery, by ascribing the chief merit to its verification.

Now three, at least, of that Board are on the list of counsellors at law in Boston; and the Chairman of the Committee for drafting the Report has for twenty years been extensively engaged in a branch of that profession. Three or more are members of the American Academy of Arts and Sciences; one of them (Mr. J. A. Lowell) being, by his position as sole Trustee of the Lowell Institute in Boston, brought more intimately into contact with scientific men and matters than almost any one in that community. He is one of the Corporation of Harvard College; and three-quarters of the Board are graduates of that institution. It is needless to add, that a more fair, intelligent, or competent jury was probably never impanelled to try an issue. It is the duty of this Board annually to lay before the Corporation a statement of the affairs of the Hospital during the past year. What should have been done on this occasion? The greatest public service ever rendered by the institution has been performed : shall it be passed over unmentioned? Certainly not. Shall the mere naked fact be stated, that these experiments were performed at the request of Dr. Morton, and all mention even of Dr. Jackson's name be omitted? This would have been the simplest, perhaps the wisest, course. But would it have been any more satisfactory to Dr. Jackson and his friends? The course actually taken was, no doubt, that by which the Committee conscientiously endeavored to do full and equal justice both to "the Dentist Morton," whom they had never seen, and to Dr. Jackson, their old acquaintance and friend. So obvious was this wish on their part, that the chief medical review of the country (Hays's), for that very reason, reprinted the Report verbatim.

It is certainly difficult to imagine any possible bias or interest, on the part either of the institution or the Trustees, to the *prejudice* of Dr. Jackson. Personal regard — his position in society — his standing as a man of science — would all seem to give him great advantages over his opponent. Dr. Jackson, indeed, very modestly suggested to the Committee of the Hospital, that a partiality was felt towards Dr. Morton, under the idea, that, if the claims of one so ignorant were eulogized, rather than his own, *the institution would thereby acquire a larger share of credit as accoucheurs of the discovery*. What possible bearing, however, can it have in the case, how Dr. Morton happened to be led to think of the subject? The operations were actually performed at *his* sole request, by surgeons who had never heard of Dr. Jackson's name in connection with the discovery. This is a " fixed fact." How is it altered or affected by the subsequent information, that Dr. Morton acted pursuant to a suggestion of Dr. Jackson? They had performed the operations on their own responsibility, unaided by a word of advice or caution from Dr. Jackson; and the credit of the " delivery," be it more or less, belongs to them, no matter who proves to be the father of the child.

To explain the position of the Massachusetts General Hospital, the Committee introduce two letters. The first is from Dr. W. J. Walker, an eminent surgeon, of Boston, or its vicinity, now retired from practice.

The second letter is from L. M. Sargent, Esq., well known as author of the Temperance Tales. This epistle is the gem of the whole collection. Mr. Sargent is a ready, playful, and caustic writer; and none can fail to be amused with this production, which exhibits, in a strong light, all his peculiarities. . . . . . .

Letters from Dr. Jacob Bigelow and Dr. George Hayward, *fully indorsing the Hospital Report*, close this list. These gentlemen are disposed of by the remark, that they are probably the persons alluded to in Dr. Walker's letter. The former is President of the American Academy. The latter is the first surgeon who ever used ether in a capital operation, and has been for many years one of the surgeons of the Hospital in Boston.

Leaving all this prolonged and useless discussion, the Committee next proceed, in great detail, to show that Dr. Jackson, after having made this induction for four years, spoke of it to various persons in the most public and decided manner. They then declare, that, "*whether Morton had been before in pursuit of this object or not*, as he failed to find it till guided in the right way by a learned chemist, the judgment of mankind as to the chief merits of the discovery will be the same in either case." Why, then, it may be asked, did the Committee think it important to make an elaborate effort to prove that Dr. Morton *had in fact made no prior experiment?* And here it is worthy of notice, that there is not the slightest attempt made to reconcile those fatal discrepancies, or to obviate those stringent objections which had been set forth in the Majority Report, in its comments upon the witnesses in the case. Don Pedro Wilson and Dr. Keep here jog along together most harmoniously. The half-dozen personal enemies of Dr. Morton prove most satisfactorily, that he unbosomed himself to them by admissions fatal to his own claims, and entirely at variance with his course publicly pursued with everybody else, and on all other occasions; *and no attempt is made to explain this remarkable selection of confidants.** Mr. Metcalf, whose testimony (from his known intelligence and high standing) is of the greatest importance to Dr. Morton, and who is able to fix dates by the decisive circumstance of a voyage to Europe, is dismissed with the remark, that

---

* Our readers are already familiar with the provoking discrepancy between the actions of Dr. Jackson and his claim. He has set about with remarkable zeal to correct the great oversight; but we can only condole with him, while we point to the *lateness of the hour.* It is in vain that he appeals to the buried years of the past to rise, that he may stealthily write modern truths on their records ere they sink again: unheeding, they slumber on. It is in vain that he refers to the utterance of familiar facts in science: they were printed long ago. It is in vain that his friends point to his reputation and ability: we will admit it all, but it does not help his case; for his actions are in advance of every thing, and they condemn him. " His case is hopeless, who, having nothing to say for his conduct, at length appeals to his character: the mercy of the court alone can save him." — *Casket and Ribbon.*

"his statement seems too vague to possess much weight, in view of so great a mass of conflicting testimony," and with some comments on the small size of the vial of ether which he saw in Dr. Morton's hands. Mr. Wightman's testimony (equally important and conclusive) the Committee endeavor to disparage, by intimating "that there is some extraordinary confusion in his dates;" carefully avoiding all allusion to those circumstances which render the *exact time* of his interview with Dr. Morton *absolutely* and *demonstratively* certain, by written as well as *internal* evidence of the most satisfactory character.

The Committee, in a former part of the Report, had introduced in italics, and quoted with great emphasis, the statement of a new deponent (Mr. Fowle), who goes all lengths, and swears that Dr. Jackson told him in 1842, that by the use of ether you can have a tooth extracted *or a limb cut off without pain.*" But it appears that Mr. Eddy, in 1846, had asked Dr. Jackson "whether he knew that the flesh of a person asleep from ether could be cut without pain;" to which the reply was, "No; nor Morton either; he is a reckless man," &c.; "the chance is he will kill somebody yet."

These two deponents (if their testimony had been brought together) would certainly seem to be somewhat at variance. The Committee resort to the adroit hypothesis, that Dr. Jackson merely meant, on the last occasion, to say that he did not *know* the fact, — not to intimate that he did not fully *believe* it. The words actually used, it must be confessed, were oddly selected, even for the purpose of expressing belief.

In general, it may be remarked that the tone of the whole document is unworthy of the Committee. It has not, in the least, a judicial character. It is an *argument for Dr.*

Jackson, exactly such as *his* attorneys would be likely to have submitted, and which we really think must have emanated from that source, and have been adopted by the Committee, without any revision or modification. It throughout exaggerates the merit of the one, and depreciates that of the other party. Thus, it is not intimated that Sir Humphrey Davy, half a century ago, suggested the same general idea of prevention of pain, in surgical operations, — using, however, another agent (nitrous oxide); that, more than thirty years ago, a case was published to the medical world, of a man having been rendered lethargic by the use of *ether mixed with atmospheric air;* the effects produced being declared to be strikingly similar to those of nitrous oxide, and *also highly dangerous.* Not one word is said of Dr. Wells; of his experiments, conducted by means of the agent recommended by Davy; of Morton's knowledge of and participation in those experiments (prior to his purchase of sulphuric ether, sworn to by Metcalf), — not one word of all this. The reader is left, instead, to infer that, to Dr. Jackson, Morton was indebted for the whole idea or conception. To *him* is given the concentrated credit due to the united genius and labors of all who preceded him. "A great truth was hidden," say the Committee, "and by *him* was first revealed."

It is not intimated, that, during all those four years, Dr. Jackson had never tried a single experiment for the purpose of demonstrating the *safety* of the agent employed, although it was, *as he well knew*, supposed by the profession to be *extremely dangerous.* There is not the slightest mention of "the earnest or indefatigable labors of Dr. Morton" in bringing out this discovery, although we are told by one of the surgeons of the Hospital, "that he absolutely haunted them." On the other hand, not a word of comment is made on the preposterous claim of Dr. Jackson, that the *verification* of the discovery, no less than its *suggestion*, was wholly his.

There is not the slightest attempt to refute Dr. Edwards's demonstration upon this point. The minority, being unable to say any thing in favor of, and unwilling to say any thing against, Dr. Jackson, preserve, upon this branch of their inquiry, a discreet silence. *In other words, the whole Committee concur in according to Dr. Morton the first actual application of ether.* We believe, indeed, that the only rebuke administered to Dr. Jackson by the Committee is the very gentle one of not being quite justified in becoming a party to the patent, "in violation of the recognized obligation of medical brotherhood."

Upon this subject of the patent, the same disingenuous course seems to have been adopted by the Committee. No attempt is made to reconcile with the "present *exclusive* claims of Dr. Jackson the fact that he consented to become a joint patentee with Dr. Morton, and to receive only *one-tenth* part of its profits, and thereupon even took an oath that they were joint discoverers." * Commenting severely on Dr. Morton's attempt to secure the patent for his own pecuniary benefit, no intimation is given of the formal

---

* What would have been Dr. Jackson's position, if he had merely permitted this discovery to go forth to the world as — in the specification accompanying the patent, he made oath that it really was — made jointly by himself and Dr. Morton? He has only, therefore, to remain silent, and he is sure of the chief honors of the discovery. The ribbon of France and the medal of Sweden will be his, and none may challenge his right to wear them. But, alas! he sees fit to claim all, though all was virtually his before; and he realizes the fate of the dog in the fable, who "grasped the shadow, and the substance missed." He too, *opens his mouth;* and what fortune gave, folly lost. Dr. Jackson must, indeed, as it seems to us, be classed among those who have been "ruined at their own request." — *Casket and Ribbon.*

attempt of Dr. Jackson, through his legal advisers, to obtain for himself an increased share of its profits. While the Report heralds forth Dr. Morton's offer to *sell* his discovery to the Government, for the use of the army and navy, and speaks of his attempt to "extort money from the nation's sufferings," it conceals his *gratuitous* offer of its use for both those departments, on account of the existing Mexican war, and his like *gratuitous* offer for the benefit of every public charitable institution in the United States. . . .

The document closes with the following intelligence: "Note. — Before the ink with which we penned our concluding sentence was dry, a telegraphic despatch was laid before us by Joseph L. Lord, Esq., of Boston, announcing that, on the 31st of January last, the *Institute of France* awarded the Cross of the Legion of Honor to Dr. Jackson, as the discoverer of etherization. It is extremely gratifying to find, that our own views concur with the decision which has been pronounced in favor of Dr. Jackson *by the most enlightened body of scientific men in the world.*"

The Committee, unfortunately, were soon to be deprived of this gratification. Like other statements which they had made on Mr. Lord's authority, this last — most flattering one — proves to have been *very highly colored.* Dr. Jackson had indeed received a *ribbon:* but the gift was in nowise connected with the *French Institute;* and he was himself at last obliged (when pressed by various newspaper inquiries) publicly to declare in print, *that he had never stated that there had been any formal decision of that body in his favor;* and that the above announcement in the Minority Report was the result of a *telegraphic mistake.* We believe, however, that he has never attempted to explain how it happened, that his attorneys, in his name, and by his sanction, gave direct currency to the same "mistake" on various other public occasions, and *when no telegraph was used as the medium of communication.* We hardly think that Dr. Jackson will ever get a verdict in his favor from the French Academy. It seems certain, at any rate, that his claims are entirely overlooked by the American Academy; since that learned body has not even published, in its new volume, Dr. Jackson's communication, setting forth his pretensions as the discoverer of etherization.

A voluminous Appendix accompanies this Minority Report. The reader will find there all the affidavits in the case, which he has seen so often in former publications, and which must by this time have assumed a very familiar aspect. An unexpected discovery will, however, reward his patient investigations, as he draws near the close of the pamphlet. He will there find various documents upon Dr. Morton's side, which (as it would seem) must have got into their present company by accident or inadvertence on the part of the Committee. There are the depositions of Spear and Leavitt,* upon which the Majority Report had been led to speak of the "professional irregularity of one of Dr. Jackson's attorneys." A most important letter from Dr. Augustus A. Gould, of Boston, also is there, charging those gentlemen with "a breach of courtesy and confidence;" exposing various inaccuracies in their statements; and expressly averring, that Dr. Morton, on an occasion alluded to, did mention to him his early experiments, made

---

* With an entire unconsciousness of demerit, Mr. Lord, accompanied by a professional brother, waits on Mr. Leavitt, and says, " Now, Mr. Leavitt, what did you mean by swearing that I sought to bribe you?" He replied, "You or Mr. Lord told me that *I should lose nothing* by signing such a statement; and *I supposed you meant to give me something,* if I would." Mr. Lord then asked Mr. Leavitt, if that was *all* the ground for saying he had bribed him. Mr. Leavitt replied in the affirmative. — *Casket and Ribbon.*

before the interview with Jackson; adding, "*Indeed I had many reasons for believing that experiments of the nature specified by him had been performed.*" There is another most severe letter from Mr. Metcalf, charging Dr. Jackson's attorneys with "positive falsehood.". . . These latter documents throw great light upon the mode in which this controversy has been conducted on the part of Dr. Jackson and his friends. *None of them had before appeared in print; and verily we are astonished that Dr. Jackson and his friends should now wish to circulate them.* . . . An excellent letter also appears, addressed by Dr. Oliver W. Holmes (the poet-physician) to Hon. Isaac C. Morse, in which he says, "It is well known that Dr. Morton, instead of profiting by his discovery, has suffered in mind, body, and estate, in consequence of the time and toil he has consecrated to it.

"I have no particular relations with Dr. Morton, and no interest in common with him, to bias me in my opinion and feelings. But, remembering what other countries have done for their public benefactors, and unwilling to believe that a rich and prosperous republic cannot afford, and will not incline, to indulge its gratitude whenever a proper occasion presents itself, I have addressed you this line to tell you, that *I think now is the time, and this is the man.*"

Finally, a communication is published by which the high authority of Dr. James Jackson, of Boston, is claimed for Dr. Morton, whom he considers entitled to a grant from Congress for the "ether discovery, *more than any and all other persons in the world.*" And we find also a letter from Dr. Henry J. Bigelow, of Boston, one of the surgeons of the Hospital, to Mr. Winthrop, which so *ably, clearly,* and *concisely* states the *whole* argument in favor of

Morton, that we cannot refrain from quoting it entire.* Dr. B. is of the opinion of Paley, who says, "He alone *discovers* who *proves.*" . . .

* "Boston, Jan. 26, 1848.

"Dear Sir, — Learning that Dr. Morton is in Washington, and being much interested in the ether-controversy, I take the liberty to write to you.

"I believe most fully, that Dr. Morton deserves any reward Congress may grant to the discoverer; because, although many people have *thought* that a man could be intoxicated beyond the reach of pain, Dr. Morton alone *proved* this *previous possibility* to be a *certainty*, and *safe*. A diagram will make the matter plainer than words: —

Before October, 1846.	Discovery in October, 1846.	*After* October, 1846.
Who made the suggestion? Here is the only ground of dispute.	Consecutive experiments by Morton.	*Morton alone* took the responsibility of danger, and proved that ether was, 1st, *certain*; 2d, *safe*.

"The two last points, viz. the consecutive experiments and their confirmation, which *nobody disputes to Morton*, make him, in my eyes, the discoverer. The only doubt is, Who made the *suggestion*? *To me this is of no importance.* Dr. Jackson says, 'I did. I told Mr. Morton to try the experiment; and unless I had so told him, he would never have tried it.' Dr. Jackson adds, 'I first tried ether when I was suffering from chlorine in 1842. I afterwards recommended it to Mr. Peabody.' But Dr. Morton confutes even these positions. He says to Dr. Jackson, — 1st, I show by the evidence of Dr. Gould, Mr. Wightman, and Mr. Metcalf that I was experimenting with ether before the interview in which you claim to have brought it to my notice. 2d, in 1842, you only rediscovered what was before clearly in print in Pereira's Materia Medica. 3d, You claim to have told Mr. Peabody what you *knew* of ether. Now, you could not *know* it. You have stated all your grounds of deduction, and the widest inference you could draw from them is a *suspicion* of the properties of ether; and a *suspicion* in science, an *unconfirmed theory*, amounts to nothing. Finally, what you claim to have discovered in 1842 you kept to yourself during four years. Do you expect the world to believe you knew its value? Do you expect it to reward you for letting people suffer during that length of time? Besides, the suggestion of anæsthetic agencies occurred to Davy: especially was it followed out, though unsuccessfully, by Horace Wells, who, disgusted with failure, abandoned his attempts. — These and others had hypotheses, as well as Dr. Jackson. Morton alone proved the hypothesis. Without Morton, there is

Finally, then, we would express our conviction, that the positions taken by Dr. Edwards are not in the slightest degree weakened by any of the arguments in the Minority Report; but that, on the contrary, they are confirmed by various new documents, which, had they not been so unaccountably appended to that Report, would probably never have seen the light. The two Reports, indeed, as it seems to us, should be examined in the reversed order.

We believe, that, if any candid or unprejudiced person, *after reading the Minority Report*, will take up that of Dr. Edwards, he will find it to be a complete *a priori refutation* of all that has since been so plausibly advanced in Dr. Jackson's behalf.

We sincerely congratulate Dr. Morton upon the fact that the opinion is constantly becoming more and more strong and general, that to *his* efforts and labors the world owes one of its choicest blessings. Though the honors already received by him have, through Dr. Jackson's instrumentality, been turned into insults, and the compensation fairly his due from Government has, through the same instrumental-

---

no evidence that the world would have known ether till the present day. I believe this covers the ground of important argument and difference in the pamphlets.

"I beg you to allow for any inelegancies, resulting from my attempt at brevity, and to believe me, very truly and respectfully, your obedient friend and servant,

"Mr. Winthrop." "HENRY J. BIGELOW."

There is not probably a more skilful surgeon in the United States than Dr. Bigelow. He has just been appointed Professor of Surgery in the Massachusetts Medical College, on the resignation of Dr. George Hayward. To a great power of imparting information orally, he unites a condensed style of writing. He apparently entertains the opinion, well expressed by a contemporary reviewer, respecting productions moderate in bulk and *portable*, viz. that "the light skiff will shoot the cataracts of time, when a heavier vessel will infallibly go down." — *Casket and Ribbon.*

ity, been as yet withheld, we cannot doubt that his services will eventually obtain a fitting reward, and that they will command the lasting gratitude of the country and of mankind.

It seems to us that these efforts of Dr. Jackson and his friends have signally failed. On the one hand, the CASKET is, in our opinion, something MORE than "a snuff-box by way of charity;" and, on the other hand, the RIBBON is something LESS than "a unanimous decision of the French Institute, after a full sifting of all the evidence."

VI. AWARD OF THE FRENCH INSTITUTE.

In March, 1850, the French Institute pronounced an award in the matter of the ether-discovery. The first prize of medicine and surgery, for the years 1847 and 1848, was decreed to Messrs. Jackson and Morton jointly. The Committee of Medical and Surgical Prizes consisted of Messrs. Velpeau, Royer, Serres, Magendie, Duméril, Andral, Flourens, Lallemand, and Rouse. Various learned labors were considered and discussed by the Committee; but the discovery of the anæsthetic properties of ether was regarded as the most important of them all. The language of the award is as follows: "Mr. Jackson and Mr. Morton were necessary to each other. Without the earnestness, the preconceived idea, the courage, not to say the audacity, of the latter, the fact observed by Mr. Jackson might have long remained unapplied ; and, but for the fact observed by Mr. Jackson, the idea of Mr. Morton would perhaps have been barren and ineffectual."* Two thousand five hundred francs are therefore awarded to Mr. Jackson " for his observations and experiments on the anæsthetic effects of the inhalation of ether ;" † and the same sum to Mr. Morton " for having introduced this method into surgical practice, pursuant to the suggestions of Mr. Jackson." ‡

It is a gratifying circumstance, that, though ether has been used at the Hospital since its first introduction in more than six hundred cases, it has never been attended with any injurious results. Dr. Hayward has always used sulphuric ether. The Drs. Warren have preferred a preparation of chloric ether, which differs, as I understand, from chloroform only in the proportion in which it is combined with

---

* " M. Jackson et M. Morton ont été nécessaires l'un à l'autre. Sans les instances, la préoccupation, et le courage, pour ne pas dire l'audace, de celui-ci, l'observation faite par M. Jackson aurait pu rester longtemps inappliquée ; et sans le fait observé par M. Jackson, la pensée de M. Morton aurait peut-être stérile et sans effets."

† " Pour ses observations et ses expériences sur les effets anesthetiques produits par l'inhalation de l'éther."

‡ " Pour avoir introduit cette méthode dans la pratique chirurgicale, d'après les indications de M. Jackson."

alcohol. I close this chapter with the following statement, kindly furnished by Dr. Borland, one of the House Physicians: —

Massachusetts General Hospital,
May 12, 1851.

Nathaniel I. Bowditch, Esq.

Sir, — In accordance with your desire, I have examined the Surgical Records of the Hospital, and find, that, since Jan. 1, 1848, there have been performed —

Under sulphuric ether	186
„ chloric ether	138
„ chloroform	25
„ nitrous oxide gas	1
	350 operations.

During this time, in cases of out-patients, medical patients, setting of fractured limbs, dressings, &c. ether has been employed in at least . . . . 150 cases * more.

Yours respectfully,
J. Nelson Borland,
House Physician to Massachusetts General Hospital.

* Prior to January, 1848, ether had been used at the Hospital in a hundred and thirty-two cases (see p. 218); making a grand total of six hundred and thirty-two cases. It is, indeed, there resorted to in every serious operation.

CHAPTER X.

1848—1851.

WEDDING AT HOSPITAL. — GIFT OF TRUSTEES. — COST OF THE TWO NEW WINGS, &c. — DEATH OF DR. ENOCH HALE. — ALL FURTHER ETHER CONTROVERSY DECLINED. — GAS. — DEVISE OF JOHN D. WILLIAMS OF STORE WORTH SEVENTEEN THOUSAND DOLLARS. — FREE BEDS PLACED AT DISPOSAL OF HIS EXECUTORS. — BEQUEST OF B. R. NICHOLS, SIX THOUSAND DOLLARS. — BEQUESTS OF JOHN BROMFIELD, IN ALL FORTY THOUSAND DOLLARS. — MR. HOOPER RESIGNS AS CHAIRMAN, AND IS ELECTED VICE-PRESIDENT. — BEQUEST OF HENRY TODD, FIVE THOUSAND DOLLARS. — DEATH OF DR. JOHN D. FISHER. — ADDITION TO LODGE AT THE ASYLUM. — POST-MORTEM EXAMINATIONS. — DEATH OF SIGNOR SARTI. — NEW DONATION OF WILLIAM APPLETON, TWENTY THOUSAND DOLLARS. — NIGHT WATCH AT ASYLUM. — RESIGNATION OF DR. HAYWARD: HIS LONG AND VALUABLE SERVICES. — VOTES OF TRUSTEES. — VARIOLOID AT HOSPITAL. — VOTES OF TRUSTEES. — LEGACY OF DR. CHARLES W. WILDER, TWENTY THOUSAND DOLLARS. — LEE DONATIONS OF 1830. — DIX WARD AT ASYLUM NAMED IN HONOR OF MISS DIX.

AT the annual meeting, Jan. 26, 1848, Messrs. Amos A. Lawrence and Charles H. Mills were elected Trustees, in place of Charles Amory and William T. Andrews, who, having declined a re-election, were thanked for their "very faithful and acceptable services." Feb. 6, all the Medical and Surgical Officers, heads of both departments, and Standing Committees, were re-elected. The following was the organization of the Hospital at this period: William Appleton, President; Theodore Lyman, Vice-President; Henry Andrews, Treasurer; Marcus Morton, jun. Secretary;

Nathaniel I. Bowditch, George M. Dexter, Robert Hooper, Amos A. Lawrence, Francis C. Lowell, Charles H. Mills, J. Thomas Stevenson, Edward Wigglesworth, Trustees on part of the Corporation; Thomas Lamb, J. Wiley Edmands, John A. Lowell, and Henry B. Rogers, Trustees on part of the Commonwealth; Drs. James Jackson, George C. Shattuck, John Jeffries, Edward Reynolds, Board of Consultation; Drs. Jacob Bigelow, Henry I. Bowditch, John D. Fisher, John B. S. Jackson, Enoch Hale, O. W. Holmes, Visiting Physicians; Drs. John C. Warren, George Hayward, Solomon D. Townsend, Henry J. Bigelow, Samuel Parkman, J. Mason Warren, Visiting Surgeons; Dr. Wm. Henry Thayer, Admitting Physician; Richard Girdler, Superintendent of Hospital; Dr. Bell, Physician and Superintendent of Asylum; and Mr. and Mrs. Tyler, Steward and Matron. Two thousand copies of the annual report ordered. March 19, salary of the Admitting Physician was fixed at two hundred dollars. The subject of arranging a system of keeping the books of the Institution, so that the Treasurer's accounts may show the exact amount of receipts and expenditures of both departments, was discussed, and referred to Mr. Stevenson, who subsequently made a report; and the following vote was adopted, viz. "That the auditor's certificate of the correctness of the quarterly accounts of the Steward of the Asylum and of the Superintendent of the Hospital may be taken by the Treasurer as sufficient authority for entries in his books, in accordance with said accounts." May 7, Mrs. Girdler was requested to purchase a suitable wedding-gift to be presented to Thomas W. Hickford and Elizabeth M'Intire, as a token of the appreciation by the Trustees of their long and faithful services at the Hospital. May 21, the subject of autopsies was referred to Mr. Bowditch, who, on June 4, made a report, which was accepted, and ordered to be placed on file. The Building Committee reported, that the new west wing cost $29,500; east wing, $28,000; furnishing, $19,000; repairing centre, rebuilding old east wing cellar throughout, three reservoirs, copper gutters, old kitchen, outside painting, $24,000; new kitchen, $16,500; autopsy-room, sheds, chains, roads, sodding, fences, $3,000: total, $120,000. On July 2, a new ventilation of the north wing of the Asylum was ordered. Aug. 16, Drs. W. O. Johnson and R. W. Oliphant were chosen House Physicians, Dr. D. D. Slade and W. H. Thorndike House Surgeons; John E. Hathaway being re-elected Apothecary. Nov. 5, House Physicians and Surgeons were ordered to carry forward the Indexes of the Medical and Surgical Records, as recommended by Dr. Thayer. Nov. 19, "Voted, that the members of this Board have heard with profound emotion of the decease of Dr. Enoch Hale, late one of the Visiting Physicians of the Hospital." " Voted that the Trustees, while they mourn his loss, in common with their fellow-citizens, as one of the most distinguished and useful members of the profession which he adorned, have especial cause for regret in the fact, that by his loss the institution committed to their charge is deprived of one of its oldest, most useful, and most successful medical officers."

Dec. 3, 1848, the Trustees request the Admitting Physician to aim at an equality in number of male and female patients at Hospital. Dec. 17, Messrs. Lawrence and Mills were appointed to prepare the annual report. This report occupies five pages, and, with the documents annexed, forms a pamphlet of thirty-two pages. It mentions the income of the year as $17,225; the property as being $154,133.82; being a reduction of $13,959.06, caused by extensive alterations and repairs at Asylum, and the final payments for the enlargement of the Hospital. It states that the bequests of Messrs. John Redman and William Oliver have not yet been received. They probably will not be for several years to come. It mentions the donation of John D. Williams, of a store valued at $15,000; now worth $17,000, and rented for $1,050; and says, " Since the closing of the Treasurer's account, this legacy has been gratefully accepted by the Trustees, who have tendered to the representatives of the deceased their acknowledgments for this last evidence of his bounty." The report thus notices the death of Dr. Hale: —

"The institution has, within the past year, been called upon to lament the loss of one of their oldest and most valued officers. Dr. Enoch Hale, one of the Visiting Physicians of the Hospital since 1838, died on the 12th of November last, in the 58th year of his age. Dr. Hale was widely known, as well from his devotion to his own profession, in which he held a distinguished position from an early period of his life, as from his ardent zeal in the pursuit of other branches of science. In the performance of his duties at the Hospital, he evinced in a remarkable degree that fidelity and tenderness of feeling which in his private practice gained for him many friends, who regarded him with affection and respect. His whole life was graced by a purity of heart which won the confidence of all who were in any way associated with him here, and which, we may humbly trust, has won for him its high reward in heaven."

Weekly expense of each patient at Hospital, $4.73; being ninety-one cents less than preceding year. The expenses at the Asylum were $33,130.09; the receipts, $36,506.52. Its inmates at end of the year, seventy-seven males, eighty-four females: total, a hundred and sixty-one. It appears that "during the year extensive alterations have been made in the north wing of the Asylum, amounting nearly to the entire remodelling of the interior of that portion of the building," at a cost of somewhat more than six thousand dollars. Dr. Bell's report contains a detailed statement of these alterations, and some important remarks on modes of ventilation generally, and a statement of means here resorted to. In interest and importance it does not fall behind his reports of former years. Dec. 29, in Hospital, sixty-four males, thirty-nine females: Americans, thirty-nine; foreigners, sixty-four: total, a hundred and three.

Jan. 12, 1849, a letter from Dr. Charles T. Jackson, with many accompanying documents, was presented by the Chairman, and laid on the table. "A communication from Moses Williams, Esq., was received and read, informing this Board that his late brother, John D. Williams, devised to this institution the store No. 17 and 18, Blackstone Street, in Boston, upon certain conditions and for certain purposes expressed in his will, an extract from which was also sent. Whereupon voted that the Trustees gratefully accept this devise, acknowledging in it a renewed instance of that bounty to which upon other occasions the institution has been so largely indebted; the said real estate to be always retained unsold, and the income thereof applied to the support of free beds in the Hospital, as directed by said testator." Jan. 17, a printed "memorial" of the Messrs. Lord, in behalf of Dr. C. T. Jackson, was several days since transmitted to each Trustee of this institution, asking a revision of the views expressed in the last annual report respecting the ether-discovery; and a letter from Dr. Jackson, with various accompanying documents, was at the last meeting laid before the Board. And letters upon the same subject from Theodore Metcalf, Esq., and Dr. A. A. Gould, having also been received, it was "voted that any further action of the Board in relation to the ether-controversy is wholly unnecessary." "Voted also that copies of the above vote be transmitted to Dr. Jackson and to Dr. Morton respectively."

Jan. 24, Dr. Thayer presented his second volume of the Medical Index. The Steward was authorized to hire the Joy Farm for one year at five hundred dollars. Copies of the letters of Mr. Metcalf and Dr. Gould, asked for by the attorneys of Dr. Jackson, were refused; a similar request from Dr. Morton having been previously declined.

At the annual meeting of the Corporation in January, 1849, the same Trustees were re-elected; William S. Bullard, Esq., being chosen by the Visitors in place of Mr. Edmands, who had declined a re-election, and was thanked for his services. Feb. 18, all the Medical and Surgical Officers, &c., were re-elected; and Dr. D. Humphreys Storer was chosen a Visiting Physician, in place of Dr. Hale, deceased; and Dr. Samuel L. Abbot, the Admitting Physician, in place of Dr. Thayer. Fifteen hundred copies of the annual report were ordered. March 4, Messrs. Rogers and Wigglesworth were chosen a Standing Committee on the library; and fifty dollars was appropriated towards the medical library. It was also "voted that, in all cases, letters of guardianship shall be required to be taken out, or the removal of the patient from the Asylum insisted on, in all cases whenever, in the opinion of the Superintendent and the Visiting Committee, it shall be thought expedient."

May 20, the executors of the late Benjamin R. Nichols transmitted six thousand dollars, being the amount bequeathed by him to the institution. "The Trustees accept with gratitude this munificent bequest, and tender to the executors their thanks for the prompt and liberal manner in which they have carried into effect the intentions of the testator." June 8, the Visiting Committee's record states, "Told John Ferris, that, if he was again found smoking in the ward, he would be discharged immediately."

Sunday, Aug. 12, 1849, the record reads, "An adjourned meeting of the Board was held at the Hospital, after evening service. The Secretary, having recently met with a severe railroad accident, was unable to attend, and desired me to act in his behalf. At the hour appointed for the meeting, there was a violent storm; and most of the Board pass their summer months in the country. The result was, that not a single member of the Board attended, a circumstance which probably never happened before.* Many years ago, on one occasion, I was the only member present. N. I. Bowditch."

Aug. 20, Drs. Charles D. Homans and Charles G. Adams were elected House Surgeons; and, on Aug. 24, Drs. Calvin Ellis and Waldo J. Burnett, House Physicians; John E. Hathaway being re-elected House Apothecary. Sept. 16, Dr. Holmes declined a re-election as Visiting Physician. Nov. 4, a communication from the Medical Officers, as to a change in the names and qualifications of the House Officers, and as to special rooms for patients whose presence in the wards is injurious to other patients, was referred to Messrs. Bowditch and Lawrence, who, on the first subject submitted to them,

---

* It had happened once before, and has happened once since. And there have been various occasions when only one Trustee was present; viz. June 14, 1835, Mr. Bond; Jan. 5, 1836, Mr. Tuckerman; Aug. 6, 1843, Mr. Andrews; Aug. 8, 1847, Mr. Hooper, &c. &c.

reported in favor of the proposed change. Nov. 18, gas was ordered to be introduced into the Hospital, under the superintendence of Mr. Dexter. Dec. 16, Messrs. Bullard and Wigglesworth were appointed to prepare the annual report. This report occupies six pages, and, with the accompanying documents, forms a pamphlet of twenty-three pages. It states the income of the year at $22,620.51, — the property, exclusive of reversionary interests and the edifices, &c. at the two departments, at $169,466.51; the part invested and yielding income being $156,898.93. The present income is shown to be insufficient for the wants of the Hospital, without annual aid from the benevolent. It contains the following appropriate notice of two deceased benefactors: —

"During the past year, we have been called to mourn the death of the Vice-President of this Corporation, the Hon. Theodore Lyman, a gentleman whose polished manners and cultivated mind made him an ornament of the social circle; whose ability, moral worth, and public spirit, gained him the esteem and confidence of his fellow-citizens, and raised him to the head of our municipal government; whose words of kindness and acts of charity are held in grateful remembrance by many hearts; and whose munificent donations and bequests, particularly those to the State Reform School, place him in the front rank of the founders and benefactors of benevolent institutions in this commonwealth.

"The past year has also witnessed the decease of another

public benefactor, John Bromfield, Esq., whose will contained, among many other munificent bequests to public objects, one of forty thousand dollars to this institution. One half of this sum is bequeathed to the Hospital in Boston, the other half to the M'Lean Asylum. This bequest, however, like some others above alluded to, is reversionary, and does not add to the present means of the institution. Mr. Bromfield's generosity and public spirit had been already evinced in a conspicuous manner by the donation which he made, a few years since, of twenty-five thousand dollars, to the Boston Athenæum. Notwithstanding these acts of liberality, Mr. Bromfield was not a seeker of notice or of praise. His habits were retired, and his manner unpretending. He was remarkable for integrity, for sound judgment, and for quiet resolution. Whatever he believed to be his duty, he did. He is remembered for his public bounty; but he deserves as much respect for his private virtues. Those who knew him best esteemed him most."

Mr. Girdler's report contains the usual statistics, and shows the weekly expense of each patient to have been $4.55. The expenses of the Asylum were $37,601 57; the net receipts, $38,988.31; and this department has been crowded through the year. The report states that but little has been expended on the buildings. It mentions the introduction of gas into the Hospital. Dr. Bell's report is quite brief, occupying six pages. It continues the table of admissions and results from former reports. It mentions the death of no less than three heads of similar institutions, and closes as follows:—

"Left almost at the head of the list of seniority in this vocation, I realize in their premature removal not only the uncertainties of life, but the heavy weight and wearing responsibilities upon the human constitution, inseparable from the care of the insane, however fully one may be sustained by every aid of sufficient and most competent fellow-laborers; and I cannot but look forward to a period, not far removed, when, with a consciousness of a full day's work completed (a day which thus far, in all my relations to your Board, to the medical profession, and the community, has been all sunshine), I may ask a discharge from your generous and grateful service."

Dec. 28, males sixty-five, females forty-five, — total, one hundred and ten, — in Hospital. Americans, paying thirteen, free thirty; foreigners, paying ten, *free fifty-seven*.

At the annual meeting of the Corporation, in January, 1850, Robert Hooper, Esq., was elected Vice-President, in place of the lamented Theodore Lyman, deceased; and G. Howland Shaw, Esq., was elected a Trustee, in place of Mr. Hooper, who was thanked for his long and valuable services. He had been a Trustee thirteen years, and Chairman of the Board for nearly eight years; displaying a zeal, fidelity, and ability in which he has not been surpassed by any of his predecessors. Feb. 3, Mr. Bowditch was elected Chairman. All the Medical and Surgical Officers were re-elected; except that Dr. George C. Shattuck, jun., was chosen as one of the Visiting Physicians, in place of Dr. Holmes, resigned. The same Standing Committees were re-appointed. Fifteen hundred copies of the annual report were ordered to be printed.

Feb. 17, a communication from Thomas P. Cushing, Executor of Henry Todd, was received, with an extract from his will; and it was voted, " that the Trustees gratefully accept the legacy of five thousand dollars bequeathed to this institution by the late Henry Todd, upon the conditions contained in his will." The number of free beds in the institution at his death, exclusive of those supported by annual subscribers, is stated as being forty-three. The subject of the will of John D. Williams was referred to the Chairman and the Visiting Committee, to decide on the number of free beds at the disposal of the executors of his will. On March 3, the Committee made a written report, which is recorded, recommending that one free bed be placed at the disposal of each of the four executors named in the will. The extract from the will is recorded with this report.

March 17, 1850, it was " voted that in the recent decease of Dr. John D. Fisher, late a physician of the Hospital, this Board deeply regrets the loss of an officer, who, to high scientific attainments, united amiable and unassuming manners and the greatest kindness of heart; one who has uniformly discharged in a most zealous, faithful, and acceptable manner his duties toward this institution." Dr. Marshall S. Perry was elected to fill this vacancy. April 17, Dr. Bell was authorized to add a second story to the male lodge. May 5, a recent official report of the Directors of the House of Industry was discussed; and it was thought not to require any notice of this Board. May 17, an invitation to attend the next meeting of the Association of Medical Superintendents of American Institutions for the Insane, to be held in Boston, June 18, was received and read. The Association met one evening at the Asylum in Somerville. The Vice-President and several of the Trustees attended. It was a very interesting and agreeable occasion. June 22, Dr. Abbot had leave to visit Europe for a few months; Dr. J. C. Dalton, jun., being appointed to act till his return. The subject of post-mortem operations was discussed, and referred to the Visiting Committee; and, on July 22, Mr. Bowditch, in behalf of this Committee, made a report, which was accepted and recorded, suggesting precautions to be used to prevent their being performed when prohibited by the friends and family of the deceased. Aug. 13, J. Nelson Borland and Albert H. Blanchard were chosen House Pupils in the Medical department; and Freeman J. Bumstead and Charles H. Hildreth, House Pupils in the Surgical department; Mr. Hathaway being re-elected Apothecary.

Sept. 3, the Chairman and Mr. Rogers were appointed a Committee on the subject of a late post-mortem examination, which had given dissatisfaction to the friends of the deceased. Sept. 10, the Committee reported; and a special meeting was called upon the subject for Sept. 13; at which Dr. Jacob Bigelow, Dr. Dalton, the Superintendent, and Mr. Bumstead the House Surgical Pupil, were present, and stated the facts of the case alluded to; and Dr. Bigelow presented his views on the subject of autopsies in general. Five votes were then adopted, prescribing very definitely certain rules for the future. Oct. 11, a statement of the facts and opinions ascertained and expressed on this occasion, prepared by the Chairman, was read, and ordered to be placed on file.

Signor Antonio Sarti, a distinguished anatomist, and the proprietor of some very beautiful and expensive wax-preparations, who had recently been delivering public lectures, died at the Hospital, Sept. 21. The Trustees, considering his services and labors in the cause of science. preferred to make no charge for his board while in the institution. The Chairman, accordingly, waited on Madame Sarti, and communicated to her this vote.

Oct. 16, the subject of putting an appropriate inscription on the statue of Apollo, presented by Mr.

Everett, was referred to the Visiting Committee, with full powers. The claim for damages against the Grand Junction Railroad, and the right of passing Craigie's Bridge free of toll, were referred to the Chairman and the Visiting Committee.

At a special meeting held Nov. 9, the following preamble and vote, as prepared by the Chairman, were adopted and recorded: "A communication having been received from William Appleton, Esq., President of this Corporation, announcing his donation of twenty thousand dollars for the erection of buildings at the M'Lean Asylum for the Insane, designed especially for such patients as shall have previously dwelt in residences of a spacious and cheerful character, and with the view of affording, as far as possible, to this the wealthiest class of our inmates the accustomed comforts and conveniences of home, — voted that the Trustees gratefully accept this munificent gift. They recognize in it the same practical wisdom and the same true benevolence that have heretofore furnished to this institution a fund of ten thousand dollars, the income of which is to be for ever applied in aid of our poorer patients. The enlarged philanthropy which has thus provided for the equal relief of *rich* and *poor*, when suffering under the greatest of human deprivations, will ever entitle Mr. Appleton to a high rank among the benefactors of this community."

TRIBUTE TO DR. FISHER. 365

Dec. 15, Messrs. Shaw and Rogers were appointed a Committee to prepare the annual report. This report is nine pages in length, and, with its accompanying documents, makes a pamphlet of thirty-one pages. It states the income of the year from property, $16,917.99; extra dividend from Hospital Life Insurance Company, $18,000; free-bed subscriptions, $2,100; surplus at Asylum, $1,500 : total, $38,517.99. The property invested yielding income is stated at $171,119.98. It mentions the investment of fifteen thousand dollars of the income. It gratefully acknowledges the receipt of five thousand dollars from T. P. Cushing, Esq., Executor of Mr. Henry Todd, and thanks the annual subscribers for free beds. It pays the following just tribute to one recently deceased : —

" Within the past year, the institution has been called to lament the death of one of its valued officers, — the late Dr. John D. Fisher, one of the physicians of the Hospital. To high attainments in other branches of science than the one to which he especially devoted himself, he united the most amiable and unassuming manners, and the greatest kindness of heart. To this institution he uniformly discharged his duties in a most zealous, faithful, and acceptable manner."

It mentions the expenses of the Hospital department, $29,024; and, deducting $4,226.27 received from paying patients, shows that nearly $25,000 a year must be drawn from the general funds; being nearly ten thousand dollars more than our average income. The weekly expense of each patient was $4.90. One startling fact is thus recorded: "*Of the whole number of patients in the Hospital during the year, nearly two-thirds have been foreigners.*"

At the Asylum, on Jan. 1, there remained a hundred males, a hundred females; the amount charged for board being $44,183.37, and the net expenses $40,623.38; sums greater than ever before. Special notice is invited to Dr. Bell's report, as containing much of interest to the Corporation and to the public. The Committee fully concur with Dr. Bell, that this department has reached what should be deemed its full capacity; the average number of inmates for the year being two hundred and one.

The Committee say: "At the Hospital in Boston, no change of importance has been made, or is believed to be required." An extended notice of the two gifts of Mr. Appleton, ten and twenty thousand dollars, closes thus:—

"The Trustees have gratefully accepted this donation. It is unnecessary to comment upon its value, or upon the liberal philanthropy which has prompted and guided the hand of the giver. While it increases so largely the debt of gratitude which the Asylum already owed to him who has been its continued benefactor, it leaves nothing apparently wanting for the perfection of that plan for complete relief to all classes of persons, which has ever been the design of the institution."

Capt. Girdler's report occupies four pages, and contains the annual analyses. Dr. Bell's report occupies nine pages, and will be found to merit the commendation of the Committee. Dec. 27, at the Hospital, Americans, eighteen paying, twenty-six free; foreigners, thirteen paying, *fifty-six free:* total, a hundred and thirteen.

Dec. 29, the subject of the expediency of employing a night-watch at the Asylum, as a protection against fire, was referred to the Visiting Committee, to report at the next meeting. Mr. Hathaway's salary was fixed at four hundred dollars; he agreeing to remain two years on those terms, if re-elected. Jan. 15, 1851, the Committee on the subject reported in favor of the establishment of a night-watch. Dr. Bell and the Committee were of opinion, that, to a great extent, the security of a night-watch was already incidentally enjoyed; but, in view of the late melancholy destruction by fire and loss of life at the institution in Augusta, it was thought altogether advisable to have a special attendant charged with this particular duty. If not actually needed for the safety of the institution, it would serve " to ward off public opinion." Jan. 22, a letter claiming compensation for a cow killed while boarded at the Asylum was referred to the Visiting Committee, *with full powers*. Dr. Thayer presented another volume of his Index of the Medical Records, and was thanked for the satisfactory manner in which the same was executed.

At the annual meeting, Jan. 22, 1851, John A. Lowell, Esq., having been for several months absent in Europe, and intending to remain absent all this year,* the Board of Visitors elected in his stead Dr. William J. Dale to be a Trustee of the institution. It is believed that Dr. Dale is the first practising physician who has ever held a seat as Trustee; though Dr. Robbins had practised for several years, and B. D. Greene and Charles Amory, Esqs., had studied that profession. Feb. 2, all the Medical and Surgical Officers were re-elected, and those of the two departments and the Standing Committees re-appointed.

A letter from Dr. George Hayward, declining re-election as one of the Visiting Surgeons of the Hospital, was read; and it was voted, that the Chairman be requested to call upon Dr. Hayward, and express to him the unanimous wishes of the Trustees

---

* When Mr. Lowell shall have returned from his present tour, he will, on the occurrence of a vacancy, receive a cordial welcome from his old associates, should he be willing at a future day to resume his duties as a Trustee.

that he should continue his connection with the Hospital. With this request, so highly complimentary to Dr. Hayward, he decided to comply. Fifteen hundred copies of the annual report were ordered to be printed. It was also voted, " that the subject of the admission of patients, and of the existence of varioloid in the Hospital, be referred to the Visiting Committee, to inquire whether there has been any neglect on the part of the Admitting Physician, or other Medical Officers of the Hospital." The subject of instructing the Treasurer to open accounts in his books, showing all the reversionary interests of this Corporation in any property, was referred to the Committee of Finance. In consequence of " the long and faithful services" of Mrs. Mary E. Tyler as Matron of the M'Lean Asylum for the Insane, her salary was raised to four hundred and fifty dollars.* Feb. 16, the Visiting Committee were not prepared to make a full report on the subject of varioloid, &c. Mr. Stevenson was appointed to consult with the Treasurer as to keeping one account in his books which should show all the receipts and expenditures of both departments of the institution, according to the report and vote of April 2, 1848.

At a special meeting, called by request of the

---

* The salary of Miss Barber, the Female Supervisor, was also lately raised to four hundred dollars.

Chairman, Feb. 24, a letter from Dr. James Jackson, on the existing small-pox and varioloid, was read and referred to the Committee on that subject. All new admissions at Hospital were stopped till further order of the Board. It appeared that there had been nineteen cases; that two had died;* and that one patient (a little girl) was severely ill. The Committee, however, had not fully completed their labors.

March 2, the following preamble and vote, as proposed by the Chairman, were adopted: — "A communication from the executors of the will of Dr. Charles W. Wilder, of Leominster, announcing a legacy of twenty thousand dollars for the support of free beds at the Hospital, was read; and it was thereupon voted that the Trustees gratefully accept this truly munificent bequest; and, in so doing, they would notice two circumstances by which its value is especially enhanced. Large as it is in itself, the gift comes not, as might have been supposed, from one of the wealthiest of our own citizens, but has been contributed from the more moderate fortunes of one of our country-towns. It is believed

---

* One was David Cummings, who died Jan. 23. His occupation was that of tender of the furnace. He was a most industrious and worthy man, and had been in the employ of the institution several years. His sphere, indeed, was humble; but he performed well all the duties of life. And who of us can hope to be entitled to a higher eulogy?

to be the first and only bequest ever received by this institution from a member of that profession which, more than any other, is competent fully to appreciate the importance of this public charity, and to form an accurate opinion as to the judgment and fidelity with which its concerns have been administered. It is a gift, noble in itself; a gift from the country to the poor of the city, from a physician in aid of the sick and the suffering. Voted that the amount thus bequeathed be known as the Wilder Fund for Free Beds; the income thereof to be for ever applied as directed by the benevolent testator." Copies of these votes were ordered to be transmitted to the executors. An extract from the will is recorded. It makes the legacy payable, half in mortgages, half in railroad stocks, — the latter, at present, are depressed in value, — the cash-amount, perhaps, not over six thousand dollars. Dr. Wilder left four children, and about ninety thousand dollars in all; thus devoting to public uses a very large share of all he was worth.

Twenty-five dollars was voted in aid of a patient who has become blind. "A communication from the Physicians and Surgeons, suggesting that the wards be distinguished by placing on their entrances names of individuals who have been celebrated in the history of medicine and surgery, was read; and the subject was referred to a Special Committee, consisting of Messrs. Bowditch and Stevenson."

The Committee upon the subject of varioloid made their final report, — stating that one patient who probably had the disease was admitted, Dec. 16; one who certainly had it, on Jan. 8; that there was no thorough general vaccination of the patients in the whole house till Jan. 28; that the total number of cases was twenty, and of deaths two; and the following votes were adopted: "Voted that there was a positive violation of the rules of the institution on the part of Dr. Abbot, in admitting Miss Eunice B. Bridge as a patient, without having first seen her;* and the fact that the patient so admitted had the varioloid is evidence of the importance of a strict observance of said rules; and the Trustees take this occasion to urge on Dr. Abbot the necessity of the greatest caution in all cases of admission of patients, where there is the slightest reason to suppose them affected by this or any other contagious disease. Voted that Dr. Bowditch took seasonable steps to have all his patients vaccinated, and saw that his orders were executed. Voted that the other Visiting Physicians and Surgeons then on duty were the two Drs. Bige-

---

* Dr. Abbot is a vigilant and careful officer; but, in this instance, had been induced by motives of courtesy towards a brother-physician to rely on his certificate as to the fitness of a patient who was an inmate of his own family.

low and Dr. Hayward. It appears that these gentlemen gave orders for the vaccination of the patients in their wards; but the Trustees have to regret that they did not take the necessary steps to have their orders executed with the least possible delay. Voted that there was a want of due care on the part of the House Pupils, and perhaps of some of the attendants, in passing from the patients ill with the varioloid to visit patients in other parts of the house. Voted that, in the opinion of the Trustees, no pains should be spared to effect a complete separation of varioloid patients from all other patients in the house." These votes were printed, and a copy sent to each of the Medical and Surgical Officers.

The subject of erecting a separate building for contagious or offensive cases, not to exceed two thousand dollars in cost, was referred to the Visiting Committee, with full powers. March 16, fifty dollars was voted for the Medical Library. The Committee on naming the wards made a report, which was read and laid on the table for future consideration. It has not yet been accepted. It recommends the giving to the wards the names of those who have been the chief benefactors of the institution, either by donations or by professional services.

Voted that the Chairman be a Committee on the subject of the Lee donations, to consult with the Lee family, and report to the Board. The Secretary was instructed to procure a record-book, in which to enter all past and future devises and bequests made to the institution, extracts from wills, &c.

A letter from Dr. George Hayward, respecting a recent vote of the Trustees, having been received, was read, and ordered to be placed on file; and the following votes were passed: — "Voted that, whenever a case of varioloid or small-pox shall occur in the Hospital, it shall be the duty of all the attending Physicians and Surgeons to see that all the patients in the Hospital, whose cases will allow it, shall be vaccinated. Voted that the Secretary be directed to send a copy of the above vote to Dr. Hayward, and to inform him that the vote referred to in his letter was passed on the ground that the course now directed to be pursued in future should, in the opinion of the Trustees, have been pursued on the first appearance of varioloid in the Hospital, in January last." Dr. Hayward's letter had stated the fact, that no case of the disease had occurred in his wards;[*] and that, when he was informed of the disease being in the House, under such circumstances as to make him apprehensive for the safety of his own patients,

[*] No case of varioloid had occurred in the ward of Dr. Bowditch; but there was subsequently a very mild one. If the vaccination was in that instance ineffectual, it was probably owing to the constitutional temperament of the patient.

viz. on Jan. 26, he took measures for their immediate vaccination.

March 30, it was ordered that patients be admitted from and after this day. The following preamble and vote, as prepared by the Chairman, were unanimously adopted: — "A communication from Dr. George Hayward, by which he declines any longer to serve as one of the Visiting Surgeons of the Hospital, having been received and read, it was voted that the Board sincerely regret the retirement of Dr. Hayward from a situation which for twenty-five years he has filled with so much honor to himself, and usefulness to the community. It was his privilege to perform the first capital operation rendered painless by the influence of ether, thus connecting this institution with the establishment of the greatest discovery of the age. His professional skill, his good judgment, and his kindness towards the patients, manifested throughout this long period of official duty, and which so recently induced the Trustees to request a continuance of his services, justly entitle him to grateful remembrance, as having been one of the most able and faithful officers of our institution."

Messrs. Lowell, Bowditch, and the Treasurer, were appointed a Committee to receive Dr. Wilder's legacy; which duty they have performed. Messrs. Rogers and Stevenson, with Mr. Tyler, were appointed " a

Building Committee for the erection of new buildings at the Asylum, according to the terms of Hon. William Appleton's donation."* Dr. Henry G. Clark was elected successor to Dr. Hayward. April 11, Mr. Rogers declined acting on the Building Committee, on account of other pressing engagements.

April 16, "owing to a storm so severe as to render it unsafe to cross the bridges, the usual quarterly meeting was not held to-day."* April 18, at a special meeting called at the Asylum by direction of the Chairman, Mr. Lamb was appointed a member of the Building Committee, and the subject of the erection of the proposed buildings was discussed.

The Chairman presented a report on the Lee donations. It states the original gift in 1830; the separate account, hitherto kept, of the income of it; the vote of the Trustees in December, 1830; the present amount of the fund, $31,681.33; that the recent donation of Mr. Appleton had rendered it inexpedient to erect any other new buildings at the Asylum; that the Trustees were therefore desirous of conferring the name of Mr. Lee on the present building for male patients; and that the family of Mr. Lee state their disinclination to have his name given to any building, old or new, and release the institution from all obli-

---

* It was in this storm that the light-house at Minot's Ledge was destroyed, and a steeple blown down in Charlestown.

gation, legal or otherwise, by reason of the vote before referred to. They say, " While we justly appreciate this proposed tribute, we beg leave to suggest the more appropriate name of Dix; and we shall be much gratified to be so far instrumental in commemorating the services of a lady in the cause the donor meant to aid, and which are admitted to be without parallel." The report closes with recommending the adoption of the following preamble and vote: " Whereas this Board hold in the same grateful remembrance as did their predecessors the munificence of the late Mr. Joseph Lee and his family, and are desirous that it should never be forgotten by those who may come after them ; and whereas the heirs of Mr. Lee have requested that the Trustees, instead of giving his name to the building for male patients, as had been proposed, would give to said building ' the more appropriate name of Dix ; ' and as this Board entertain a very high sense of the services rendered by Miss Dix in the cause of the insane, — voted that they willingly accede to this suggestion ; and that the building for male patients at the Asylum be henceforth known as the Dix Ward." This preamble and vote were unanimously adopted.

April 22, the Treasurer was instructed to close the separate account hitherto kept of the income of the Lee donations. The subject of the new buildings proposed at the Asylum was further discussed. April 29, Dr. Bell submitted plans and estimates for the erection of two buildings, according to the terms of Mr. Appleton's donation; and it was thereupon " voted that said plans be referred to the Building Committee, with authority to make such modifications thereof as they think proper, and to proceed at once in the erection of buildings according to said plans." These plans were drawn up with much taste and judgment. They are for two-story buildings, about fifty feet square; in their exterior resembling houses recently erected in Brookline by Messrs. J. D. Russell and F. Standish. These plans seemed to meet with the general approval of the Trustees.

May 8, this afternoon, his Excellency Governor Boutwell, with the Honorable the Board of Visitors, made the annual visitation. They were received by the President of the Corporation and the Chairman of the Trustees. It was a visit made in a simple, informal manner, and seemed highly gratifying to all present. Nothing was the subject of unfavorable comment, except the Hospital fence.

On May 18, the Secretary laid before the Board the volume prepared by him, containing a record of all bequests to this institution. It is executed with great accuracy and elegance. June 2, the subject of the Hospital fence was referred to the Visiting Committee. June 17, fifteen hundred dollars was awarded as damages for land in Somerville taken by the Grand Junction Railroad and Depot Company.

At this meeting, the following letter from Miss D. L. Dix was read, and ordered to be entered on the records: —

" St. John's River, Florida East,
" May 22.

" DEAR SIR, — At this remote point and late date, your communication of April 18, addressed to Thomas Lee, Esq., has reached me. This will at once explain and apologize for a seemingly uncourteous delay in acknowledging the receipt of a copy of the preamble and vote which, by request of the Messrs. Lee, and unanimous assent of the Trustees of the General Hospital, gives my name to a department of that institution. Profoundly moved by a distinction so unexpected, I own, that, while I would ever avoid notoriety and popular applause, — while I would make the *cause* I labor to advance, and not myself, the centre of attention, I cannot but be as much gratified as I am honored by this evidence of esteem from those whose good opinion is so kindly illustrated. The *name* which they have united to distinguish it must be my care to make more and more worthy the place assigned to it on the walls of that noble and Christian institution, which unfolds its portals to admit the sick and heavy-laden, which gives healing influences to many, and blessed protection to all who seek its shelter.

" Very respectfully,
" D. L. DIX.

" To Marcus Morton, jun., Esq.
" Secretary of the Massachusetts General Hospital."

July 5, John P. Reynolds and Joshua J. Ellis were elected Medical House Pupils, and Thomas H. Gage and Albert F. Sawyer Surgical House Pupils, for the year ensuing. July 11, the Superintendent was "authorized to buy two dozen silver forks for use of the Hospital;" also to cause the wooden sidewalk to be relaid. On July 15, the Chairman, Dr. Bell, and Mr. Tyler were appointed "a Committee to carry the Cochituate water to the Asylum, with full powers." This measure, when consummated, will be found highly important to the health and comfort of our patients. The thanks of the Corporation are due to the Cochituate Water Board, and to the city of Boston, for the promptness with which this application was complied with. The stipulations required by the city of Charlestown for leave to lay the pipes through their streets (such as constructing six hydrants, &c.) were of so onerous a character, and the necessity of crossing flats owned by individuals whose consent could not probably be in all instances obtained, seemed so objectionable, that the Committee were led to ask permission to introduce the water along the line of the Lowell Railroad. The liberality and courtesy with which this Corporation at once acceded to their request, while they lightened the immediate labors of the Committee, have placed our institution under great and lasting obligations. It is, indeed, quite doubtful whether this beneficial arrangement could otherwise have been carried into effect. — Mr. Tyler was authorized to employ a clerk at the Asylum, at a salary not exceeding three hundred dollars.

Among the most important changes of this final period of the Hospital-history, were the deaths of Dr. Hale and Dr. Fisher, and the retirement of Dr. Hayward. The stream of public liberality has still continued to flow towards the institution in an undiminished current. The munificent bequests of John Bromfield, John D. Williams, Benjamin R. Nichols, Henry Todd, and Dr. Charles W. Wilder, and the additional donation of Hon. William Appleton, amounting in all to one hundred and eight thousand dollars, have all occurred within the last four years. The precautions respecting varioloid, recommended for the future, will, it is hoped, prevent that disease from again spreading as extensively through the Hospital as it did a few months ago.

This compilation, itself designed as a slight commemoration of the benefactors of the institution, finds its appropriate close in the vote passed in honor of Miss Dix, and by her so gracefully and feelingly acknowledged. In all the annals of philanthropy, there is not to be found the record of a life of more active effort, unwearied self-denial, and entire devotedness, than hers. It is a gratifying reflection, that the first building erected in New England as an Asylum will henceforth bear the name of one who has so nobly earned for herself the title of the Friend of the Insane.

CHAPTER XI.

VISITS OF TRUSTEES: THEIR GREAT REGULARITY. — INCIDENTS AND ANECDOTES OF LIFE IN THE ASYLUM AND IN THE HOSPITAL. — DEATH OF A LITTLE ITALIAN BOY AND OF A FEMALE ATTENDANT.

A WEEKLY visit of a Committee of the Trustees has always been made with great regularity to both departments of the institution; only a dozen omissions having occurred in respect to each of them during this long period of years.

The following is believed to be a correct list of all these instances: —

AT THE ASYLUM.	AT THE HOSPITAL.
1. April 2, 1821.	1. Sept. 9, 1831.
2. Dec. 31, 1828.	2. April 12, 1833.
3. March 15, 1831.	3. Nov. 1, ,,
4. ,, 22, ,,	4. Sept. 4, 1835.
5. June 7, ,,	5. Sept. 1, 1836.
6. Feb. 5, 1833.	6. Aug. 15, 1837.
7. Nov. 12, ,,	7. ,, 22, ,,
8. January, 1834.	8. March 19, 1840.
9. July 14, 1835.	9. April 23, 1841.
10. Sept. 1, ,,	10. March 13, 1846.
11. Aug. 3, 1837.	11. Feb. 3, 1848.
12. ,, 10, ,,	12. Jan. 19, 1849.
13. ,, 24, ,,	

It may be remarked, that, during the three or four first years, at the Asylum, two visits were made every week, and sometimes even more; and that one or more of the Trustees have always been in the habit of visiting at the Hospital on other occasions, whenever inclined so to do. The supernumerary visits thus made at each institution have doubtless been much more numerous than the total of the above instances of omission. Indeed, it has happened, on no less than six occasions,* that the casual presence of another Trustee at the Hospital has saved the credit of the Visiting Committee. On examination of the foregoing list, it will be seen, that, while only two omissions occurred prior to 1831 (say during ten years for the Hospital, and fourteen for the Asylum), no less than five omissions occurred during one single month of the year 1837; and that, for the last thirteen years, not one omission of the weekly visit at the Asylum has occurred; a proof that the present Board of Trustees have at least discharged this part of their duties with great fidelity.

No Trustee of the Hospital can fail duly to appreciate the two choicest of life's blessings, a sound mind and a sound body. To more than one of those who have held that office, the sight of physical suffering

---

* March 23, 1844; March 28, 1846; Feb. 3 and March 31, 1849; March 23, 1850 (during a severe snow-storm); and in April, 1851.

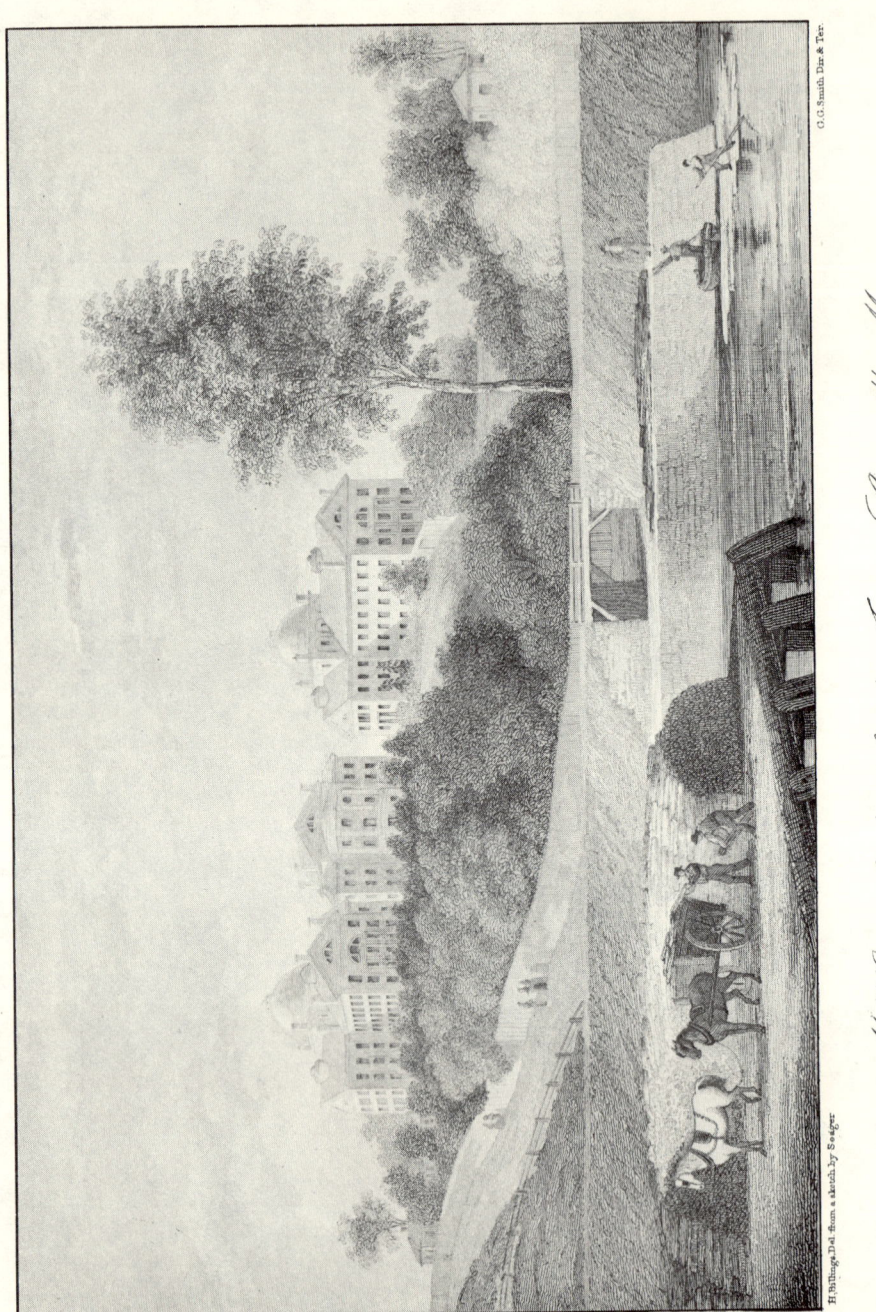

McLean Asylum for the Insane, Somerville, Mass.

and of mental alienation has rendered it so distasteful and painful as to lead to its speedy resignation; while others, in view of so much done to alleviate and remove those evils, find a visit to each of our institutions always agreeable, — sometimes even delightful.

At the M'Lean Asylum, for instance, one may see in summer five or six of our patients, with their scythes, mowing in as dexterous and orderly a manner as those employed in any farmer's field. We mingle without apprehension among five or six more, who, with axes, beetles, and wedges, are engaged in splitting wood. The billiard-table has its party of scientific and expert players. Many a spare ball is gained in the ninepin-alley. Lovers of whist are seen strictly observant of the rules of Hoyle; while others are entirely absorbed in the game of draughts, or in the deeper mysteries of chess. A circle of ladies are perhaps seated around their centre-table, with its vase of flowers, engaged in their favorite occupations of reading or needlework. Manly strength and female grace and beauty have alike, from time to time, made a temporary sojourn among us. Intellect of a very high order has here been restored to a healthy tone. The brilliant and varied plumage of the humming-bird has been traced by one of our inmates with a life-like truthfulness and delicacy not surpassed by the pencil of Audubon. Flowers in wax have been executed by another with such a minute and exact imitation of nature as almost to deceive the senses, and lead the beholder to expect the perfume of the lily, the pink, or the rose. "The last interview of Charles I. and his children," *in worsteds*, the handiwork and the gift of one of our patients, hangs beside the picture of John M‘Lean. The exquisite voice of the singer, and the skilful touch of the musician, have been heard within our halls. Poetry has here had its votaries.* There is much of serenity and cheerfulness among the convalescent; and, amid the occasional displays of melancholy and despair, or the vacant look of idiocy, which it is distressing to witness, the visitor's attention is agreeably attracted to an infinite variety of amusing and interesting eccentricities, which are either voluntarily displayed or easily drawn forth.

* In the "Christian Examiner" for January, 1855, were published some lines by the Rev. N. L. Frothingham, D.D., on the M‘Lean Asylum. One of these verses thus speaks of the institution : —

"O House of Sorrows! sorer shocks
Than can our frame or lot befall,
Are hid behind thy jealous locks; —
Man's Thought an infant, and his Will a thrall."

In the "Boston Transcript" of Jan. 6 appeared a beautiful reply "by one of its inhabitants," in five stanzas, the first being as follows : —

"Oh! call me not a house of woe and sorrow,
For human souls a final, fatal tomb!
Slowly perchance may dawn the blessed morrow,
That wakes the drooping flowers to brighter bloom."

The closing stanza begins : —

"Oh! House of Miracles, *not* house of Sorrow."

Sallies of wit are uttered more keen and lively than are heard under the restraining influences of social life. Epithets are bestowed which, though sometimes discourteous, are often signally appropriate. A preternatural degree of shrewdness and cunning is sometimes manifested. We notice everywhere an almost entire personal freedom, and a pervading air of comfort and enjoyment, which make it difficult for one to imagine that he is in a mad-house.

The last quarter of a century has done much, very much, for the insane. It seems to me, that between the restraints which were at first thought indispensable, and the present improved system of management, there is almost as wide a difference as our first patient must have felt when he found himself suddenly transferred from the cruel " flagellations " of home to the cautious and considerate, but kindly, care and treatment of Dr. Wyman.

A few anecdotes may serve to illustrate my own experience as a visitor at this department of our institution. A Trustee once asked a patient if she did not remember him, and said, " Does not my face look natural?" She replied, " Your face, sir, looks as natural as a natural *fool's*." — " Don't tell *me* about your not having time to hear my story. If you haven't, you ought to have. It is the very thing you were sent here for," — was the equally unanswerable rejoinder of another patient to a Trustee who had attempted to escape from the repetition of his already twice-told tale. We once had a " glass " patient, who was afraid of being *broken*, and took curious precautions on account of his imaginary brittleness. Another thinks the air full of spirits, which get in at his ears, and, after making a great disturbance in his brain, come out at the roots of his hair. He kept his ears closed with his hand so long, that they remained, for a considerable period, bent forward, having lost their natural elasticity. Some personal comments on his Excellency once disturbed the equanimity of the Honorable the Board of Visitors, at an annual visitation. — One of our oldest patients never utters two sentences together, no matter on what subject, without introducing at its close an ejaculation of great emphasis, followed by the words " Look out." His speech is slow and distinct, but generally wholly incoherent. The right words do not come at his bidding. The following is a specimen: " I have a commission as justice of the peace, and an asparagus-bed. I like lightning best at a distance. Whoever puts his name on paper in the Wiscasset Bank has a mark on his forehead, and is worse off than if he was dining with one of the selectmen: — Look out." *

---

* A patient escaped, and succeeded in getting to San Francisco, from which place he sent to one of the Trustees a bill charging the institution

A young man who had been in a government-office in Canada came among us. For years and years he read a Latin dictionary, making critical comments in the margin of its leaves, and putting paper-marks in the book, almost as numerous as its pages. At last, back and covers became detached. Each leaf was separate. The whole, however, was always placed in an orderly pile. I asked him if he should not like a new dictionary. He said, "Yes." I told him I would procure one. He insisted on paying for it. I gravely accepted his draft on his former employer, whose service he had left some dozen years before. At my next visit, I brought a copy of Leverett's Lexicon. He was highly pleased, but hesitated about using it till he was sure that his draft was accepted and paid. I told him, however, that this was a needless hesitation, as that would undoubtedly be "all right." He has read and re-read this volume, like its predecessor. Like that, it has its three or four hundred marks in it; but it has been preserved with most scrupulous nicety, though somewhat embellished by

"for four months' wrongful detention, $50,000, and for a pair of pantaloons destroyed, $10,—total, $50,010,"—and asking an immediate remittance of the amount by the bankers, Wells & Co. The same patient subsequently sent to the physician of the Asylum *a large halter by mail*, though, fortunately, it was transmitted from a less distant locality.

A patient who had been once remanded on a hearing before Chief Justice Shaw, was, on a second hearing, discharged. He sued the institution "for 1,450 days' wrongful detention, $525,000," and directed an attachment for $650,000, estimating the probable costs of Court at $125,000.

marginal annotations. He will always reply in Latin to any question asked him, though his language is not Ciceronian. Thus, to a question as to his health, he said, " Meus salus, Domine, est *tolerabilis*."

Another of our patients, an inveterate walker, actually trod down the grass into a pathway of the shape of a pair of mammoth suspenders; the buttonholes at the ends being elaborated with great skill and care.

An inmate once said to Dr. Wyman, " I have you in my power. If you kill me, you'll be hung. But I can kill you with safety; for I am crazy, and therefore not responsible." — One patient fancied himself to be General Jackson, and received us with appropriate dignity and courtesy. He had also the whim of pronouncing all his vowels; thus, of course, often dividing words of one syllable into two. On being asked how he did, he replied, " I hav-e a-ches from the top of my he-ad to the ends of my to-es "

A Russian sailor, whose name alike defied chirography and pronunciation, was styled on the books John Williams. Accustomed to a life of toil and active exertion, ennui and listlessness seemed to oppress his spirits. He was a perfect Hercules, and yet naturally gentle and amiable. When addressed by his fictitious name, however, his fury was at once aroused. He imagined that he was detained by mistake, instead of the veritable John Williams. I once inadvertently addressed him by that name. He instantly struck his fists together with tremendous force, and sprang to the door-way, effectually barring my egress from the room. My courage immediately sank to zero. A summary close of my official duties seemed to be at hand. But, fortunately, the Physician, with one glance of his eye and a few quiet words, readily soothed him. We were generally on quite a friendly footing. He had much skill and ingenuity, especially in plaiting straw. He once worked for me a little gift. It was a sad embodiment of his prevailing idea of a wrongful detention, — a small straw chain, with fetters at each end.

Another patient thought himself so large that he could not get out of the doors, and invariably kicked and struggled and bruised himself at each attempt of the attendants to get him through. The bruises thus received he always exhibited as a complete demonstration of his theory. — One inmate was overwhelmed by the dreadful delusion that he was a convict under sentence of death, awaiting execution He was so much distressed, that Dr. Wyman thought a full and free pardon from the executive might be a prescription worth administering. A document of that purport, with a large seal attached, was accordingly prepared, and delivered to him. It at first worked to a charm. But in a few days he became, if possible, more desponding than ever. "For," said he, "I have repeated the same offence, and nobody ever heard of a person being twice pardoned. I shall now certainly be hung."

An educated patient asked a Trustee to listen to some oratorical rehearsals. He immediately commenced his recitation. The assistant approached to listen. When the speaker came to the phrase, "and smote him thus," he suited the action to the words, and served the unsuspecting attendant exactly like his prototype of old, "the circumcised dog." I have had my book * and pencil snatched from my hand by one of our inmates, who, before it could be recovered, broke the one, and tore the other to pieces. A patient, who, after the lapse of thirty years, is still with us, once aimed a blow, with a carpenter's hammer which he happened to pick up, at the head of Dr. Wyman, who was standing with his back towards him, and a step or two below him. It crushed through the crown of his hat, and wounded his forehead, so that the blood flowed copiously. This patient, though generally harmless, I have heard express, with truly diabolical earnestness, the wish that he could have cut off the Superintendent's head, before he had

---

* By which the Visiting Committee check the name of each patient when seen.

drawn the first breath of life. A few years ago, a large jack-knife was found snugly concealed about his person, which he had probably also abstracted from a carpenter who had recently been at work.

A female, who had only been with us one day, broke a window, and, taking a triangular piece of the glass, concealed it in her hand, and came out and joined the Trustees and Dr. Bell. She watched her chance, and struck at the doctor's eye, but fortunately only slightly cut his cheek, just beneath it. — A patient, mad with delirium tremens, was brought to the institution. He was placed for a moment or two in a room where there was a bed ripped open, and in a process of being filled. He thrust into this bed a large horse-pistol, loaded with ball and primed. He was then forthwith removed to another apartment, nothing dangerous being found about him. The bed was finally filled up, and did service for a year or so; when one day this truly mysterious inmate was discovered. In view of these and similar incidents, a visitor cannot but feel a profound sentiment of wonder and admiration, alike at the entire fearlessness and self-possession of the officers, and at the quiet harmlessness of those who might, as it would seem, destroy life in an instant.

We turn now to the Hospital for the sick. Its advantages have been enjoyed by all, — the highest and the humblest. Every class in the community, alluded to in the circular letter of 1810 as likely to need its aid, has received it. Every profession and occupation in life has, from time to time, here had its representative. It is seldom that there are not in this institution several interesting patients, particularly among the children and females. I have often known six or eight little girls made for the moment forgetful of all their ailments, and perfectly happy, by a few cheap toys, or playthings, which altogether cost but the merest trifle.* Many a lesson of patient endurance may be learned at our visits. Many a bright vision recurs to my imagination, of sufferers who, by their truly Christian resignation and fortitude, through long, tedious months, warmly enlisted the sympathy and regard of all who saw them. By a general rule, incurable free-patients are, after a trial of three months, discharged to make room for cases of acute disease or recent accident. One free patient I recollect, a young girl who had been with us a year, hopelessly ill, and whom the Visiting Committee reluctantly discharged on this ground. She had no home, and was much distressed at the thought

---

* A little boy of five years old, who had been gratified by an occasional picture-book, asked his nurse *why she did not let Mr. Bowditch come every day?* And a young girl, who was a great sufferer from a disease of the heart, once stopped me as I was passing her bedside, and, with much concern, informed me that she *had broken her glass dog.*

of her desolate situation. One of our number told her that she might remain, as long as she pleased, a *pay*-patient, at his expense. She gladly availed herself of this offer, and died among us more than a year afterwards; having been uniformly cheerful, and always grateful beyond expression for the benefits which the institution had conferred upon her.

A young girl with an incurable disease (an internal tumor) remained with us five years and nine months; and when, in January, 1855, the Trustees felt that they could no longer make her case an exception to the general rule, they individually subscribed $100 a year, for five years, to defray her board in the house of a relative. She felt deep regret at leaving what had become to her a *home*, where her periodical sufferings were skilfully alleviated; and where, in her intervals of ease, she enjoyed as much as an invalid like her could do anywhere, devoting herself to reading and needlework, and receiving constant proofs of sympathy and regard.*

A young and delicate woman, a mother, the wife of a mechanic in this city, seeing her child, of a few years old, in danger of being run over by a heavily loaded truck, threw herself on the ground before the

---

[* It will be observed from the date in this paragraph that it is one of the marginal additions made by Mr. Bowditch in his private copy of his History.]

approaching wheel, and succeeded in snatching her infant from certain death; but had her own arm terribly crushed in this heroic act, performed under the divine impulse of maternal affection. Her case excited universal interest. Every thing was done to relieve her anxiety about her little ones at home, as well as to alleviate her own sufferings. She was at last discharged without any danger of permanent injury resulting from her accident. May filial gratitude and obedience in coming years be her fitting, her all-sufficient reward! The spirit of self-sacrifice, thus shown in a *humble* station, would have adorned the *highest*. Our institution may well rejoice that it had the opportunity of giving aid and relief to so deserving an inmate. In 1851, several years after our heroine's discharge, a young daughter of hers was run over and was brought to the Hospital, with a broken limb which was successfully treated. She had much of her mother's beauty. All of us who remembered *her*, became attached to *her* pretty child.

One face of surpassing loveliness comes back to my remembrance. A patient young in years, but who had borne a large share of the ills of life, was received among us. She had buried husband and child, and was herself soon to follow them, a victim to consumption. With features whose regularity and beauty I have seldom seen equalled, and a brunette-complexion through whose delicate tinge the hectic flush of disease was painfully visible, hers was always an expression of mingled vivacity and sweetness. No visitor could behold without emotion a being so bright and so graceful, standing all unconsciously on the very verge of the grave. She was poor; yet she did not remain many weeks in the Hospital. In a large ward there is unavoidably much to annoy and disturb an invalid. She longed for the loving presence of her who had cared for her childhood, for the quiet of her own home, " be it never so homely." And so she left us. But till her death she was attended, without charge, by a physician of the institution; and the delicacies of the passing summer were daily procured for the gratification of one who was never to taste the fruits of another season. She was to the last a great sufferer.

"Beating heart and burning brow, ye are very patient now!"

One of the most distressing cases ever received within our walls was that of a lad from the Farm School. He had playfully attempted to swing, by means of an iron hook suspended from the ceiling, over a large open vessel of boiling water set in brick-work. His hands were burned by the hook; he involuntarily let go his hold, and fell into the water beneath; and the whole lower part of his body was frightfully scalded. His mother, one of the most experienced of nurses, was constantly with him in an apartment where he was separated from all the other patients. He lingered for some time, amid much pain and restlessness, till he was finally released. How vividly does that scene come again before me, — that remote room; that unfortunate boy, thus dying, as it were, by inches; and that devoted parent, who, through the wearisome days and the long nights, still hoped against hope, to be so grievously disappointed at last! As I look back through the long period of my connection with the Hospital, I can recall nothing more harrowing at the time, or more sad in the remembrance. And yet there is a melancholy satisfaction in the thought, that I have seen even that poor boy's eyes lighted up by a momentary gleam of pleasure at some slight act done to afford him consolation or relief.

A sweet little girl of seven years old, picking up chips in a basket in the Maine Railroad enclosure, was run over by a train of cars, and had her foot cut off. It was after the ether-discovery. While the surgeons were amputating her limb, visions of beauty and splendor seemed to pass before her mind's eye. She exclaimed, "What superb dresses! what elegant ear-rings!" As soon as she became well enough, I ascertained the time of a directors' meeting of the Maine Railroad, and took the child there to argue her own cause. In this instance at least, the maxim proved false, that "Corporations have no souls." They gave her case a merciful consideration, granting three hundred dollars to be held in trust for her sole, personal use, at the discretion of the Superintendent and myself. Through the kindness of the Matron (Mrs. Girdler), it was also arranged that she should be allowed to live at the Hospital, to attend school in its vicinity, and finally become a seamstress in the establishment. A future of usefulness and happiness seemed secured for her. Her parents, however, were Irish. They over-persuaded her to return to them; at the same time, indeed, informing her that within twenty-four hours she would be hungry, cold, and dirty. That she left her adopted home was a source of deep regret to her protectors; but the trust specially assumed in her behalf will still be sacredly fulfilled.

In the spring of 1854, a beautiful orphan girl, of eleven years of age, was found by a benevolent lady, evidently in the last stages of consumption, in a cellar in Boston, where she had passed the long months of a most severe winter, suffering from insufficient food and clothing. She was admitted into the Hospital, where, during the remaining fortnight of her life, some slight atonement was made for the previous social neglect to which she had been so fatally exposed. That thin, pale face; those soft blue eyes; that voice never heard above a whisper; and that sad smile, — had about them a strange fascination. They have lived in my memory, and the joyous scenes of happy childhood have to me more than once been darkened by the painful vision.

One case is remembered which is probably unique in the history of the Hospital. An entire family, natives of Boston, husband and wife and three very pleasing young daughters, were admitted into the institution. The father died there. The others all recovered from the fever by which they had been simultaneously attacked and prostrated. The convalescent daughters visiting their mother, still very ill, in a distant ward, and she in her turn carried down to the ward beneath her own to see and converse for a few moments with a dying husband, were circumstances alike novel and interesting.

Two cousins* from Maine, — bright, blooming girls, — domestics in the same family in this city, and dear to each other as sisters, were admitted as fever-patients, and placed in adjoining beds. One, becoming quite seriously ill, was removed to a different ward, lest the other should suffer from anxiety on her account.

---

* At the Hospital, they were supposed to have been sisters.

The latter became convalescent. The attending physician, on making his visit, expressed his pleasure at seeing her so much better, and, alluding to her diet, said, " Now, what is there to-day that you would most wish to have?" She looked up at him with great earnestness, and replied, " What I most wish is, that I could see my mother." A day or two afterwards, in answer to her earnest inquiries respecting her friend and relative, she was inconsiderately informed of her death. The shock of this intelligence overwhelmed her. A fatal relapse shortly afterwards ensued; not, however, — it is to be hoped, — the result of this indiscretion.

A young and beautiful girl from Salem, that city of fair faces, was admitted, suffering intense pain in the ball of her foot. A local disease of the bone was finally developed; and amputation was resorted to. Her firmness and uncomplaining gentleness were beyond all praise. She possessed a native refinement that rendered her highly attractive. The disease re-appeared on her return home; and she died there, some months afterwards, exhausted by protracted sufferings. A message of grateful remembrance was sent by the dying one to her friends in our institution; who, on their part, will assuredly never forget her lovely person, her interesting manners, or her sad fate.

A young girl, the daughter of a German clergyman of this city, and a teacher in his Sunday-school, died among us, after a severe illness of but a few days. She was an edifying example of that equanimity and resignation with which the young and the happy are sometimes enabled to meet their approaching end. The funeral services were performed at the Hospital. There was quite a numerous attendance of her friends and fellow-worshippers. None could fail to be solemnly impressed by the touching and plaintive melody of their united voices, as they poured forth a hymn of sorrow and of triumph in their native tongue.

A young man of limited means, but of studious habits, who had hoped to obtain an education, and eventually to devote himself to the ministry, was, by the tornado at Medford, in August, 1851, crushed beneath his father's house, so that it was half an hour or more before he could be extricated. He was brought to the Hospital, where it was found necessary to amputate both his limbs, — one above, the other below, the knee. As I witnessed there his uniform patience and calmness, his unfaltering trust and confidence, I felt that he was already a most eloquent preacher of God's word, consecrated to his high office by this dreadful calamity.

But a visit to the Hospital has also a cheerful side.

How delightful is it to see the pale cheek gradually regaining its color, and the feeble frame its strength; to witness the exhilaration of spirit resulting from returning health, the instantaneous relief from agony, the rescue from the very grasp of death! And joyful indeed to all beholders are the daily miracles of ether, that " sweet, oblivious antidote" to pain.

But a few years ago, and on one occasion of almost every week at the Hospital, deep groans of distress or sharp cries of agony penetrated into the innermost recesses of the building, and were often distinctly audible through the neighborhood. Now, the performance of the severest and gravest duties of the surgeon awakens only the faint murmur of a dreamy unconsciousness.

I will mention but one instance, perhaps as striking as the lapse of coming years can ever produce. A young lady was admitted with a tumor extending from the upper to the under surface of the tongue, which it had become necessary to extirpate. Dr. Hayward administered ether. A steel hook was then inserted into the tongue, to prevent its being withdrawn by any involuntary muscular movement. Next the tumor was cut out. To stop the effusion of blood, a red-hot iron was then passed three successive times into the cavity, which was finally filled with a piece of sponge. The patient was then asked how she felt; and her reply was, "Very comfortable." She had known nothing of all that had been done. What would otherwise have been torture indescribable had been by her unfelt. In a few days, she was well enough to leave us.

One young girl, of about seventeen, was long confined by a tedious and discouraging complaint. She was a universal favorite, and was at last discharged, well. A year or two afterwards, I saw her standing at the altar, in a church brilliantly lighted, a bride in all the bloom of youth and of renovated health and beauty. A former House Physician was there with me. Her recollections of the Hospital were so agreeable that she wished to have it represented on this, the most joyous occasion of her life. She was certainly one of the most interesting of all the "graduates" of our institution.

A young Hungarian lady had shared her husband's fatigues and privations, and, after a temporary sojourn in the dominions of the Sultan, had been obliged to seek here a new home. Her health having become impaired, she was for several months the occupant of one of our private rooms. Of a noble and commanding stature, remarkable alike for dignity and grace, her beauty and her misfortunes gathered around her friends from among the young and the fair of our city, who were unwearied in the kindest and most delicate attentions. Thus it was determined that, as far as possible, this interesting invalid should have a merry Christmas. And a Christmas tree was prepared according to the customs of her native land, and with its tapers lighted was borne into her room, with various gifts for use or ornament, of the value of several hundred dollars. This incident, as may readily be believed, afforded her great delight, as it did likewise to such of the other female patients as were well enough to be present on the occasion.

Several years since, I passed my summer-months in the country, being dependent on an omnibus for my daily ride into the city. I was the first passenger called for. On one occasion, we stopped at a neighboring house. A young Irish girl was assisted by two of her countrymen into the vehicle. She was suffering from acute rheumatism. I asked her where she was going. She said, "To the Hospital." To my several questions, whether she had seen the Physician, or got any permit, and whether she had any means of paying her board, she replied in the negative. "How, then," said I, "do you expect to get into the Hospital?" She answered, "*I trust in Providence.*" Now, by a singular coincidence, it happened that no one in the whole county except myself had power to give her the desired admission. I at once determined to do so, and thus to justify the trust which she had so confidently expressed. When, therefore, I left the vehicle, I told the driver to take her directly to the Hospital, giving him a note to the Admitting Physician, which secured her reception on a free bed. She was cured in a few weeks, and was always known as the " Providential Patient."

Such, and so varied, is the experience of a Trustee in the discharge of his official duties. I will close this review by the mention of three incidents, the first two of which occurred in 1846, and were brought peculiarly within my notice as a member of the Visiting Committee. Of one of them I inserted the following account in a newspaper of the day: — " Died, at the Massachusetts General Hospital, July 25, after a painful illness of ten months, Angelo Lathwer, aged fifteen years. He was a small, interesting Italian lad, who had exhibited a white mouse in London, and afterwards in this city. Separated from home and kindred, his patience and gentleness won the regard of strangers. The sympathy of the officers and of the inmates of the institution showed itself in various little attentions and acts of kindness. One of the Trustees gave him a number of a recent English publication, which contained a representation of himself exhibiting a white mouse. He contemplated it with as much gratified ambition as Napoleon would have felt on viewing an engraving of the battle of

Austerlitz. The day before he died, a beautiful, young white mouse was found in the garden of the Hospital, and brought to Angelo. He was delighted. The bitterness of death was for the moment forgotten. The night which followed was solemn and melancholy to all his fellow-sufferers, as they listened to his touching ejaculations: 'I cannot die! I am afraid to die! I want my mother!' But the weary one was soon to be at rest; —

> 'For when the morn came, dim and sad,
> And chill with early showers,
> His quiet eyelids closed: he had
> Another morn than ours.'"

One of the attendants at the Hospital, a young girl with a sunny face, a kind heart, and agreeable manners, the very picture of health and beauty, was, in the spring of the same year, attacked by a cough, which, in a few weeks, was ascertained to be attended with disease of the lungs. She did not wish to go to her distant home. She declined the opportunity of breathing the purer air of a neighboring country-town. She preferred to die among those who, for the several last years, had been her companions, and amid the scenes of her recent labors. The Trustees, at the close of the quarter, directed that she should be paid in full; though, for the last half of the time, she had been wholly unable to perform her duties. I witnessed her gratitude at this expression of interest on the part of the Board. On the morning of the fourth of July, I left a gay and happy scene, — the Floral Festival at the Warren-street Chapel, — and walked to the Hospital to see her. She had just died.* The companions who, throughout her illness, had watched over her with the utmost tenderness and assiduity, had now completed their sad offices. She was clad in the white robes of death. Grapes, which were to be tasted by other lips than hers, lay upon the table. On her shrouded breast were flowers, to whose fragrance she was insensible. All traces of suffering and illness had passed away from her countenance, which had resumed its habitual serenity. The struggles of worn and exhausted nature were at last over. She rested —

> "—— as sweetly as a child,
> Whom neither thought disturbs nor care encumbers,
> Tired with long play, at close of summer-day
> Lies down, and slumbers."

We gathered around her bedside in silence. The scene formed a truly striking contrast with that which I had just left. But it was not a painful one. "For," thought I, "what more could have been done for that poor girl, even by the hands of

---

* The close of her brief and blameless career was thus chronicled in the records of the Visiting Committee: — "Emeline Wright died of consumption on the 4th instant, aged twenty-four, after an illness of about three months. She had been for several years an attentive and faithful nurse in the institution."

sisters beneath the domestic roof? Surely, on this occasion, at least, the Hospital has well performed its mission of kindness and love."

In 1851, there died a young woman, twenty-one years of age, who a few months before had been brought to the Hospital, burnt by the breaking of a camphene lamp, in an assault committed upon her in a house of ill repute where she was an inmate. On her bed of pain, she had leisure to reflect on her former life. The retrospect filled her with horror. The severest physical sufferings were as nothing to the agonies of an awakened conscience. The past had become hateful; the present was full of anguish and distress; and the future held out no promise. Young as she was, life and all its opportunities had passed irrevocably away. She died in the Hospital; and yet the last moments of that poor, degraded Magdalen were soothed and cheered by words and acts of encouragement and compassion, such as the world seldom accords to its fallen children. To her contrite spirit may they have proved a foretaste of that Father's mercy which she so deeply needed and so earnestly sought!

> "Were not the sinful Mary's tears
> An offering worthy Heaven,
> When o'er the faults of former years
> She wept, and was forgiven?"

CHAPTER XII.

THE MEMBERS OF THE CORPORATION. — LIST OF TRUSTEES. — REMARKS AND ANECDOTES.— LIST OF OFFICERS. — LIST OF SUBSCRIPTIONS.— SUMMARY OF THE SAME TO 1843. — ENLARGEMENT OF HOSPITAL IN 1844. — FREE-BED SUBSCRIPTION LIST. — LEGACIES, DONATIONS, AND DEVISES. — RECEIPTS FROM LIFE OFFICE, &C. — GRAND SUMMARY OF ALL THESE DONATIONS. — TABLES OF ADMISSIONS AND DISCHARGES AT THE ASYLUM AND AT THE HOSPITAL. — CONCLUDING REMARKS.

THE Act of Incorporation names as members the following fifty-six gentlemen : —

Adams, John	Fowler, Samuel
Adams, John Q.	Gerry, Elbridge
Amory, Jonathan	Gore, Christopher
Amory, Thomas C.	Gray, William
Bowdoin, James	Greene, Benjamin
Bridge, Matthew	Hallowell, Robert
Brown, Samuel	Harris, Jonathan
Bussey, Benjamin	Hazard, Thomas, jun.
Cabot, George	Heath, William
Childs, Timothy	Hill, Aaron
Coolidge, Joseph	Jones, John Coffin
Craigie, Andrew	Kilham, Daniel
Crowninshield, Benj. W.	King, William
Cutts, Thomas	Kirkland, John Thornton
Dana, Samuel	Kittredge, Thomas
Davis, Jonathan	Lincoln, Levi
Dawes, Thomas	Lowell, John
Dearborn, Henry	Mann, James
Derby, Elias Hasket	Melville, Thomas
Eustis, William	Morton, Perez

Otis, Harrison Gray
Parker, Isaac
Parsons, Theophilus
Payne, William
Perkins, James
Perkins, Thomas H.
Phillips, William
Prince, James

Spring, Marshall
Story, Joseph
Sullivan, Richard
Thorndike, Israel
Tilden, David
Varnum, Joseph B.
Warren, John
Welles, Arnold.

The right to elect members has been but very rarely exercised. Six of the gentlemen constituting the first Board of Trustees were chosen members, to make them eligible to that office (1813): —

Barnard, Tristram
Bradford, Gamaliel
Lee, George G.

May, Joseph
Sargent, Daniel
Sullivan, John L.

In June, 1825, were chosen —

Edes, Robert B. . . . ⎫
Tilden, Bryant P. . . ⎬ through whom the donation of a mummy had been made;
Van Lennep, Jacob, ⎭

Swett, Samuel, ... to render him eligible as a Trustee; and
Wyman, Rufus, Dr., Superintendent of the M'Lean Asylum, who was already a member by a donation of over a hundred dollars.

In June, 1827, two members were elected, —

Bowditch, Nathaniel, who was Actuary of the Massachusetts Hospital Life Insurance Company;
Codman, Henry, to render him eligible as a Trustee.

It is believed that not a single member has been since elected, say for a period of twenty-five years. All, however, who have served as Trustees of the

LIST OF TRUSTEES.

institution are, by a subsequent vote, made members; also all donors to the amount of a hundred dollars and upwards. Those who have become members in this latter mode will be found in the alphabetical list of donors. The following is an alphabetical list of the Trustees of the Institution: —

Amory, Charles
Andrews, William T.
Appleton, Samuel
Appleton, William
Armstrong, Samuel T.
Barnard, Tristram
Belknap, John
Bond, George
Bowditch, N. I.
Bradford, Gamaliel
Brimmer, Martin
Bullard, William S.
Chadwick, Ebenezer
Chapman, Jonathan
Codman, Henry
Coolidge, Joseph
Curtis, Thomas B.
Dale, William J.
Dexter, George M.
Edmands, J. Wiley
Edwards, Henry
Eliot, Samuel A.
Francis, Ebenezer
Gardiner, William H.
Gray, Francis C.
Greene, Benjamin D.
Greene, Gardiner

Guild, Benjamin
Hallet, George
Head, Joseph
Higginson, Stephen, jun.
Hooper, Robert, jun.
Jackson, Patrick T.
Lamb, Thomas
Lawrence, Abbott
Lawrence, Amos
Lawrence, Amos A.
Lawrence, Samuel
Lee, George G.
Loring, Charles G.
Lowell, Francis C.
Lowell, Francis C.
Lowell, John
Lowell, John A.
Lyman, Theodore, jun.
May, Joseph
Mills, Charles H.
Oliver, Francis J.
Otis, William F.
Parker, Daniel P.
Perkins, Thomas H.
Phillips, Jonathan
Prescott, William H.
Quincy, Josiah

LIST OF TRUSTEES.

Quincy, Josiah, jun.
Robbins, Dr. Edward H.
Rogers, Henry B.
Sargent, Daniel
Sargent, Ignatius
Sears, David
Shaw, J. Howland
Shaw, Robert G.
Stevenson, J. Thomas
Stone, William W.
Storrow, Chas. S.

Sturgis, William
Sullivan, John L.
Sullivan, Richard
Swett, Samuel
Thorndike, John P.
Ticknor, George
Tilden, Joseph
Tuckerman, Edward
Ward, Thomas W.
Wigglesworth, Edward.

On this list of Trustees will be found the names of two individuals who, as authors, have acquired a European reputation in the respective departments of history and of Spanish literature; one President, three Treasurers, and four other Fellows, of Harvard College; one minister to the Court of St. James; two members of Congress; one Lieutenant-Governor of Massachusetts, and no less than six mayors of Boston; the two fathers of American manufactures, — the late noble-spirited Patrick T. Jackson, and the late Francis C. Lowell, whose name has been conferred upon our manufacturing emporium; and also one who in his day was the head of the Suffolk Bar, and afterwards the most scientific agriculturist of the Commonwealth. Associated with these are found many of our wealthiest and most liberal merchants, — Mr. Sears, Col. Perkins, and others. It will not, I am sure, be thought invidious if mention is made of two of these as our "Brothers Cheeryble," — Samuel Appleton and Amos Lawrence,* so generally known and so universally respected as among the most amiable and benevolent of our citizens. Both have been the architects of their own fortunes. Mr. Appleton tells a humorous story, that, when a young man, he kept a school, during the winter-months, in a country-town, where he *was put up at auction*, to be boarded out in the family that would consent to take him at the lowest rate. Mr. Lawrence tells an equally good story of the small shop first opened by himself and his brother, and of a purchase of some trifling article once made by a sailor, who was so pleased with his bargain that he returned in a few days with several of his messmates, and began spelling out the sign-boards in the street, at last exclaiming with a loud voice, as the modest sign of which he was in search met his eye, "That's it, *A. and A. Lawrence;* that's the place;" an instance of humble patronage which at the time was more gratifying than the most brilliant success that has ever crowned the enterprise and industry of a firm now known throughout the commercial world.

* Mr. Lawrence died Dec. 31, 1852, in the 67th year of his age. Mr. Appleton died July 12, 1853, having just entered on his 88th year. He placed $200,000 at the disposal of his three executors, for public uses. To have been thus selected as one of the almoners of his bounty I regard as the most gratifying incident of my professional life. — [*Marginal Note by Mr. B.*]

The former, in advanced age, and unable to walk from his house, continues, in the highest and best sense, to enjoy life. He has, indeed, no children; but a numerous band of nephews and nieces look up to him with truly filial regard. Indeed, the community itself ventures to apply to him *their* familiar and affectionate appellation of "Uncle Sam." This name, in the abstract so dear to every patriot, could not be more worthily bestowed. The latter, also for some years past an invalid, and unable to attend at all to business, is yet at heart as young as ever, finding leisure and strength for innumerable good works and kind offices. He, too, has thus won from the public a corresponding title of respect and regard. Everybody loves "Uncle Amos," and he loves everybody. He is particularly fond of the young. For a considerable time, and at a cost, doubtless, of several thousand dollars, he defrayed the entire expenses of a private Hospital for children, under the charge of his son, Dr. W. R. Lawrence. On a bright winter's day, he was passing a primary school just as recess began. One of the little girls cried out, "How I should like a sleigh-ride!" He at once filled his vehicle with as many of them as could get into it. In my visits at the Asylum, I occasionally find that, as an amateur, he has preceded me. Mr. Lawrence is the elder brother of Hon. Abbott Lawrence, who, high as is his present official station, has gained a yet prouder distinction as founder of the scientific school of Harvard College.

[The Lists of Officers, of Subscribers, &c., which follow, are reprinted as prepared by Mr. Bowditch, — terminating with the date of the publication of his History. The additions to them appear in their proper place, as a part of the Continuation.]

OFFICERS OF THE HOSPITAL

FROM ITS FOUNDATION.

PRESIDENTS.

William Phillips . . . . from 1814 . . through 1826 . . 13 years.
Thomas H. Perkins . . from 1826 . . through 1827 . . 2 ,,
John Lowell . . . . . . from 1828 . . to Jan. 1830 . . 2 ,,
Gardiner Greene . from June, 1830 . . through 1832 . . $3\frac{1}{2}$,,
Joseph Head . . . . . . from 1833 . . through 1835 . . 3 ,,
Ebenezer Francis . . . . . . 1836 . . . . 1 ,,
Edward Tuckerman . . from 1837 . . through 1843 . . 7 ,,
William Appleton . . . from 1844 . . through 1851 . . 8 ,,

VICE-PRESIDENTS.

Samuel Parkman . . elected 1814 . . . . . . and declined serving.
James Perkins . . . . 1815 . died Aug. 1822 . . . $7\frac{1}{2}$ yrs.
Thomas H. Perkins . . from 1823 . . to June, 1826 . . . $3\frac{1}{2}$,,
John Lowell . . . from June, 1826 . . to June, 1829 . . . 3 ,,
Gardiner Greene from ,, 1829 . . to June, 1830 . . . 1 ,,
Joseph Head . . from ,, 1830 . . through 1832 . . . $2\frac{1}{2}$,,
Ebenezer Francis . . . from 1833 . . through 1835 . . . 3 ,,
Samuel Appleton . . . . 1836 . . . . 1 ,,
Jonathan Phillips . . . from 1837 . . through 1845 . . . 9 ,,
Theodore Lyman . . . . . . 1846 . . died in 1849 . . . 4 ,,
Robert Hooper . . . . . from 1850 . . through 1851 . . . 2 ,,

TREASURERS.

James Prince . . . . 1813 . died Feb. 1821 . . . $8\frac{1}{6}$ yrs.
William Cochran . Feb. 28, 1821 . died in 6 months . . $\frac{1}{2}$,,
N. P. Russell . . . . Sept. 14, 1821 . . through 1834 . . $13\frac{1}{4}$,,
Henry Andrews . . . . from 1835 . . through 1851 . . 17 ,,

SECRETARIES.

Richard Sullivan . . . from 1811 . . through 1816 . . 6 years.
Henry Codman . . . . . from 1817 . . through 1826 . . 10 ,,
N. I. Bowditch . . . . . from 1827 . . to June, 1836 . . 9½ ,,
William Gray . . from June, 1836 . . through 1841 . . 5½ ,,
Marcus Morton, jun. . . from 1842 . . through 1851 . . 10 ,,

TRUSTEES.

Thomas H. Perkins . . from 1813 . . through 1818 . . 6 years.
Josiah Quincy . . . . . from 1813 . . through 1820 . . 8 ,,
Daniel Sargent . . . . . from 1813 . . through 1821 . . 9 ,,
Joseph May . . . . . . from 1813 . to Nov. 5, 1826,
                                            nearly . . . . . 14 ,,
Stephen Higginson, jun. from 1813 . . through 1815 . . 3 ,,
Gamaliel Bradford . . . from 1813 . . through 1823 . . 11 ,,
Tristram Barnard . . . from 1813 . . through 1818 . . 6 ,,
George G. Lee . . . . . from 1813 . . through 1816 . . 4 ,,
Francis C. Lowell . . . from 1813 . . through 1815 . . 3 ,,
Joseph Tilden . . . . . from 1813 . . through 1815 . . 3 ,,
John L. Sullivan . . . . from 1813 . . through 1816 . . 4 ,,
Richard Sullivan . . . . from 1813 . . through 1822 . . 10 ,,
Jonathan Phillips . . . . from 1816 . . to July, 1832 . . 16½ ,,
John Lowell . . . . . . from 1816 . . through 1819 . . 4 ,,
Joseph Coolidge . . . . from 1816 . . through 1831 . . 16 ,,
David Sears . . . . . . from 1817 . . through 1819 . . 3 ,,
Eben Francis, part of 1817;
  chosen by Corporation, 1818
  (resigned for part of 1820) . . . . . through 1831 say 14 ,,
Peter C. Brooks . . . elected 1819 . . . . . . but declined serving.
Joseph Head, elected by Trus-
  tees in 1819; by Corporation, 1820   to June, 1829 . . . 8½ yrs.
Thomas W. Ward, elected by
  Trustees in 1819; by Corpo-
  ration, 1820 . . . . through 1823 . . . 4 ,,

OFFICERS OF HOSPITAL.

Samuel Appleton, elected by
  Trustees in October, 1819 ;
    by Corporation, 1820 . . . . to Dec. 1822 . . 3 years.
John Belknap . . . . . from 1820 . . through 1822 . . 3 „
Daniel P. Parker . . . from 1821 . to July 26, 1825 . . $4\frac{1}{2}$ „
Theodore Lyman, jun. . from 1822 . to July 26, 1825 . . $3\frac{1}{2}$ „
Benjamin Guild . . . . from 1823 . . to Jan. 1834 . . 11 „
William H. Prescott . . from 1823 . to July 26, 1825 . . $2\frac{1}{2}$ „
Gardiner Greene . . . from 1823 . . to July, 1830 . . $7\frac{1}{2}$ „
Samuel Swett . . from May, 1823 . . to July, 1826 . . $3\frac{1}{6}$ „
Edward Tuckerman . . from 1824 . . through 1836 . . 13 „
George Ticknor . from July, 1826 . . to July, 1830 . . 4 „
Edward H. Robbins from „ 1826 . . through 1834 . . $9\frac{1}{2}$ „
William Sturgis . from „ 1826 . . to July, 1827 . . 1 „
Amos Lawrence from Dec. 5, 1826 . to Feb. 26, 1831 . . $5\frac{1}{4}$ „
P. T. Jackson . . from July, 1827 . . to July, 1828 . . 1 „
Henry Codman . from „ 1827 . . . to Jan. 1835 . . $7\frac{1}{2}$ „
Wm. H. Gardiner from „ 1828 . . . . 1 „
Francis C. Gray . from „ 1829 . to Oct. 30, 1836 . . $7\frac{1}{4}$ „
Josiah Quincy, jun. from „ 1830 . . through 1836 . . $6\frac{1}{2}$ „
Benj. D. Greene from Aug. 26, 1830 . . to Oct. 8, 1833 . . 3 „
James Bowdoin, elected Aug. 1830 . . . . declined serving.
Heman Lincoln, elected . Jan. 1831 . . . . declined serving.
George Bond, elected . Feb. 1831 . died May 23, 1842 $11\frac{1}{4}$ yrs.
George Hallet, elected . July, 1831 . . through 1833 . . $2\frac{1}{2}$ „
Thomas W. Ward, re-elected 1832 . . . . . . and declined serving.
Abbott Lawrence from July, 1832 . . through 1835 . . $3\frac{1}{2}$ yrs.
Francis J. Oliver . . . . from 1833 . . through 1835 . . 3 „
Samuel A. Eliot . . . . from 1834 . . through 1838 . . 5 „
Charles G. Loring . . . from 1834 . . through 1837 . . 4 „
Rufus Wyman . . . . 1835 . elected and declined serving.
Thomas B. Curtis . . . from 1835 . . through 1838 . . 4 years.
Charles Amory . . . . . from 1836 . . through 1847 . . 12 „
Henry Edwards . . . . from 1836 . . through 1845 . . 10 „
Samuel Lawrence . . . from 1836 . . through 1838 . . 3 „
Robert G. Shaw . . . . from 1836 . . through 1838 . . 3 „

John P. Thorndike . . from 1836 . . through 1837 . . 2 years.
Martin Brimmer . . . . from 1837 . . through 1842 . . 6 „
Robert Hooper, jun. . . from 1837 . . through 1849 . . 13 „
N. I. Bowditch . . . . . from 1837 . . through 1851 . . 15 „
William Appleton . . . from 1838 . . through 1841 . . 4 „
Thomas Lamb . . . . . from 1838 . . through 1851 . . 14 „
George M. Dexter . . . from 1839 . . through 1851 . . 13 „
Francis C. Lowell . . . from 1839 . . through 1851 . . 13 „
Henry B. Rogers . . . from 1839 . . (omitting 1840)
                                      through 1851 . . 12 „
Ebenezer Chadwick . . from 1840 . . through 1842 . . 3 „
Ignatius Sargent . . . . 1841 . . . . 1 „
William T. Andrews . from 1842 . . through 1847 . . 6 „
Jonathan Chapman . . . . . 1843 . . . . 1 „
William F. Otis . . . . 1843 . . . . 1 „
John A. Lowell . . . . from 1843 . . through 1850 . . 8 „
Charles S. Storrow . . from 1844 . . through 1845 . . 2 „
Edward Wigglesworth . from 1844 . . through 1851 . . 8 „
William W. Stone . . . . . . 1846 . . . . 1 „
J. Wiley Edmands . . . from 1847 . . through 1848 . . 2 „
J. Thomas Stevenson . from 1846 . . through 1851 . . 6 „
Charles H. Mills . . . . from 1848 . . through 1851 . . 4 „
Amos A. Lawrence . . from 1848 . . through 1851 . . 4 „
William S. Bullard . . from 1849 . . through 1851 . . 3 „
G. Howland Shaw . . . from 1850 . . through 1851 . . 2 „
William J. Dale . . . . 1851 . . . . 1 „

CHAIRMEN OF THE TRUSTEES.

Thomas H. Perkins . . . . . 1818 . . . . 1 year.
Joseph May . . . . 1819 . . to Nov. 1826 . . 8 „
Joseph Head . . . . . Dec. 5, 1826 . . to July, 1829 . . 2½ „
Ebenezer Francis . . . July, 1829 . . to July, 1831 . . 2 „
Edward Tuckerman . . July, 1831 . . to Feb. 1835 . . 3½ „
George Bond . . . from Feb. 1835 . . to May, 1842 . . 7¼ „
Robert Hooper, jun. June 19, 1842 . . to Jan. 1850 . . 7½ „
N. I. Bowditch . . . . 1850 . . through 1851 . . 2 „

SUPERINTENDENTS OF HOSPITAL.

Capt. Nathl. Fletcher, April 21, 1821 . died May 1, 1825 . 4 years.
Nathan Gurney . . . June 12, 1825 . . . to Nov. 1833 . 8 „
Gamaliel Bradford . Oct. 11, 1833 . died Oct. 23, 1839 . 6 „
Charles Sumner . . . Dec. 17, 1839 . to Mar. 21, 1841 . $2\frac{1}{4}$ „
John M. Goodwin . March 21, 1841 . . to Nov. 2, 1845 . $4\frac{1}{2}$ „
Richard Girdler . . . Nov. 16, 1845 . . . . to 1852 . 6 „

PHYSICIANS OF ASYLUM.

Dr. George Parkman conditionally elected Oct. 4, 1816 . . . . never served.
Dr. Rufus Wyman, March 23, 1818 . . to May 31, 1835 . 17 years.
Dr. Thomas G. Lee, chosen . . . . Jan. 16, 1835 . . died Oct. 1836 . 2 „
Dr. Luther V. Bell . Dec. 11, 1836 . . . . . . to 1852 . 15 „

STEWARDS, &c., OF ASYLUM.

John M. Goodwin . . Nov. 23, 1823 . . to June 4, 1826 . $2\frac{1}{2}$ yrs.
G. W. Folsom . . . . died in Oct. 1827 . 1 „
Henry Pierce . . . . Oct. 9, 1827 . office abolished, Nov. 11, 1828 . 1 „
Oliver V. Bond (as supervisor), ... Nov. 23, 1828 . . to Oct. 5, 1830 . 2 „
Columbus Tyler (as supervisor) . . . . Oct. 8, 1830 . . . .
Luke Bigelow, chosen Oct. 3, 1832 . to March 9, 1834 } 4 „
„   „   „   May 18, 1834 . to Nov. 23, 1836 }
William Wyman . . . Dec. 2, 1834 . . . . 2 mos.
Columbus Tyler . . Jan. 16, 1835 . . . . to 1852 . 16 years.

ATTENDING PHYSICIANS AND SURGEONS AT HOSPITAL.

Dr. James Jackson . . April 6, 1817 . . to Oct. 13, 1837 . $20\frac{1}{2}$ yrs.
„ John C. Warren .   „   6, 1817 . . . . . . to 1852 . 34   „
„ Walter Channing . Oct. 4, 1821 . . . . to Jan. 1839 . $17\frac{1}{4}$ „
„ John B. Brown . Nov. 23, 1823 . to Feb. 26, 1826 . $2\frac{1}{4}$ „
„ George Hayward, March 19, 1826 (first chosen assistant-surgeon; then junior, Feb. 21, 1830; then chief, Jan. 1838) . . . . . . to April, 1851 . 25 years.
„ Edward Reynolds, Aug. 3, 1828 . . to April 7, 1829 . 8 mos.
„ George W. Otis .   „   3, 1828 .   to new organization in Feb. 1830 . $1\frac{1}{2}$ year.
„ John Ware, assistant, Sept. 27, 1829; and resigned July 8, 1836; chosen Feb. 10, 1839 . . . . and served 1 year . 8   „
  Jacob Bigelow . July 8, 1836 . . . . . . to 1852 . 15   „
„ Enoch Hale . . . Oct. 13, 1837 . . died Nov. 1848 . 11   „
„ Solomon D. Townsend, February, 1839 . . . . to 1852 . 13   „
„ J. B. S. Jackson . Jan. 22, 1840 . . . . to 1852 . 12   „
„ H. I. Bowditch . „   28, 1846 . . . . to 1852 . 6   „
„ John D. Fisher .   „   28, 1846 . died March, 1850 . 5   „
„ O. W. Holmes . .   „   28, 1846 . . . to end of 1849 . 4   „
„ H. J. Bigelow . .   „   28, 1846 . . . . to 1852 . 6   „
„ Samuel Parkman   „   28, 1846 . . . . to 1852 . 6   „
„ J. Mason Warren   „   28, 1846 . . . . to 1852 . 6   „
„ D. H. Storer . . . . Jan. 1849 (in place of Dr. Hale) 3   „
„ G. C. Shattuck, jun.   „   1850 („   „ Dr. Holmes) 2   „
„ M. S. Perry . . . March, 1850 („   „ Dr. Fisher) 2   „
„ Henry G. Clark .   „   1851 („   „ Dr. Hayward) 1   „

LIST OF ORIGINAL SUBSCRIBERS

OF ONE HUNDRED DOLLARS AND UPWARDS.

Prepared by Joseph May, Esq., in 1828; continued by Henry B. Rogers, Esq., to July 10, 1843; those marked (*) having been added by Mr. Rogers.

Adams, Benjamin and Caleb	$100.00
Allen, Joseph	100.00
Amory, Hannah R.	100.00
Amory, John	200.00
Amory, Jonathan	200.00
Andrews, Ebenezer T.	300.00
Appleton, Nathan	500.00
Appleton, Samuel	2000.00
*Appleton, William, for himself	100.00
Appleton, William, for an unknown	200.00
*Armstrong, Samuel T.	100.00
Austin, Nathaniel	100.00
Babcock, Adam	300.00
Baker, Brown, and Co.	100.00
Baldwin, Aaron	110.00
Barnard, Charles	100.00
Bartlett, John	100.00
Bartlett, Thomas	300.00
Bean, Stephen	100.00
Belknap, Jeremiah	100.00
Belknap, John	100.00
Bellows, John	100.00
Binney, Amos	300.00
Bishop, John	100.00
Blake, George	100.00
Bond, George	180.00
Boott, Kirk, and Sons	300.00
Boott, Mary	300.00

ORIGINAL SUBSCRIBERS.

Bradbury, Charles	$100.00
Bradford, Gamaliel	100.00
Bradlee, Josiah	200.00
Bradlee, Thomas D.	100.00
Bridge, Nathan	100.00
Brimmer, Andrew	100.00
Brooks, Peter C.	2000.00
*Brown, Moses	100.00
Brown, Samuel	100.00
Bryant, John	100.00
Bumstead, Thomas	125.00
Bussey, Benjamin	1000.00
Cabot, George	100.00
Cabot, John	150.00
Cabot, Sarah and Susan	100.00
Cabot, William	100.00
Carnes, Francis	200.00
Chamberlain, Richard	100.00
Channing Walter	100.00
Channing, William E.	100.00
Chapman, Henry	100.00
Chelsea, town of	145.42
Child, David W.	100.00
Cobb, Samuel	200.00
Cochran, William	100.00
Codman, Charles R.	100.00
Coffin, Margaret (and Ann Smith)	100.00
Collections in Ward 4	340.00
Collections in Ward 10	373.00
Coolidge, Joseph	2000.00
Coolidge, Joseph, jun.	1000.00
Cordis, Thomas	100.00
Cotting, Uriah	100.00
Crocker, Allen	100.00
*Crowninshield, Benjamin W.	200.00
Crowninshield, George	500.00

ORIGINAL SUBSCRIBERS. 425

Curtis, Thomas	$100.00
*Cushing, John P.	5000.00
Cushing, Thomas, a share in Exchange Coffee House, worth	300.00
Dall, William	100.00
Dana, Benjamin	100.00
*Dane, Nathan	200.00
Davis, Amasa	100.00
*Davis, A. and C.	150.00
Davis, Charles	100.00
Davis, Daniel	100.00
Davis, Eleanor	200.00
Davis, Joshua	100.00
Davis, Thomas	100.00
Davis, William	150.00
*Dearborn, H. A. S.	150.00
Degrand, P. P. F.	175.00
Dennie, Thomas	100.00
Derby, John	300.00
Derby, Richard	100.00
Derby, Richard C.	300.00
Devereux, Humphrey	100.00
Dexter, Aaron	100.00
Dexter, Katharine	100.00
Dodge, Pickering	300.00
Dorr, John	110.00
Dorr, Samuel	100.00
Eliot, Catherine	200.00
Ellery, John S.	100.00
Ellis, David	100.00
Endicott, Samuel	100.00
*Exhibition of Mummy	1257.87
Fales, Samuel	100.00
Farley, Ebenezer	125.00
Female Association	753.08
Field, Joseph	100.00

ORIGINAL SUBSCRIBERS.

Fisher, Joshua	$100.00
Forrester, Simon	2000.00
Francis, Ebenezer	200.00
French, John	100.00
French and Weld	120.00
Gardiner, Robert H.	200.00
Gardiner, Samuel P.	100.00
Gibson, Abraham	100.00
Goddard, Nathaniel	200.00
Gore, John	200.00
Gray, Francis C.	100.00
Gray, Henry	1000.00
*Gray, Horace	1000.00
Gray, John C.	100.00
*Gray, John C.	1300.00
Gray, William	500.00
Greene, Gardiner, $1000 in three per cents	650.00
Greenough, David	200.00
Greenough, David S.	200.00
*Hall, Dudley	200.00
Hammond, Samuel	200.00
Hancock, John	200.00
*Harvard College	213.32
Hayward, Lemuel	100.00
Head, Joseph	1000.00
Head, Joseph, jun.	100.00
Heard, Augustine	100.00
Hedge, Barnabas	150.00
Hinckley, David	1000.00
Hingham, Third Parish	504.44
Holland, John	200.00
Homer, Benjamin P.	100.00
Homes, Henry	100.00
Howe, John	100.00
Hubbard, Henry	100.00
Hubbard, John	200.00

ORIGINAL SUBSCRIBERS.

Humane Society of Massachusetts	$5140.56
Humane Society (Merrimack)	2000.00
Hunnewell, Jonathan	100.00
Hurd, John	100.00
Hurd, Joseph	200.00
Jackson, Charles	400.00
Jackson, James	420.00
Jackson, Patrick T.	220.00
Jaques, Samuel, jun.	100.00
Jones, John Coffin	500.00
Jones, Thomas Kilby	200.00
Joy, Abigail and family	300.00
Joy, Benjamin	250.00
Kidder, John, jun.	100.00
Knapp, Josiah	100.00
Knowles, Seth	100.00
Lambert, William	100.00
Lawrence, Amos and Abbott	200.00
Lawrence, William	100.00
Lee, Francis	100.00
Lee, George	150.00
Lee, Joseph	300.00
Lee, Thomas, jun.	100.00
Lewis, Winslow	100.00
Lincoln and Wheelwright	100.00
Lloyd, James	1000.00
Loring, Caleb	100.00
Lowell, Francis C.	300.00
*Lowell, Francis C.	100.00
Lowell, John	450.00
Lyman, George W.	150.00
Lyman, Theodore	2000.00
Lyman, Theodore, jun.	150.00
Marshall, Josiah	100.00
Massachusetts Charitable Fire Society	900.00
May, Perrin	100.00

May, Samuel	$100.00
Miller, Samuel R.	100.00
Minot, William	100.00
Morse, John	100.00
Motley, Thomas	100.00
Munson, Israel	1000.00
*Oakes, Caleb	100.00
Odin, John	200.00
Odiorne, George	100.00
Orne, Joseph	200.00
Orne, Samuel	200.00
Osborn, John	200.00
Otis, H. G.	500.00
Parker, Daniel P.	500.00
Parker, John	500.00
Parkman, Samuel	2000.00
Parkman, Samuel, jun.	200.00
Parsons, Nehemiah	200.00
Parsons, William	1500.00
Payne, M.	100.00
Payne, William	100.00
Peabody, Joseph	2000.00
Perkins, James	5000.00
Perkins, Samuel G.	100.00
Perkins, Thomas H.	5000.00
Perry, John	100.00
Phillips, John	100.00
Phillips, Jonathan	100.00
Phillips, Stephen	200.00
Phillips, Wm., including $5000 legacy of his father	20,000.00
Pickering, Henry	100.00
Pickman, Benjamin, jun.	1000.00
Pickman, Dudley L.	150.00
Pickman, William	300.00
Pope, Paschal P.	100.00
Pratt, John	135.00

ORIGINAL SUBSCRIBERS.

Pratt, William	$400.00
Prescott, William	150.00
Prince, James	250.00
Prince, John	200.00
Quincy, Josiah	200.00
Rand, Isaac	100.00
Randall, John	100.00
Reed, John T.	100.00
Revere, Paul	100.00
Revere, Joseph W.	100.00
Rice, Henry G.	100.00
Rich, Benjamin	300.00
Richards, John	100.00
Ritchie, Andrew	500.00
Robinson, Nathan	200.00
Rogers, Daniel D.	1000.00
*Ropes, William	150.00
Russell, Nathaniel P.	500.00
Salisbury, Samuel	500.00
Salisbury, Samuel, jun.	100.00
Sanford, Samuel	300.00
Sargent, Daniel	200.00
*Sargent, Ignatius	400.00
Sawyer, William	100.00
Sears, David	5000.00
Sewall, Joseph	500.00
Shaw, Robert G.	500.00
Shepherd, Michael	100.00
Shimmin, William	100.00
Silsbee, Nathaniel	100.00
Skinner, John	100.00
Smith, Barney	400.00
Snelling, Samuel	100.00
*Society, Washington Benevolent, Charlestown Branch	200.00
* „ Hollis-street	148.05
* „ First Church	100.67

430 ORIGINAL SUBSCRIBERS.

*Society, King's Chapel	$114.44
* " West Church	190.06
* " Roman Catholic	100.40
* " First Parish, Dorchester	168.48
* " Dr. Bancroft's, Worcester	140.60
* " Dr. Pierce's, Brookline	173.38
Soley, John	100.00
Spear, Samuel	100.00
Spelman, Phineas	100.00
Spooner, William	100.00
Stanton, Francis	100.00
Sturgis, Russell	200.00
Sturgis, William	100.00
Sullivan, George	200.00
Sullivan, Richard	400.00
Sullivan, William	200.00
Tappan, John	350.00
Tappan, Lewis	100.00
Taylor, Charles	300.00
Theatre, Boston	1190.00
Thompson, Abraham	100.00
Thorndike, Israel	2000.00
Thorndike, Israel, jun.	100.00
Tilden, Joseph	100.00
Torrey, Catherine	200.00
Torrey, John G.	100.00
Torrey, Samuel	100.00
Touro, Abraham	300.00
Trott, George	100.00
Tucker, Gideon	200.00
Tucker, Richard D.	100.00
Tuckerman, Edward	100.00
Tuckerman, Edward, jun.	500.00
Tuckerman, William and Gustavus	100.00
*Town of Concord	200.00
*Town of Malden	193.80

ORIGINAL SUBSCRIBERS.

*Tufts, Cotton	$135.00
Tufts, Nathan	100.00
Upham, Phineas	100.00
Vose, Coates, and Co.	100.00
Waldo, Daniel	200.00
Wales, Thomas B.	100.00
Walker, Timothy	150.00
*Walker, William J.	400.00
Ward, Artemas	100.00
*Ward, Nahum	100.00
Ward, Thomas W.	150.00
Ward, William	100.00
Warren, John C.	400.00
Webster, Redford	153.00
Welch, Francis	200.00
Weld, Benjamin	500.00
Welles, John	300.00
West, Nathaniel	1000.00
Wetmore, Eliza	200.00
Wheeler, Elisha	100.00
Wheeler, Moses	100.00
White, James	300.00
Whitney, Asa	100.00
*Wiggin, Benjamin (Exhibition of Picture)	1604.07
Wigglesworth, Thomas	200.00
Williams, John D.	1000.00
Williams, Moses	100.00
Williams, Samuel G.	100.00
Williams, Thomas	100.00
Williams, Timothy	100.00
Winchester, Amasa	100.00
Winthrop, Thomas L.	100.00
Wood, John	100.00

NOTE. — Some of these subscriptions Mr. Rogers ascertained to be the same which were made to free beds; say in all, $3,712.

SUMMARY AND ANALYSIS.

SUMMARY OF SUBSCRIPTIONS TO JULY, 1843.

Total for Hospital $101,619.21
Total for Asylum 45,373.34
$146,992.57

SUBSCRIPTIONS ANALYZED.

1 of $20000 is $20000.00
4 of 5000 are 20000.00
8 of 2000 . . . . 16000.00
1 of 1604.07
1 of 1500.00
12 of 1000 . . . . 12000.00
1 of 650.00
14 of 500 . . . . 7000.00
1 of 450.00
1 of 420.00
7 of 400 . . . . 2800.00
1 of 350.00
21 of 300 . . . . 6300.00
2 of 250 . . . . 500.00
1 of 220.00
44 of 200 . . . . 8800.00
1 of 180.00
1 of 175.00
1 of 153.00
13 of 150 . . . . 1950.00
2 of 135 . . . . 270.00
2 of 125 . . . . 250.00
1 of 120.00
2 of 110 . . . . 220.00
151 of 100 . . . . 15100.00
1 of 94.89
1 of 60.00
6 of 75 . . . . 450.00

SUBSCRIPTIONS ANALYZED.

101 of 50	$5050.00
1 of	45.00
1 of	44.50
10 of 40	400.00
1 of	37.50
31 of 30	930.00
43 of 25	1075.00
114 of 20	2280.00
1 of	18.00
25 of 15	375.00
1 of	13.00
1 of	12.00
1 of	11.00
178 of 10	1780.00
2 of 7	14.00
257 of 5	1285.00
16 of 4	64.00
36 of 3	108.00
1 of	2.50
42 of 2	84.00
21 of 1	21.00
3 of $0.50, and 1 of $0.25	1.75
	131269.21
Ward Collections $847.50	
Exhibitions, Concerts, &c. 2782.69	
Five Benevolent Societies 8993.64	
Twenty-four Religious Societies 2349.97	
Twelve Towns 749.56	
	15723.36
	$146992.57

SUBSCRIPTIONS FOR ENLARGEMENT OF HOSPITAL, 1844.

Amory, Charles $500
Amory, James S. 250
Amory, William 500
Andrews, Ebenezer T. 1000
Appleton, Nathan 1000
Appleton, Samuel 2000
Appleton, Samuel A. 100
Appleton, William 2000
Armstrong, Samuel T. 100
Austin, Edward 100
Aylwin, Richard 100
Bacon, Daniel C. 100
Bangs, Benjamin 200
Barnard, Charles 500
Bassett, Francis 100
Bates, John D. 250
Binney, Amos 200
Blake, Mrs. Joshua 200
Blanchard, Edward 500
Boardman, William H. 100
Bowditch, J. Ingersoll 100
Bowditch, N. I. 500
Boyden, Dwight 100
Bradlee, Josiah 1000
Bradlee, James B. 200
Brimmer, Martin 500
Brooks, P. C. 2000
Brooks, P. C., jun. 500
Bromfield, John 100

ENLARGEMENT OF HOSPITAL. 435

Bryant, John, jun.	$250
Cabot, Henry	200
Cary, Thomas G.	100
Carney and Sleeper	100
Chace, Caleb	200
Chadwick, Eben	500
Chandler, Abiel	100
Chickering, Jonas	500
Codman, Charles R.	100
Codman, Henry	100
Colby, Gardner	100
Crowninshield, B. W.	300
Cunningham, A. and C.	100
Curtis, Charles P.	100
Curtis, Thomas B.	100
Dalton, Peter R.	100
Dana, Samuel	100
Dixwell, John James	100
Edmands, J. W.	200
Eliot, Samuel A.	500
Everett, Moses	100
Fales, Samuel	200
Fletcher, Richard	100
Forbes, John M.	100
Francis, Ebenezer	1000
Gardner, George	100
Gardner, John L.	1000
Goodenough, John	100
Goddard, Benjamin	500
Goodwin, Ozias	500
Gray, Francis C.	500
Gray, Horace	300
Gray, John C.	1000
Gray, Samuel C.	100
Gray, William	100
Greene, Elizabeth C.	500

Greene, Sarah	$1000
Greenough, David S.	100
Hall, Henry	100
Hallet, George	200
Hayward, George	100
Hooper, Nathaniel	100
Hooper, Robert	250
Hooper, Robert C.	100
Hooper, Samuel	250
Howe, George	500
Howe, Jabez C.	200
Iasisi and Goddard	100
Jackson, P. T.	100
Johnson, James	100
Johnson, Samuel	100
Joy, Abigail	100
Kendall, Abel, jun.	100
Kuhn, George H.	100
Lane and Reed	100
Lawrence, Abbott	2000
Lawrence, Amos	1000
Lawrence, Amos A.	100
Lawrence, William	1000
Lawrence and Stone	500
Lee, George	1000
Lee, Thomas	500
Livermore, Isaac	100
Loring, Elijah	100
Loring, Francis C.	100
Low, John J. and Francis	100
Lowell, Francis C.	500
Lowell, John A.	1000
Lyman, Charles	500
Lyman, George W.	500
Lyman, Theodore	1000
Marland, John	100

ENLARGEMENT OF HOSPITAL. 437

Mason, Robert M.	$100
Mason, William P.	500
Mills, Charles H.	100
Milton and Slocumb	100
Nichols, Benjamin R.	100
Oliver, William	100
Otis, William F.	100
Parker, Daniel P.	500
Parker, James	500
Parker, John	1000
Parkman, George	150
Parsons, William	100
Perkins, William P.	100
Peters, Edward D.	100
Phipps, William	100
Pickman, C. Gayton	100
Pope, Paschal P.	500
Pratt, Mary	500
Prescott, William	500
Prescott, William H.	100
Putnam, Samuel R.	100
Quincy, Josiah, jun.	1000
Revere, Joseph W.	100
Rice and Thaxter	100
Richardson, Jeffry, and Brother	100
Robbins, Edward H.	100
Rogers, Henry B.	500
Russell, James D.	100
Richardson, Burrage, and Co.	100
Salisbury, Stephen	500
Sargent, Ignatius	1000
Sargent, Lucius M.	100
Savage, James	100
Sayles, Willard	500
Sears, David	2000
Shaw, R. G.	1000

Skinner, Francis	$250
Stickney, Josiah	100
Stoddard, Charles	100
Sturgis, William	1000
Thayer, John E.	500
Thayer, Nathaniel	100
Tilden, Joseph	100
Timmins, Henry	500
Upham, Phineas	1000
Waldo, Daniel, and sister	200
Wales, Thomas B.	1000
Walker, William J.	200
Waterston, Pray, and Co.	100
Warren, John C.	500
Welles, John	500
Wetmore, Thomas	100
Whitney, William F.	100
Wigglesworth, Edward	100
Wigglesworth, Thomas	300
Williams, John D.	2000
Williams, Moses	100
Total	$62550

ANALYSIS OF THESE SUBSCRIPTIONS.

6 of $2000	$12000
19 of 1000	19000
33 of 500	16500
3 of 300	900
6 of 250	1500
14 of 200	2800
78 of 100	7800
2 of 75	150
37 of 50	1850
2 of 25	50
	$62550

FREE-BED SUBSCRIPTIONS.

Adams, Horatio, 1848–49	$258.00
Amory, Charles, 1845–46	200.00
Amory, James S., 1845–48	400.00
Amory, William, 1844	100.00
Appleton, Nathan, 1826 and 1840	200.00
Appleton, Samuel, 1850	100.00
Appleton, William, 1837–40, 1847–49	800.00
Belknap, Jeremiah, Life-bed, 1827	654.00
Boston and Lowell Railroad, 1848–49	150.00
Boston and Maine Railroad, 1849	100.00
Boston and Providence Railroad, 1848–49	150.00
Bowditch, H. I., 1847	100.00
Bowditch, N. I., 1841–51	1000.00
Bradlee, Josiah, 1843–50	800.00
Bradlee, Thomas D., 1828	100.00
Brimmer, Martin, 1837–39	300.00
Brooks, Peter C., 1826, $100; 1828, Life-bed, $810	910.00
Bryant, John, 1849	100.00
Bullard, William S., 1850	100.00
Bumstead, John, 1828	100.00
Codman, Henry, 1833–36	400.00
Coolidge, Joseph, 1827–31	500.00
Cushing, John P., 1829–43, 1845–47	2900.00
Cutler, Pliny, 1836	100.00
Cutler, William C., 1837–38	200.00
Dixwell, John James, 1841	100.00
Dwight, Edmund, 1828–33, 1845–49	1100.00
Eliot, Catherine, 1826	100.00
Eliot, Samuel A., 1826, 1828, 1840, 1845–47	600.00
Fales, Samuel, 1828	100.00
Ferriera, L. G., 1839	100.00

Francis, Ebenezer, 1826–32	$700.00
Gray, Francis C., 1828–31, 1840–41	600.00
Gray, John C., 1828–32	500.00
Greene, Gardiner, 1828–32	500.00
Greene, J. S. C., 1843–48	600.00
Hallet, George, Life-bed, 1836	600.00
Hallet, Mrs. George, Life-bed, 1846	600.00
Head, Joseph, sen. and jun., Executors, 1826	1200.00
Head, Joseph, 1827–28	200.00
Howard Benevolent Society, 1828	100.00
Howe, George, 1840, 1841	200.00
Hubbard, Samuel, 1837	100.00
Humane Society, 1825–50	9700.00
Ives, R. H., 1847	100.00
Jackson, Charles, 1826–43	1800.00
Jackson, Patrick T., 1822 and 1827–40	1460.00
Jeffries, John, 1835 and 1844–47, 1849–50	800.00
Joy, Elizabeth, 1847–48	166.67
Joy, Hannah, 1833–34, 1836–42	900.00
Lambert, William, 1823	400.00
Lawrence, Abbott, 1828	100.00
Lawrence, Amos, 1826–32 and 1841	800.00
Lawrence, William, 1828	100.00
Loring, Abby M., 1847–50	400.00
Lowell, Francis C., 1845–50	500.00
Lowell, John A., 1843 and 1846–49	500.00
Lyman, Theodore, 1839, 1840–42	900.00
Massachusetts Charitable Fire Society, 1832, 1845–50	2325.00
Munson, Israel, 1826–28, 1831–38, 1843	1200.00
Oxnard, Henry, 1843	100.00
Parker, Daniel P., 1828	100.00
Parker, John, 1826–40	1500.00
Parker, J. B., 1845–47	237.50
Parsons, William, 1826	100.00
Perkins, James, 1826	200.00
Perkins, Thomas H., 1825–33	820.00

FREE-BED SUBSCRIPTIONS.

Phillips, Jonathan, 1828–32, 1843–50	$1200.00
Phillips, William, 1826–27	300.00
Pratt, Elizabeth, 1849–50	200.00
Pratt, Sarah P., 1848–50	300.00
Pratt, William, 1828, 1840–42	400.00
Prescott, William, 1828	100.00
Raymond, E. A., 1848	100.00
Redman, John, 1844–46	300.00
Reed, Hannah, 1844–50	700.00
Robbins, Edward H., 1827–29	270.00
Rogers, Henry B., 1844–46, 1849–50	500.00
Salisbury, Elizabeth, 1833–43, 1846–50	1600.00
Sears, David, 1825 and 1840	200.00
Shattuck, George C., 1829	100.00
Shaw, Robert G., 1828, 1840, 1842–43, 1845–50	1000.00
Stanton, Francis, 1835	100.00
Stone, William W., 1847	100.00
Sturgis William, 1827–32, 1840–43, 1845–48	1300.00
Tappan, John, 1826	100.00
Thorndike, Israel, 1826	100.00
Ticknor, George, 1826–30	500.00
Tuckerman, Edward, 1828–32	500.00
Waldo, Daniel, 1839	100.00
Waldo, E. and S., 1827, 1829–50	2300.00
Wales, Thomas B., Life-bed, 1828	825.00
Williams, John D., 1826–48	2300.00
Williams, Moses, 1847–50	400.00
Total to 1851	$65,069.17

LEGACIES, DONATIONS, DEVISES.

Dec.	1843.	Appleton, William, for relief of indigent patients at Asylum	$10000.00
Aug.	1830.	Belknap, Jeremiah, for free beds	10000.00
Nov. 1832, to Jan. 1833.		Belknap, Mary	89882.60
Jan.	1841.	Brimmer, Mary Anne, for free beds	5000.00
July,	1845.	Brown, John (lost in the "Lexington")	100.00
March,	1847.	Clough, Sarah, a domestic	599.84
Feb. &c.	1811,	Commonwealth of Massachusetts: Old Province House $40000.00 And for labor of convicts at Hospital . . $30893.84 At Asylum . . . 4176.43 ———— 35070.27	75070.27
Dec.	1838.	Courtis, Ambrose S., $10,000, compromised with heirs for	2500.00
March,	1826.	Crocker, Allen	100.00
Feb.	1825.	Davis, Eleanor, for free beds	900.00
April,	1820.	Eliot, Samuel, for the Asylum	10000.00
July,	1844.	Everett, Moses, donation of	116.00
Oct.	1830.	Lee, Joseph, heir of Francis Lee, a deceased patient, stocks, valued at	20000.00
June,	1813.	Lucas, John, six shares in Worcester Turnpike, worth	900.00
Feb. 1, 1824, to Nov. 1827.		M'Lean, John $94858.20	
Oct.	1834.	And after his widow's death 25000.00	119858.20
Aug.	1834.	Moseley, Jonathan	753.46
March,	1844.	Munson, Israel	20000.00
May,	1849.	Nichols, Benjamin R.	6000.00
Jan.	1826.	Oliver, Thomas	22438.70

LEGACIES, DONATIONS, DEVISES.   443

Sept.	1827.	Phillips, William, for free beds . . .	$5000.00
July,	1836.	Richardson, Susan, for female free beds	250.00
Nov.	1819.	Russell, Polly	400.00
May,	1845.	Russell, W.	100.00
Jan.	1829.	Savage, James	100.00
Aug. 1831, to July, 1843.		Thomas, Isaiah, bequest . $4599.81	
May,	1845.	„ „ 182.02	
Aug.	1846.	„ „ 235.00	
Oct. 1847, to Dec. 1850.		„ „ 240.00	
			5256.83
Feb.	1850.	Todd, Henry	5000.00
July,	1823.	Touro, Abraham	10000.00
Sept.	1820.	Tucker, Beza, House in Boylston Place, sold for	5350.00
Aug.	1842.	Tucker, Margaret, his daughter, for free beds	2929.97
Dec.	1845.	Waldo, Daniel	40000.00
Nov.	1841.	Warren, John C., fund for books to be given to Hospital patients	1000.00
Nov.	1822.	Webber, Seth	1000.00
March,	1841.	Westerfield, Peter, for poor patients .	165.67
April,	1851.	Wilder, Dr. Charles W., of Leominster, for free beds	20000.00
March,	1849.	Williams, John D., store, which now rents for the interest of $17,000 . .	13000.00
		Making in all . .	$503,922.86

The valuations in this list are those on the books of the Hospital. The Province House, appraised at $40,000, brought only $33,000. On the Lee donation there was perhaps a loss of $7,000 more. From the Wilder donation there should be a deduction of $4,000 more; the M·Lean $25,000 was also deficient. These deductions (about $20,000) are probably balanced by the increased value of other items; say, at least, $12,000 or $15,000 on Mary Belknap's bequest, and $4,000 on Mr. Williams's devise.

To the amount in page 443 . . . . $503,922.86 should be added the receipts from the Massachusetts Hospital Life Insurance Company, under the agreement referred to in page 79: —

Jan.	1829.	. . . .	$687.50
,,	1830.	. . . .	2500.00
,,	1831.	. . . .	2500.00
,,	1832.	. . . .	2500.00
,,	1833.	. . . .	2500.00
,,	1834.	. . . .	5000.00
,,	1835.	. . . .	5000.00
,,	1836.	. . . .	5000.00
,,	1837.	. . . .	5000.00
,,	1838.	. . . .	5000.00
,,	1839.	. . . .	5000.00
,,	1840.	. . . .	5000.00
June,	1840.	Extra	15000.00
Jan.	1841.	. . . .	5000.00
,,	1842.	. . . .	5000.00
,,	1843.	. . . .	5000.00
,,	1844.	. . . .	5000.00
,,	1845.	. . . .	5000.00
June,	1845.	Extra	20000.00
Jan.	1846.	. . . .	5000.00
,,	1847.	. . . .	5000.00
,,	1848.	. . . .	5000.00
,,	1849.	. . . .	5000.00
,,	1850.	. . . .	5000.00
June,	1850.	Extra	15000.00
Jan.	1851.	. . . .	5000.00

———— 150,687.50

Total $654,610.36

GRAND SUMMARY OF SUBSCRIPTIONS, &c.

Total donations, &c.			$654,610.36
Original subscriptions for Asylum	$45,373.34		
Original subscriptions for Hospital	$101,619.21		
Subscriptions for enlargement of Hospital	62,550.00		
		164,169.21	
			209,542.55
			864,052.91
Free-bed subscriptions			65,069.17
			929,022.08
Deduct the error noticed by Mr. Rogers, p. 431			3,712.00
			925,510.08
William Appleton's new donation			20,000.00
			945,510.08
Reversionary interests, say —			
Present value of Province House, leased till 1916		$10,000.00	
John Redman's bequest, at least		100,000.00	
Thomas Oliver's bequest		50,000.00	
John Bromfield's bequest		40,000.00	
John Parker's bequest		10,000.00	
			210,000.00
			1,155,510.08
Estimated value of the rights under the charter of the Massachusetts Hospital Life Insurance Company, at least			100,000.00
Grand Total			$1,255,510.08

SAY, A MILLION AND A QUARTER OF DOLLARS.

RESULTS OF ADMISSIONS AND DISCHARGES AT THE M'LEAN ASYLUM FROM ITS ESTABLISHMENT.

Year.	Admitted.	Discharged.	Recovered.	Dead.	All other Discharges.	Remaining at end of year.	Average.
1818 } 1819	58	35	11	5	19	23	
1820	44	40	11	1	28	27	
1821	47	46	10	3	33	28	
1822	64	50	14	5	31	42	
1823	73	61	20	2	39	54	
1824	53	56	23	5	28	51	
1825	59	56	21	8	27	54	
1826	47	46	20	5	21	55	
1827	58	56	34	5	17	57	
1828	77	65	23	5	37	69	
1829	73	77	26	9	42	65	
1830	82	78	34	10	34	69	
1831	83	84	30	8	46	68	
1832	94	98	43	10	45	64	
1833	103	100	42	8	50	67	
1834	107	95	41	7	47	80	
1835	83	84	45	11	28	77	
1836	106	112	64	10	38	71	
1837	120	105	72	8	25	86	80
1838	138	131	74	12	45	93	95
1839	132	117	69	10	38	108	112
1840	155	138	75	13	50	125	128
1841	157	141	75	11	55	142	135
1842	129	138	80	15	43	133	143
1843	127	126	63	18	45	134	131
1844	158	140	68	19	53	152	146
1845	119	120	74	13	33	151	149
1846	148	126	65	9	52	173	164
1847	170	170	87	33	50	173	172
1848	143	155	82	23	50	155	171
1849	161	137	64	15	58	184	177
1850	173	157	78	28	51	200	201
Total	3341	3140	1538	344	1258		
Since Dr. Bell	2030	1901	1026	227	648		
Before ,,	1311	1239	512	117	610		
	3341	3140	1538	344	1258		

RESULTS OF ADMISSIONS AND DISCHARGES AT THE HOSPITAL FROM ITS ESTABLISHMENT.

Year.	Admitted.	Discharged.	Well.	Relieved.	Not relieved.	Dead.	Unfit, and not treated.	Eloped.	By request, and for all other causes.
1821 . .	18	12	7	4	1				
1822 . .	115	103	60	28	3	12			
1823 . .	188	174	81	69	7	12	1	4	
1824 . .	349	338	152	103	4	29		7	43
1825 . .	407	404	158	166	16	34	5	2	23
1826 . .	553	550	228	221	68	30		3	
1827 . .	428	428	189	148	67	18	3		3
1828 . .	544	548	269	172	59	29	5	3	11
1829 . .	535	527	299	135	51	32	6	1	3
1830 . .	423	429	221	124	46	33	2	2	1
1831 . .	448	444	213	153	38	28	2	3	7
1832 . .	447	448	259	100	38	44	1	4	2
1833 . .	515	522	272	152	53	31	7	7	
1834 . .	481	486	242	137	57	45	2	2	1
1835 . .	505	492	193	175	67	44	4	6	3
1836 . .	485	482	224	155	55	44	2	2	
1837 . .	440	453	206	152	54	32	7	2	
1838 . .	380	384	174	121	48	35	3	3	
1839 . .	369	360	128	161	40	19	11	1	
1840 . .	362	355	144	137	43	22	7	2	
1841 . .	404	403	151	152	53	26	18	3	
1842 . .	347	344	121	137	45	25	13	3	
1843 . .	365	364	136	115	55	41	16	1	
1844 . .	435	431	183	137	41	47	22	1	
1845 . .	453	454	205	130	37	54	26	2	
1846 . .	459	447	211	137	30	36	30	3	
1847 . .	674	626	340	145	54	57	27	2	1
1848 . .	804	813	400	219	52	103	35	1	3
1849 . .	870	866	436	218	75	84	45	1	7
1850 . .	746	744	363	200	56	76	47		2
	13549	13431	6265	4203	1313	1122	347	71	110
	13549 13431								
In house	118								

Total admissions on the books to
Dec. 31, 1850 13533   Do. to Sept. 1, 1851 14091
Total discharges on books to
Dec. 31, 1850 13420   ,,   ,,   ,, ... 13984
Remaining Dec. 31, 1850 . . . 113   ,,   ,,   ,, ... 107

This Table is formed from the official Quarterly Reports. There are books of admission and books of discharge, in which the numbers opposite to each name have been continued from the beginning. So that the difference between the numbers opposite the names of the patient last admitted, and of the patient last discharged. ought to show the total remaining in the Hospital. Accidental mistakes have, however, occurred from time to time, so that these numbers are not precisely accurate, either positively or relatively.

How much of joy and of sorrow, of life and of death, is compressed within this little table of admissions and discharges! An *army* of more than *thirteen thousand* sufferers received, comforted, and cared for in our institution; six thousand of these at last discharged well, and four thousand more, to a greater or less extent, relieved: on the other hand, more than eleven hundred of them borne from within our walls to their long home!* What can surpass the eloquence of statistics!

In view of the facts now presented, one or two concluding remarks may, with propriety, be made; and, first, the question may perhaps fairly be asked, whether an institution which has been already thus liberally endowed needs, or can ever need, any further aid. To this I answer, that our two estates for the sick and the insane have cost over $500,000; that our present invested funds, as stated in the last annual report for 1851, were $171,119.98, to which add Mr. Wilder's legacy, since received, and the amount is about $200,000, yielding an interest of $12,000,— making, with the annual payment of $5,000 from the

* This excessive mortality is explained by the fact that many are brought to the Hospital in a dying condition from recent accidents.

NEED OF FURTHER AID. 449

Massachusetts Hospital Life Insurance Company, a total income of $17,000. The reversionary property to which the Hospital is eventually entitled, on the decease of certain tenants for life, &c., will not probably be received for many years, nor until the increasing wants of the institution will exhaust all the additional income thus derived.* The number of patients at the Asylum is now two hundred, — as many, it is believed by the Trustees, as should ever be under the care of one physician. This department,

---

* If from the total donations, &c. $1,257,510.08
We deduct the amounts hitherto received from
   the Life Insurance Company $150,687.50
Also the free-bed subscriptions 65,069.17

The same having been received and expended
   as income $215,756.67
Also the estimated value of the life-office charters, which may be at any time annulled by
   the Legislature 100,000.00
Also the reversionary interests not receivable for
   many years 210,000.00
                                                                                             525,756.67

There will remain for the cost of Hospital and Asylum, and
   the invested funds yielding income $731,753.41
The actual balance on the Treasurer's books, January, 1851, is
   $700,029.38, which, of course, does not include Dr. Wilder's legacy of $20,000, &c.
By the Treasurer's books, it appears that the —
   Cost of Hospital to January, 1851, was . . $269,463.92
   Cost of Asylum to January, 1851, was . . 246,345.98
   Cost of Mr. Appleton's new buildings will be 20,000.00
                                                                              535,809.90

The balance is the value of the whole invested property . . . $195,943.51
           Or say about $200,000.

therefore, will never be materially enlarged. The amount charged for board of its inmates was, during the last year, $44,183.87. It fully supports itself, or defrays its own current annual expenses.* But there are no free beds in that department, and no means available for reducing the expenses of its patients, except the six hundred dollars a year derived from Mr. Appleton's ten thousand dollar fund. Now, it is obvious that the sum of six or even twelve thousand dollars a year could be advantageously applied for that object. This alone would absorb the income of an additional hundred and fifty thousand dollars. Further, the grounds of the Asylum are by no means sufficiently extensive. There should be a small farm for cultivation, besides more spacious enclosures for gardens, &c. One hundred thousand dollars more would perhaps be judiciously expended for these objects. Though this department, therefore, is at present carried on without being a burden to the general funds of the Corporation, an additional donation of two or three hundred thousand dollars could be most usefully applied in reducing the expenses and increasing the comforts of its large band of unfortunate inmates.

* Any apparent annual surplus of *receipts* from the Asylum is believed to be less than the salaries of the officers, which, being paid by the Treasurer from the general funds, increase to that extent the *expenses* of this department.

NEED OF FURTHER AID.

At the Hospital in Boston, there are eighty free beds; and, of the remaining patients, few pay over three dollars, — about half the actual cost. The result is, as stated in the last report, that its annual expenses exceed its annual receipts by the large sum of twenty-five thousand dollars; while, as we have just seen, our whole yearly income is but seventeen thousand dollars.* This deficiency has hitherto been made good by private subscriptions for free beds, and by those occasional bequests, &c., from year to year, by which the diminished property of the institution has been replaced. The permanent supply of this deficiency would require an additional donation of a hundred and fifty thousand dollars. A separate building for the accommodation of contagious, offensive, or delirious patients, is at this very time urgently pressed upon the notice of the Trustees. The mere cost

---

* The salaries of the institution are as follows: —

Treasurer	$500
Secretary and Auditor	200
Physician of Asylum, including annual grant of $500	2000
Steward and Matron of Asylum	1450
Assistant Physician of Asylum	700
Male Supervisor of Asylum	500
Female Supervisor of Asylum	400
Superintendent of Hospital	1500
Admitting Physician of Hospital	200
Apothecary of Hospital, say (average)	300
Four Medical and Surgical House-pupils at Hospital, $50 each	200
	$7950

of a suitable fence is estimated at ten or fifteen thousand dollars; and the Board have not hitherto felt themselves justified in ordering one, though well aware that the present unsightly structure disfigures and disgraces the institution. Besides, the Hospital at present accommodates only about a hundred and twenty patients,— a number extremely small, when compared with that in any similar establishment of the Old World. The necessity of another separate Hospital has been, for this reason, already strenuously and ably urged upon the consideration of the City Government. There can be no doubt, indeed, that, with the growing necessities of an advancing population, additional buildings must and will be eventually erected within our enclosure, — greatly increasing the cost of this portion of our fixed property, and also its future annual expenses. An additional donation of two or three hundred thousand dollars for the ultimate extension of this department would probably be a most judicious and useful charity.

One other question also perhaps remains to be asked, viz., Have the large sums already given by the community been faithfully managed and applied? and have the results of our two departments been commensurate with the magnitude of the means placed at our disposal? To this inquiry, I trust that the present publication will afford a satisfactory reply. It has certainly been the constant endeavor of the Trustees to check, and, if possible, prevent, all abuses. In their appointments to office, they have always aimed at selecting, without fear or favor, those individuals whom they conscientiously believed to be best qualified. The general fitness and wisdom of these appointments they fearlessly leave to the judgment of an intelligent public. Where, indeed, can be found physicians more wise or more kind than those who, from year to year, have stood by the bedside of our patients? or surgeons more skilful than those to whose firm and cautious hands, we have, from year to year, entrusted their lives and limbs as, if need were, we would have unhesitatingly submitted our own? Where are nurses more faithful and devoted than our own "sisters of charity"? Who could have better "ministered to the mind diseased" than those who have successively been called by us to that highest of human trusts, — the cure of insanity? How ably have the complicated details of our two establishments been managed by those to whom, from time to time, we have confided that difficult and delicate task! That deficiencies exist, indeed, in each department of the institution, its Trustees are well aware. For instance, inadequate opportunities for air and exercise afforded to the female patients at the Asylum,* and a tendency to an excess of foreigners among the patients at the Hospital, they feel to be evils; and the latter especially one of the greatest magnitude, tending to the entire violation of the intent of its original founders. The Admitting Physician has been requested to use the utmost vigilance on this point, that none may be received who should properly be sent to the city institutions at South Boston. The admission of such patients creates in the minds of our own citizens a prejudice against the Hospital, making them unwilling to enter it,— and thus tends directly to lower the general standing and character of its inmates. Some such admissions must unavoidably take place. Thus there has always existed a most excellent rule, that every case of sudden accident may at once be brought to the Hospital. A broken arm or leg is a plenary certificate, entitling the *bearer* to all its benefits. Of these sufferers by accidents, — laborers on railroads, canals, buildings, &c., — a very large proportion are Irish. Some of them are, in all respects, most deserving and suitable persons; while others are so repulsive in their personal habits and appearance

[* It would have afforded Mr. Bowditch the highest satisfaction to have known how this deficiency has been met since his death by extensive purchases of additional land.]

as to be disgusting and offensive to those near them, and most unwelcome and unfit guests for our neat and orderly establishment.*

On the whole, however, it is believed that both institutions have been uniformly managed with great fidelity and success. Massachusetts has, indeed, within her borders no nobler monuments than her General Hospital for the sick, and her M'Lean Asylum for the insane. Glorious memorials of Christian charity, teachers of the great lesson of man's brotherhood to man! long may ye stand, an honor to the ages past, a blessing throughout the ages to come!

* In such cases, the primary medical prescription is a warm bath; and, in many instances, a bath of any kind is obviously an entire novelty. An Irishman of this class was received into a sister institution, and made perfectly clean. As he emerged from the unwonted process, the physician said to him, "Well, Patrick, how do you feel?" His reply was, "Och faith! yer honor, and sure I can't tell ye till to-morrow; for 'tis the first time in me life I ever tried it."

CONTINUATION OF THE HISTORY

FROM 1851 TO 1872.

PREPARED BY REQUEST IN A VOTE OF THE TRUSTEES, CHIEFLY FROM THE RECORDS AND ANNUAL REPORTS.

CHAPTER XIII.

From August 5, 1851, to March 16, 1856.

Mr. Bowditch's History: Its Value. — Thanks of the Committee of Trustees. — Claim of the Corporation on a Life Insurance Company. — Pipes for the Cochituate Water. — Visitors to the Railroad Jubilee. — Charges for Out-of-Town Patients. — Dr. Warren's Gift of Surgical Instruments. — Indexes to Hospital Records. — Contract for Water. — Office of Chemist and Microscopist. — Dr. J. Bacon, jun., elected thereto. — Case of Alleged Abuse at Asylum Investigated. — Bequest from Mrs. Salisbury. — Report for 1851. — Improvements at the Asylum. — Organization for 1852. — Tribute to Mr. Rogers. — A Question of Prerogative. — Legacy from J. Ingersoll. — Sad Occurrence at the Hospital. — Resignation of Dr. J. C. Warren. — Annual Meeting. — Organization for 1853. — Report for 1852. — Resignation of Mr. Goodhue. — New Supervisors at the Asylum. — Another Offering from Mr. Bowditch. — Tribute to Hon. S. Appleton. — Hospital Index. — Additional Physician at Asylum. — Annual Meeting. — Organization for 1854. — Report for 1853. — Bequest of Judah Touro. — Death of Dr. Shattuck. — Building of a Foul Ward. — Dr. J. Homans elected a Consulting Physician. — Dr. M. Ranney, Assistant-Physician at Asylum. — Pathological Museum. — Gift from S. Appleton's Estate. — Gift of J. B. Bradlee. — Dr. C. Ellis, Curator of the Pathological Cabinet. — Death of Dr. S. Parkman. — Dr. G. H. Gay elected a Visiting Surgeon. — Annual Meeting, 1855. — Organization. — Report for 1854. — Tribute to J. P. Bigelow. — Microscopist at the Hospital. — Resignation of Dr. J. Bigelow. — Additional Rooms at Hospital. — Bequest of Miss E. Pratt. — New Fence at Hospital. — Annual Meeting. — Organization for 1856. — Report for 1855. — Resignation of Dr. Bell: his Farewell.

The report to the Trustees of the Hospital, made by the Committee for the year 1851, closes with the following acknowledgment of the labor of love and zeal done by Mr. Bowditch in behalf of the Institution, which he had served with such fidelity in very many ways : —

"Your Committee would also, among the important events of last year, notice the publication of a most valuable and interesting History of the Hospital, by the private liberality of the Chairman of this Board, who has for so many years aided the government of the Institution by his counsel and experience, and cheered its inmates by his kindness and encouraging sympathy."

Mr. Bowditch was at that time Chairman of the Board of Trustees, which office he held till 1856, when, at the annual meeting of the Corporation, he was elected Vice-President, being annually re-elected as such till his death in April, 1861.

It will be most fitting to defer to the summary of the History of the Institution for the year last mentioned an appropriate tribute to that honored man, whose large and beautiful culture, added to fine natural endowments, whose sensibility of feeling, whose wise practical judgment and varied labors of love and ingenuity were devoted to its welfare.

The last abstract in Mr. Bowditch's History is of the business of the Board of Trustees at its meeting on July 15, 1851. Several matters of interest and importance engaged the action of the Board before the close of that year. At the meeting on Aug. 5,

Rejoice Newton, Esq., was authorized to take proper legal steps for collecting of the State Mutual Life Insurance Company the proportion of profits to which this Corporation is entitled. An instrument, executed by the President, William Appleton, Esq., with the Boston and Lowell Railroad Corporation respecting the laying of the Cochituate water-pipes along a portion of the line of that road, was adopted and ratified. At the meeting of the Board on Sept. 16, an invitation was extended to the expected guests of the city, from Canada and elsewhere, for the approaching Railroad Jubilee, to visit both departments of this institution, in Boston and Somerville, at their convenience. Messrs. Appleton, Hooper, and Bowditch were chosen a Committee to receive such visitors.

At the meeting on Oct. 10, it was voted that when the Admitting Physician is called to visit patients, applicants for admission to the Hospital, who reside outside of the limits of the city proper, he is authorized to charge such patients the usual fee for his services; and if they are unable to pay, he is to charge the same to the Hospital. A letter was received by the Board at its meeting, Nov. 2, from Dr. John C. Warren, accompanying the gift from him of a valuable case of surgical instruments, when it was voted, " That the Trustees gratefully accept the same; and that they would present to Dr. Warren their sincere thanks for this new instance of his continued interest in this institution." The Physicians and Surgeons made a communication to the Board, which was referred for report to Messrs. Dale and Stevenson, relative to the appointment of a Chemist and Microscopist for the Hospital.

At the meeting on Nov. 16, the Board, continuing its care for securing proper Indexes to its Medical and Surgical Records, acknowledged the receipt of a fifth volume of the Index prepared by Dr. Thayer; and the Treasurer was authorized to pay him one hundred and twenty-five dollars therefor. The Chairman, Mr. Bowditch, was authorized to execute, on the part of this Corporation, with the Cochituate Water Board of Boston, an instrument concerning the privilege allowed of connecting with the water-pipes, and drawing therefrom for the use of the Asylum, and also regulating the rates of payment. The Committee on the appointment of a Chemist and Microscopist made a report, which was accepted; and the votes recommended by them were passed, — that such an officer should be elected annually by the Trustees, at the first meeting succeeding the annual meeting of the Corporation, with a statement of the scientific qualifications which should be required, and a defining of the duties to be exacted of him, in the Medical and Surgical Departments, in attendance on autopsies within the walls of the Hospital, and in the preparation of records of his observations, with the privilege, when matters of sufficient importance have accumulated as results, of publishing them to the world, under the patronage of the Hospital, and at the discretion of the Surgeons and Physicians. At the next meeting of the Board, on Nov. 30, Dr. John Bacon, jun., was chosen Chemist and Microscopist for the remainder of the year.

Dr. Bell reported another of the cases occasionally arising at the Asylum, of a complaint on the part of a patient of alleged maltreatment, and requested the appointment of a committee to investigate the case. Messrs. Bowditch, Rogers, Lawrence, and Stevenson were accordingly appointed as such a committee. The matter is regarded as worthy of mention here only as it illustrates the care and patience and fidelity which have uniformly been engaged on the part of the Trustees in the thorough examination of every similar complaint brought against the officials in charge of either branch of this institution, or against any subordinate or attendant. As might be expected, the report of the Committee, made at the next meeting, Dec. 14, asserted that, after the most minute and impartial investigation of the case, the charge alleged was wholly groundless. The Secretary was instructed to read this report to the attorneys of the complainant if they should be desirous of hearing it.

Messrs. Dale and Dexter were appointed to examine the Treasurer's accounts and to prepare the annual report.

At the meeting of the Board Dec. 28, a letter was read which was received by the Treasurer from Stephen Salisbury, Esq., of Worcester. The writer informed the Board that his mother, recently deceased, left no will, but that he found among her papers a memorandum expressing her wish that $4,000 of her property should be given to the Massachusetts General Hospital. In conformity with this wish, Mr. Salisbury enclosed a check for that sum. In accepting and acknowledging this gift, the Board recognized the interest which the late Mrs. Salisbury had for many years manifested in this institution by the maintenance of a free bed at the Hospital, and lamented in her death the loss of a benefactress. The Board also recognized " in the prompt and cordial fulfilment of her benevolent intentions a graceful and an honorable act of filial piety." A vote was passed making it the duty of the House Pupils, in the Medical and Surgical Departments respectively, to make up and present at the quarterly meetings of the Board the Indexes to the Medical and Surgical Records. The Superintendent was directed, under the advice of the Chairman, to procure tablets to be placed on or under each of the portraits in the Hospital, each tablet to contain the name and date of the death of the original of the portrait. This direction was carried into effect in November of the next year. At the quarterly meeting of the Board, held at the Asylum, Jan. 21, 1852, the salary of Homer Goodhue, the male Supervisor, was raised to $600 a year.

The report of the Trustees for 1851 — of which it was ordered that fifteen hundred copies should be printed — was presented to the Corporation at the annual meeting, Jan. 28, 1852. It appeared from the Treasurer's accounts that the whole income of the year had been $21,391.32, and that the expenses had been $45,619.13. The report makes grateful mention of the munificent bequest of Dr. C. W. Wilder, and of the gift, through the son, of Mrs. Salisbury; it refers to the loss of the valuable services of Dr. George Hayward, through his resignation, and to the appointment of Dr. H. G. Clark, as his successor; — these, with the election of new House Pupils and of Dr. J. Bacon, jun., as Chemist and Microscopist, being the only changes in the Medical Staff for the year. From the report of Mr. Girdler, the Superintendent of the Hospital, it appeared that the whole number of patients for the year was 839, at an average weekly expense for board of $4.84. Attention was again urged to the necessity of a new building for the reception of contagious, foul, and other disorders; and notice was taken of an accompanying communication from Dr. Samuel Parkman, one of the Surgeons, on the advantages of an additional wing with separate rooms for single patients.

Dr. Bell reported the whole number of patients that had been under treatment at the Asylum during the year as 364, and as remaining at the close of the year, 191. Dr. Bell renews his reference to the fact that the Asylum is generally filled to its utmost capacity, and that, though he is constantly obliged to refuse applications for admission, he never does so except the number of patients would exceed two hundred. He regards it as never permissible or justifiable to put two patients in one room.

After a reference to the commencement and progress of the new Appleton wards, Dr. Bell gives an elaborate account of the introduction of the Cochituate water. The Asylum had suffered from its commencement from the want of an adequate supply of water for bathing and laundry purposes: the deep wells through the diluvial gravel of the hill, while affording what was exceedingly fine for drinking, were so highly impregnated with sulphate of lime as to interfere with their uses for cleansing. Though by conduits from the roofs and capacious cisterns, the rain-water which fell upon an acre and a half of surface was availed of, it proved insufficient; and this had to be raised to the tops of the buildings, and distributed by expensive methods. On the introduction of the Cochituate water into Boston, and the subsequent provision for the supply of East Boston by crossing Charles River into Charlestown through pipes and an inverted syphon under the channel, a successful application was made by the Board to the Water Commissioners for permission to convey the water from Charlestown Square, through its territory, for about two thousand feet, to the flats at the State Prison, whence, by about the same additional distance, it might be carried to the Asylum. Permission was then asked of the Charlestown authorities to lay the necessary pipes, — all costs and risks, of course, being assumed by the Hospital Corporation. "With a degree of surprise beyond the power of language to express," says Dr. Bell, the authorities of Charlestown made the granting of the privilege conditional upon the provision by the Hospital of a series of hydrants for the use of the city. The Trustees, not being inclined to make from their funds this contribution to the fire apparatus of Charlestown, turned, as an alternative, to a route by the Lowell Railroad and its bridge. Full and unconditioned permission was granted on application for this privilege, though the necessary works had to be carried for more than a mile on the crowded track of that road. The full, pure stream poured into the Asylum in December, rising in the domes to a level about twelve feet below its surface in the Beacon-hill Reservoir. Dr. Bell describes very minutely the processes and the materials used in this enterprise. Block-tin pipes were preferred, from 2 to $2\frac{1}{4}$ inches in diameter, in lengths of about 15 feet, united at the joints by melting the metal, instead of by soldering. The pipes cross a main bridge and three minor bridges, and are led under water in strongly ironed oak logs, the interstices being filled with plaster of Paris, and, where there was danger of freezing, enclosed in wooden boxings filled with melted resin. Though the cost of the undertaking was near $6,000, it was still found to be a saving one.

Dr. Bell again refers to that steady adaptation by which the furnishings, the arrangements, and the management of the Asylum have fitted it to afford the fullest means of comfort, and even of luxury, to a class of patients who had been used to a generous mode of life, and who with their friends were able and willing to pay more than remunerating charges therefor. In this way the Asylum is enabled to receive many patients in very restricted circumstances, either gratuitously or at rates much below the actual expense. In fact the major portion of its inmates, being charged much less than the actual outlay for their support and oversight, are receivers not only from the general fund of benevolence contributed to the institution, but also from the annual contributions in their behalf made by the friends of a few of the patients.

Dr. Bell closes his report by adverting briefly to those results of his experience so faithfully and intelligently acquired by him, which he sustains by a quotation from an eminent author and director of a similar institution, relating to the occasional complaints of discharged patients, or their unwise or uninformed or credulous friends. He had learned to bear patiently all the annoyances visited upon him from these sources, trusting, as he might, to the confidence reposed in him by the Trustees in their constant routine of inspection, and to the thorough investigation of each and every case, however mistaken or groundless the allegations of complaint or rumor.

The annual meeting of the Corporation was held on Jan. 28, 1852, and the first meeting of the Board of Trustees after it was held on Feb. 22. It appeared that the following officers had been elected for the ensuing year: viz., William Appleton, President; Robert Hooper, Vice-President; Henry

Andrews, Treasurer; Marcus Morton, jun., Secretary; Messrs. N. I. Bowditch, G. M. Dexter, A. A. Lawrence, F. C. Lowell, C. H. Mills, G. H. Shaw, J. T. Stevenson, and E. Wigglesworth, Trustees on the part of the Corporation; and Messrs. J. P. Bigelow, W. S. Bullard, W. J. Dale, and T. Lamb, Trustees on the part of the Commonwealth. N. I. Bowditch was elected, by ballot, Chairman of the Board for the ensuing year. The officers of the Hospital and Asylum for the year were chosen as follows: Drs. J. Jackson, J. Jeffries, G. C. Shattuck, and E. Reynolds, as a Board of Consultation; Drs. J. Bigelow, J. B. S. Jackson, G. C. Shattuck, jun., H. I. Bowditch, M. S. Perry, and D. H. Storer, Visiting Physicians; Drs. J. C. Warren, S. D. Townsend, J. Mason Warren, S. Parkman, H. J. Bigelow, and H. G. Clark, Visiting Surgeons; Dr. J. Bacon, jun., Chemist and Microscopist; Dr. S. L. Abbot, Admitting Physician; R. Girdler, Superintendent of the Hospital; Dr. L. V. Bell, Physician and Superintendent of the M'Lean Asylum; Columbus Tyler, Steward; and Mrs. M. E. Tyler, Matron. The Standing Committees of the Board were appointed, and the Visiting Committees were arranged for the year. Henry B. Rogers not having been re-appointed a Trustee on the part of the State, the Board, by a preamble and vote, unanimously passed, presented to him its thanks for his twelve years of devoted service.

"In the annals of this charity," reads the vote, "there will hardly be found an instance of more devoted official fidelity. To his personal influence and exertions, more than to any other cause, we are indebted for that noble public subscription, which, by the enlargement of the Hospital, has doubled its means of usefulness. He was vigilant in enforcing a prudent economy in the expenditures of the institution. Our records bear witness to his clear and able reports on the various important subjects which, from time to time, were submitted to his consideration. The donation book has been under his exclusive control. His votes have always been given in accordance with his convictions of duty, even when they involved the sacrifice of personal feelings."

Happily the Board was not to be long deprived of the services of this faithful member of it.

At the next meeting of the Trustees, on May 7, a letter of reply from Mr. Rogers was received and read. On the nomination of Dr. Bell, Dr. C. Booth was elected Assistant Physician; Homer Goodhue, male Supervisor; and Miss R. R. Barber, female Supervisor of the Asylum.

A communication from the Physicians and Surgeons was laid before the Board, asking whether they should not return a negative answer to an inquiry made of them by the House Pupils, — "If they are to consider themselves amenable in matters purely medical and surgical to any officer of the Corporation, other than the attending Physicians and Surgeons?" The action of the Trustees, when this "inquiry" came before them, might well be inferred from their own sense of their duties, rights, and responsibilities, from their ready and courteous recognition of the professional and official claims of those to whom they delegated authority within the walls of the Hospital, and from their intention to retain their own reserved authority, even if the assertion of it involved a rebuke to any who might bring it under question. It was —

Voted, "That every officer of the Hospital, in the discharge of his duties, is responsible to the Board of Trustees. In matters purely medical or surgical, indeed, the Board confide in the ability and discretion of gentlemen selected by themselves, and would not think of interfering with their prescriptions or practice. But should a specific charge be made against any Physician or Surgeon, either of a want of competency and skill, or of humanity or delicacy in the treatment of a patient, the Trustees would feel it to be not only their right, but their duty, to investigate the circumstances of the case, and to act as in their opinion should be required by a due regard to the interests of the Institution and of the community. So likewise the Trustees will not interfere with the professional duties prescribed to medical and surgical pupils by their immediate superiors, but will, nevertheless, at all times, hold them accountable for the performance of those duties in an exact, kind, and proper manner."

Voted, "That the Trustees cannot refrain from expressing their surprise at the inquiry thus submitted by the medical and surgical pupils, — an inquiry which would seem to be founded on an entire misapprehension of their own true position, and an unwillingness to recognize the paramount authority of this Board, or of its duly constituted committees."

A copy of the foregoing votes was ordered to be sent to each of the Physicians and Surgeons, and a Committee of the Trustees was instructed "to inquire whether there has been any want of due subordination and propriety on the part of any of the House Pupils," and especially to investigate the circumstances of a case which had been brought to the notice of the Visiting Committee. The same Committee was to consider and report whether it was expedient to make any change in the rules and regulations in regard to House Pupils. As was to be expected, frankness and a mutual understanding disposed of this question. Up to this time, the semi-monthly meetings of the Trustees had been held at the Hospital, after the close of the second service on Sunday. The meeting on Monday, June 7, 1852, was held at the American Insurance Office, in State Street, as were also several subsequent meetings. At the meeting on June 21, a communication was received from Jacob A. Dresser, announcing a legacy of $2,000 to the Hospital, by the will of James Ingersoll, deceased. Grateful acknowledgments were passed for this bequest. The Board, at its meeting on Aug. 17, elected George G. Tucker Hospital Apothecary.

At the meeting of the Trustees on Nov. 21, action was taken on an occasion the occurrence of which was the cause of painful interest within the walls of the Hospital and to the community outside of it. At the meeting of the Board on Nov. 7, the case of James Clancey, who had died on that day in the Hospital, had been referred for full investigation and report to a special Committee. The report, which was submitted at a meeting on Nov. 10, and then laid upon the table for future consideration, was acted upon at a meeting on Nov. 15, and, after being amended, was unanimously accepted, and ordered to be recorded at this meeting, on the 21st. It appeared from the report, after a most thorough investigation, that by a mistake which had occurred, without, however, involving any culpable neglect on the part of the Hospital Apothecary, the Surgeons accidentally administered chloroform for the usual preparation of chloric ether, to three subjects of operations. The third of these patients, James Clancey, whose arm had been amputated, after the use of the anæsthetic, sunk into a state of insensibility, from which he was recovered only to die in a few hours afterwards; and also, that when he was apparently in a dying condition, one of the Surgeons " accidentally poured into his mouth a quantity of undiluted caustic ammonia."

The Committee considered the circumstances as disclosed to be of a very serious character. After a very full discussion, the Board, " having good reason to believe that every precaution will be taken to prevent such deplorable accidents in future," voted, " That no further action be had in the premises." Also voted, " That this event is a solemn warning to all persons connected with the Hospital to exercise the greatest care in the performance of the delicate and difficult duties which devolve upon them."

At the meeting on Dec. 5, Messrs. Bigelow and Lawrence were appointed a Committee to examine the Treasurer's accounts, and to prepare the annual report.

At the meeting on Jan. 2, 1853, Messrs. Dexter and Lowell gave notice that they should decline a re-election as Trustees.

The Trustees received at their meeting on Jan. 19, 1853, the following letter of that date from Dr. John C. Warren : —

"Gentlemen, — For some years I have contemplated resigning the office of Surgeon in the Massachusetts General

Hospital. The desire of transmitting to others the results of my experience has hitherto prevented the execution of this design. Having accomplished the proposed object as well as I could, I would now request that my name be not included among the candidates at your next election; desiring you at the same time to accept my thanks for the confidence which you have so long extended to me. And I would further ask leave to add that, in the performance of my professional duties, that to the Hospital has ever stood paramount in my mind to all others."

The preamble and vote which were thereupon passed by the Trustees must be copied here, alike on the score of their historical as of their personal character: —

"More than forty years ago Dr. Warren, and his associate, Dr. James Jackson, by an admirable circular letter, first called the attention of the public to the necessity of a Hospital. Becoming thus one of our original founders, he was appointed our first Surgeon, and has been annually re-elected to that office ever since.

"His name has become illustrious in the annals of American Surgery, and reflects honor on the Institution which is so deeply indebted to him for its establishment and success. Finding here those opportunities of professional practice by which his own skill and experience were from year to year increased, he has, in return, devoted to the gratuitous performance of his official duties among us much time and thought during a long life. By pecuniary donations and otherwise, he has manifested a continued interest in the welfare of the Hospital. And now that, having completed his labors, he is about to retire from this honorable and responsible situation, the Trustees would assure him of their best wishes for his future health and happiness. And they would congratulate the Institution and himself on the circumstance that he leaves behind him in our service, and, as we hope, for many years to come, a son whose high professional skill and attainments are universally recognized as worthy of his parentage.

" *Voted*, That Dr. Warren be requested to sit for his bust or portrait, to be preserved at the Hospital, and that Messrs. Lowell and Dexter be a Committee to communicate to him this wish of the Trustees."

The report and documents for the year being received were ordered to be laid before the Corporation at the coming annual meeting.

At the meeting of the Board on Feb. 6, 1853, after the annual meeting of the Corporation held on that day, it appeared that the same officers of the Hospital had been elected as in the last year on the part of the Corporation and of the Board of Visitors; except that, on the part of the former, Messrs. Dexter and Lowell having declined further service, Messrs. Henry B. Rogers and Charles H. Warren were chosen in their places. All the members of the Board were present, and Mr. N. I. Bowditch was re-elected Chairman. It was voted so to amend a rule both of the Hospital and the Asylum that the Board of Consultation should henceforward consist of three, instead of two, Physicians and Surgeons.

Drs. J. Jackson, Jeffries, Shattuck, Reynolds, Hayward, and J. C. Warren, were by ballot elected a Board of Consultation; Drs. Bigelow, Storer, J. B. S. Jackson, Bowditch, Shattuck, jun., and Perry, Visiting Physicians; Drs. Townsend, J. Mason Warren, Parkman, H. J. Bigelow, Clarke, and Cabot, Visiting Sugeons; Dr. John Bacon, jun., Chemist and Microscopist; Dr. S. L. Abbot, Admitting Physician; R. Girdler, Superintendent of the Hospital; Dr. Bell Physician and Superintendent, and Columbus Tyler Steward, and Mrs. Mary E. Tyler Matron, of the Asylum. The Standing Committees were appointed, and the Visiting Committees were arranged for the year.

It was ordered that two thousand copies of the report be printed. The portion of it coming from the Committee covers seven pages. The property of the Institution, exclusive of reversions, grounds, and buildings, is set at $197,257, and the income at $23,727. Acknowledgment is made of the bequest of the late James Ingersoll, of Boston, of $2,000. The number of patients admitted to the Hospital had been 826. The expenses had been $30,173, of which $5,359 had been repaid by paying patients. The weekly expense of each patient had been $4.54. The necessity of a foul ward is again mentioned. Reference of a very earnest character is made to the sad case already related, of the death of a patient, caused apparently by mistake in the administration of appliances, which was "the subject of public comment and inquiry." The retirement of Dr. J. C. Warren is noticed.

Dr. Bell reports the number of patients in the Asylum, in the course of the year, as 336; remaining, 201. He is again obliged to speak of the over-demand upon the accommodations of the Asylum, involving the rejection of as many patients as had been received, with the pain of constantly turning back from the doors anxious, exhausted, and hopeful friends, who had brought their charges trusting for relief. The other New England Asylums, public and private, he says, are filled, while insanity is probably an augmenting form of disease. The proportion of incurable cases under his charge naturally increases from the kind care they receive, when, from year to year, they are the residuum of the whole number. Dr. Bell reiterates his protest against any refuges for the insane, save those over which the community legally, or by a Board of Visitors, exercises control. Philanthropy, by generous gifts and bequests, must henceforward, as heretofore, provide what the public cannot be expected to furnish for those having means of their own. Even after the Appleton wards, which are in progress, shall be completed, the fair extent of accommodations, looking at the highest order of arrangements, will not admit of more than 160 patients, though, by the use of attics and corners, 210 have been within the walls. Dr. Bell found seventy patients when he came to his charge, so that the number had trebled. Considering it a settled point that this is as large a number as ought to be under one supervision and in one institution, he proceeds, at some length, to suggest a plan of expansion and relief. He recommends the establishment, in another place, near to Boston, of a duplicate institution for the insane, under the patronage and management of the same Corporation, either for patients of both sexes, or, as he should advise, for female patients exclusively, — that at Somerville being retained for male patients. He argues that, depending upon the generosity, munificence, and philanthropy, which had heretofore so lavishly sustained the objects of the Corporation, they might expect the means to be furnished them for the first establishment of such a duplicate institution. Afterwards, he thinks, it would be self-supporting; the richer class of patients covering much of the expense of maintenance beyond the actual cost for them, and the experience of the past being availed of to make all the outlays for the new constructions much less than had been spent upon the alterations, adaptations, extensions, and patchings up of the buildings at Somerville. Of course, Dr. Bell offered these suggestions with the allowance that they were of such a nature, and involved so many serious conditions, that the Trustees could not be expected at present to do more than give them a hearing.

At the same meeting of the Board, the Chairman was "requested to collect, if possible, a complete set of the reports and other documents of the Hospital, and to have them bound and placed in the library." Mr. Bowditch had already earnestly devoted his researches to that object; and the Trustees committed the matter to one most willing and competent to effect it.

At the meeting of the Board, Feb. 20, a letter was received from Homer Goodhue, resigning the office of male Supervisor at the Asylum. In accepting his resignation, the Trustees instructed the Visiting Committee to express "their regret at parting with one who had so long and faithfully performed the responsible duties of his office, and to request his acceptance of a gold watch, with a suitable inscription upon its case, as a testimonial of their appreciation of his services."

The Trustees, at their meeting on March 6, sanctioned an arrangement made by Dr. Perry with his associates, for the performance of his duties during his proposed visit to Europe. A change was made in the term of service of the House Officers, so that henceforward they should enter upon their duties on the first day of May of each year.

At the meeting of the Board, on March 20, at the nomination of Dr. Bell, George C. Lincoln was elected male Supervisor, and Miss Relief R. Barber female Supervisor, of the Asylum, — the salary of the former being fixed at $500. The Visiting Committee were authorized to procure a new operating chair for the Hospital. The Chairman, Mr. Bowditch, received the thanks of the Board for the bound volumes of reports and other Hospital documents, which he presented at this meeting.

On May 22, the Trustees, at their meeting, acted on the report of a Committee, to whom had been referred the consideration of a proposed change in the regulation concerning House Pupils. It was then voted that but one of them each, in the Medical and Surgical Departments of the Hospital, should reside within the walls, and live in the family of the Superintendent, — neither of them more than six months in any one year, nor less than three months consecutively. One of the House Pupils was to be within the walls at all times.

After the business of the Board, at its meeting

on July 15, had been done, the Chairman proposed the following preamble and vote, which were unanimously adopted: —

"The funeral of the late Hon. Samuel Appleton takes place this afternoon, and the bells of the city are now tolling as a public expression of respect for one of its worthiest sons and its noblest benefactors, who, at the advanced age of eighty-seven years, has died universally beloved and regretted. Formerly a Trustee of this institution, and always cherishing a lively interest in its welfare, we are happy to acknowledge our indebtedness to him, alike for his valuable personal services, and for a large share of that bounty which he has always so wisely and so liberally bestowed.

"This Board would present to the widow of the deceased, by whose affectionate attentions and devoted care his life has been for so many years prolonged and rendered happy, the assurances of their profound sympathy, now that she has lost a companion and friend by whom she was ever most tenderly beloved. *Voted*, That this Board do now adjourn to attend the funeral of the deceased."

An Analytical Index of the Surgical Records of the Hospital, made by Dr. Samuel Kneeland, jun., had been laid before this meeting, for which thanks and compensation were voted, with a request to Dr. Kneeland to continue the Index.

At the meeting of the Board, Nov. 20, 1853, a letter was received from Dr. S. L. Abbot, accompanying the Index of the Medical Records, made up by him to vol. 186, inclusive, for which compensation was voted.

At the meeting of the Trustees on Dec. 4, Messrs. Warren and Dale were appointed a Committee to examine the Treasurer's accounts, and to prepare the annual report. At their meeting on Dec. 18, the Trustees authorized Dr. Bell to employ an additional Assistant Physician at the Asylum, at a salary not exceeding that paid to Dr. Booth.

The annual meeting of the Corporation was held at the Hospital on Jan. 25, 1854. The first subsequent meeting of the Trustees was held on Feb. 5. It then appeared that the officers of the last year had been re-elected, except that, in place of Mr. A. A. Lawrence, Mr. Robert M. Mason had been chosen a Trustee on the part of the Corporation. Mr. Bowditch was re-elected Chairman for the ensuing year. The same members of the Board of Consultation, the same Visiting Physicians and Surgeons, Chemist and Microscopist, Admitting Physician, Superintendent of the Hospital, Physician and Superintendent, and Steward and Matron of the Asylum, were re-elected, as had already proved their ability and fidelity in previous service. The Standing Committees were appointed, and the Visiting Committees were arranged for the year. It was voted that two thousand copies of the annual report be printed. From this report it appeared that the income of the Corporation for the last year had been $21,672.48; the pecuniary property of the institution being $182,212.88. There had been admitted into the Hospital 925 patients. The average weekly expense of each patient was $4.87. The expenses of the Hospital were $32,615.30, of which sum only $5,562.27 were paid by patients. Dr. Samuel Cabot, jun., had been elected a Visiting Surgeon on the resignation of Dr. John C. Warren. The Hospital is pronounced to be in good condition, as regards economy and discipline; and the officers are spoken of with high approval.

Dr. Bell reported that 114 new patients had been received into the Asylum, 195 remaining at the end of the year. This was also the average number of patients within the walls, being more than was consistent with the best care and comfort of the inmates. The pressure on the Asylum had been such that it was probable that three times as many applicants had been refused as had been accepted. Dr. Bell is obliged to remonstrate with his professional brethren for not ascertaining in each case, before sending a patient thither, whether there is a chance of accommodation. The responsibility thrown upon him has been very painful, either of incommoding and injuring all those within the walls, or of sending away an applicant in a state of prostration and danger. He reports most of the rooms in the new Appleton ward for males as occupied, and congratulates the Trustees on this provision of luxurious apartments for such as have been used to like privileges, — by a method, too, which so directly reduces the charges for support and oversight to the less favored in pecuniary resources. He renews his suggestion, founded on present and prospective needs, for the provision of another Asylum to be devoted to female patients. The Committee in the annual report look favorably on this suggestion, but do not feel able to promote it.

The Chairman in a letter to the Board communicated memoranda, which he had made and gathered in preparing matter for the tablets under the portraits, — of the dates of the birth and death of the benefactors of the Hospital. These memoranda are entered upon the records.

At the meeting of the Board on Feb. 19, the Visiting Committee presented a surgical operating chair invented by Dr. Henry J. Bigelow, and constructed under his supervision; and it was voted, "That in consideration of the excellence of the chair, and the ingenuity displayed by Dr. Bigelow in its construction, it be called 'The Bigelow Operating Chair,' in honor of the inventor."

The Trustees, at their meeting on March 19, received a communication from the executors of the late Judah Touro, of New Orleans, announcing a legacy in his will of $10,000 to the Hospital; whereupon the following preamble and votes were unanimously adopted: —

"More than thirty years ago there died in this city one, of Jewish faith and parentage, who bequeathed to this institution the sum of $10,000. The name of Touro has thenceforth been familiar to us as that of one of our chief benefactors. And now another of the same name and lineage, an eminent merchant, who for fifty years has resided in the distant city of New Orleans, has, by like liberal bequests, remembered the home of his own youth and its various charitable institutions which were the objects of his brother's bounty: therefore —

"*Voted*, That the Trustees, in accepting the legacy of the late Judah Touro, recognize in it an act prompted by fraternal love and a philanthropy not confined within the narrow bounds of time, place, or sect."

Another vote authorized the Treasurer to receive and make discharge for this generous legacy.

The death of Dr. George C. Shattuck, for many years one of the Consulting Physicians of the institution, having been announced by Dr. Dale, it was —

"*Voted*, That the Board have received the intelligence of the decease of Dr. Shattuck with deep regret. That they remember with grateful satisfaction his long and useful connection with the institution as one of the Board of Consultation. That in common with the citizens of Boston they deplore his loss as one who through a long and eminent career in his profession was distinguished for acts of disinterested benevolence to the poor, making his memory dear to this community. That his munificent donations to the cause of learning and science entitle him to the distinction of a public benefactor; and that in honor of his memory a record of these proceedings be made and transmitted to the family of the deceased."

After the subject had frequently been before the Board at its meetings, a Committee to whom it had been referred reported at this meeting in favor of erecting a building for patients suffering under offensive diseases, near the north-west corner of the Hospital grounds, at a cost of about $10,000. A remonstrance against said location from those residing near the Hospital was read; and it was voted that Messrs. Bullard, Rogers, and Wigglesworth be a Building Committee to erect a building according to the report of the said Committee.

At the meeting of the Trustees on April 22, Dr. John Homans was elected a Consulting Physician, in place of Dr. George C. Shattuck, deceased. Dr. Bell reported, at a meeting of the Board on July 18, that he had engaged Dr. Mark Ranney of the Butler Asylum as additional Assistant Physician. The salary for this new officer was fixed, at the meeting of the Trustees on Oct. 18, at $600.

The Physicians and Surgeons offered a communication to the Board at their meeting on Nov. 5, recommending the establishment of a Pathological Museum at the Hospital, and the Visiting Committee were instructed to report upon the subject. The Treasurer was authorized to execute, acknowledge, and deliver a legal instrument covenanting with the Boston and Lowell Railroad Corporation to establish no claim on the score of the privilege — which, by courtesy, had been granted the Hospital — of laying a gas-pipe from Boston across the track of said railroad to the Asylum; and agreeing at any time, when so requested, to remove the pipe at the charge of the Hospital. The Visiting Committee reported at the meeting, Nov. 19, that it was expedient to establish a Pathological Museum at the Hospital. Whereupon it was " voted that the report be accepted, and that the subject be referred back to the Committee to report a system of rules for the management of the Museum, and to nominate a suitable person as Curator."

At the meeting of the Board on Dec. 3, the following communication, from the trustees under the will of the late Samuel Appleton, was read, dated Boston, Nov. 18, 1854: —

"As trustees under the will of the late Samuel Appleton, and in accordance with what we believe would have been his wish, we have transferred to the Massachusetts General Hospital the following stocks, appraised according to the inventory of his estate, as nearly as may be, at the sum of ten thousand dollars; viz., five shares in the Amoskeag Manufacturing Company, one share in the Stark Mills, two shares in the Merrimack Manufacturing Company, and one share in the Appleton Manufacturing Company. This donation is made in trust to constitute a fund the income of which shall be applied to the relief of poor, curable patients at the M'Lean Asylum for the Insane. In other words, it is to be added to the existing 'Appleton Fund' of that department of the Institution."

Signed by N. Appleton, Wm. Appleton, and N. I. Bowditch. It was then —

"*Voted*, That the donation be accepted upon the terms mentioned in the said communication, and that the Secretary be directed to return the thanks of this Board to the trustees under the will of the late Samuel Appleton."

Mr. J. B. Bradlee having sent to the Treasurer $1,000, for the purpose of procuring a life free bed, it was —

"*Voted*, That art. 1, chap. 8, of the Rules and Regulations of the Hospital be so amended as to read as follows: 'All subscriptions for free beds shall date from Jan. 1, in each year, and any individual subscribing $100 shall be entitled to a free bed at the Hospital during that year; and on payment of $1,000, or of such a sum as the applicant would be required to pay for an annuity of $100 on the principles of life insurance, he shall be entitled to a free bed for life.'"

Messrs. Mason and Rogers were appointed a Committee to examine the Treasurer's accounts and prepare the annual report. A report from the Visiting Committee on a Pathological Cabinet was accepted, with its recommendations, which were as follows: that $100 be appropriated for commencing such a Cabinet; that a Curator for it should be chosen annually by the Trustees; that it should be his duty to preserve morbid specimens and arrange them in the way best fitted to make them useful; and that he should make all the autopsies excepting such as shall be made by the attending Physicians and Surgeons, and shall observe all the regulations now in force or that may be made respecting them. Upon the nomination of the same Committee, the Board then elected Dr. Calvin Ellis Curator of the Pathological Cabinet.

At the meeting of the Board on Dec. 31, the death of Dr. Samuel Parkman having been announced, it was —

"*Voted*, That this Board have heard with deep regret of the decease of Dr. Samuel Parkman, one of the Surgeons of the Hospital. Appointed to this high trust at the time of the enlargement of our building in 1846, he has, by professional skill and ability of the very highest order, reflected honor on the institution, while by his agreeable manners and amiable disposition he has won the sincere and universal regard of the officers and inmates. And now that his life of usefulness and virtue has been suddenly closed by severe disease while he was in the strength of manhood and in the full maturity of his powers, the Trustees deem it proper to place upon record an expression of their profound sense of the loss which they and our whole community have sustained by this bereavement."

The following votes of the Trustees, passed at this meeting, may be inserted here, as manifesting the pains taken to perfect the internal discipline of the Hospital: —

"*Voted*, That the Superintendent and House Officers be directed to see that the nurses of the Hospital are in their several wards each morning, ready for duty, before the night-watchers leave the ward-rooms for the day, in order that there may be no period of time when the patients shall be without attendants, and to report all cases of remissness to the Visiting Committee."

"*Voted*, That the Physicians, Surgeons, and other officers of the Hospital, be particularly requested to take notice of every thing which occurs within the building that, in their judgment, is detrimental to the health or comfort of the patients, inconsistent with the rules and regulations, or adverse in any way to the best interests of the establishment, and report the same to the Visiting Committee."

The Secretary was instructed to communicate these votes to all the officers, and the Superintendent was directed to impart them to the nurses and other attendants of the Hospital. Dr. George H. Gay was elected a Visiting Surgeon, in the place of Dr. Samuel Parkman.

At the annual meeting of the Corporation, Feb. 4, 1855, all the officers of the preceding year were re-elected, except that on the part of the Commonwealth Mr. Henry M. Holbrook was chosen a Trustee, in place of Mr. John P. Bigelow. At the subsequent meeting of the Board of Trustees, Mr. N. I. Bowditch was chosen Chairman. With the exception of Dr. John Homans, in place of Dr. G. C. Shattuck, deceased, on the Board of Consultation, and of Dr. G. H. Gay, in the place of Dr. Samuel Parkman, deceased, as one of the Visiting Surgeons, those Boards, and also that of the Visiting Physicians, remained as in the last year. Dr. J. Bacon, jun., was elected Chemist and Microscopist; Dr. Calvin Ellis, Curator of the Pathological Cabinet; Dr. Samuel L. Abbot Admitting Physician, Richard Girdler Superintendent, of the Hospital; and Dr. Luther V. Bell, Physician and Superintendent of the Asylum; Columbus Tyler Steward, and Mrs. Mary E. Tyler Matron, of the same. The Standing Committees were chosen, and the Visiting Committees were arranged for the ensuing year.

The Committee were authorized to print two thousand copies of the annual report. In this report the property of the Corporation from which income is derived is set at $206,042.02. The whole income of it for the year had been $25,291.40. There had been admitted to the Hospital 922 patients: the whole number under medical advice or treatment had been 1,041. The expenses of the Hospital had been $40,654.78, of which patients had paid $6,128.49. The average weekly expense of each had been $5.46. The internal condition of the Hospital was highly satisfactory, the Superintendent and all the officers having faithfully performed their duties. The successful establishment of a Pathological Cabinet is remarked upon. In view of preventing any serious encroachment on the funds, the Committee think that an effort should be made to reduce the number of patients supported wholly at the expense of the Hospital. The urgent need that had long been felt of a separate ward for cases of a foul and dangerous nature, to relieve and secure other patients from discomfort and risk, had during the year been supplied. At the cost of $12,000, including that for a necessary sea-wall, a commodious building of two stories, west of the main edifice, had been erected, containing sixteen rooms, with every needful convenience. Mr. Judah Touro's generous bequest recalls the remembrance of the like munificence of his brother, Abraham. Renewed gratitude is expressed to the trustees of the late Samuel Appleton, a former Trustee and Vice-President, for directing, in the exercise of the discretion left to them, so generous an apportionment of his estate to this institution. Attention is called to the dilapidated state of the fence, and the opportunity for embellishing and improving by walks, shrubbery, flowers, and culture, the extensive grounds of the Hospital, reaching as they do to low-water mark. Heartfelt tributes are rendered to the memory and devoted services of Drs. Parkman and Shattuck. From some statistical facts embodied in a table, it appeared that during the last seventeen years $295,074 had been gratuitously expended by the Hospital, and that there had been received into it in twenty years nearly twelve thousand patients.

The expenses of the Asylum for the year had been $46,724.31; the receipts for the board of patients being $53,821.43. Dr. Bell makes a very brief report, having so fully in previous years treated the general subjects of his experience. He had received during the year 120 patients; had had under his care 315, of whom 195 remained. He again bears testimony to the fidelity and earnest co-operation of all the subordinates of the Asylum.

The Board at its meeting on Feb. 18, taking notice of the fact that Mr. J. P. Bigelow had not been re-elected as a Trustee on the part of the Commonwealth, voted to him their thanks —

"For the faithful performance of those duties for which he was so well qualified by his general intelligence and by his experience acquired in other high public trusts; and that while he has gained the good-will of the patients by the interest he uniformly manifested in their behalf, his amiable disposition and pleasant manners have always been highly appreciated by his late colleagues, the members of this Board."

At the meeting of the Trustees on March 18, the Visiting Committee reported on a communication received from Dr. Bacon, and referred to them, that the duties of a Microscopist more appropriately belong to the office of Curator of the Pathological Cabinet, and advised that hereafter the said duties should be performed by that officer instead of by Dr. Bacon, who shall remain Chemist. The report was accepted. The Visiting Committee also received full power to engage the services of Mr. Hermogen S. Balcom, as Apothecary, in place of Mr. Tucker, resigned.

The salary of the male Supervisor of the Asylum was raised to six hundred dollars by the Board of Trustees, at their meeting on April 18.

At the meeting of the Board on Aug. 7, a communication was received from Dr. Jacob Bigelow, resigning his office of Visiting Physician, on which it was —

"*Voted*, That the resignation be accepted, and that a Committee be appointed to report resolutions expressive of the sense this Board entertains of the valuable services of Dr. Bigelow."

Messrs. Dale, Rogers, and Stevenson were appointed such Committee. Dr. Augustus A. Gould was, by ballot, chosen to fill the vacancy as a Visiting Physician.

The report of the Committee on the resignation of Dr. Bigelow, made at the meeting on Aug. 15, was as follows: —

"That Dr. Bigelow was elected as one of the Consulting Physicians of this Hospital in 1827; that he has been immediately connected with the institution since that date; that he has brought to its service great skill, a large experience, deep knowledge, and an unusual degree of good judgment; that his services, invaluable as they are known to have been, and occupying much of his time, as they are known to have done, have been requited only by the consciousness on his part of devotion to humane duties, and by the respect and affection of those who have known how faithfully those duties have been performed. And the Committee recommend that he be requested by the Trustees to permit his bust or portrait to be taken by a competent artist, to be preserved in the Hospital."

In accepting this report, the Board authorized and instructed the same Committee to take the necessary steps for carrying their recommendation into effect.

On Sept. 15, a Committee, to whom had been referred the converting of the Lecture and Reception Room in the Hospital into rooms for patients, reported to the Board that they had attended to that duty, and that, through the changes they had made, the number of beds for patients had been increased by twenty-three, at an expense, including the furniture, of $3,009.45. The new wards thus formed were appropriated to male patients.

At the meeting of the Board on Oct. 12, Mr. George T. Lyman, as executor of the will of the late Miss Elizabeth Pratt, communicated to the Trustees that she had left ten thousand dollars for the use and benefit of the Hospital in Boston, and the same sum for the use and benefit of the Asylum at Somerville. The Treasurer was authorized to receive and receipt for these legacies, and was instructed to enter them in his books to the credit of each department. A special Committee was empowered to contract for a new fence around the grounds of the Hospital, at an expense not exceeding $5,500.

At the regular quarterly meeting of the Board, held at the Asylum on Oct. 17, a communication having been received from Dr. Bell resigning his office at the close of the year, it was —

"*Voted*, That it be referred to a Committee consisting of Messrs. Stevenson, Lamb, Warren, and Bullard, to express to Dr. Bell the deep regret which the Board feels, and to confer with him upon the general state of the institution."

At the meeting of the Board on Dec. 16, Messrs.

Wigglesworth and Shaw were appointed a Committee to examine the Treasurer's accounts, and to prepare the annual report. Satisfactory arrangements had been made during the year with the Fitchburg Railroad Company, for land of the Corporation taken by them to widen their track. At the meeting on Jan. 11, Mr. N. I. Bowditch declined, by letter, a re-election as Trustee, as did also Mr. G. H. Shaw, at the meeting of the Board on Jan. 23.

At the annual meeting of the Corporation, on Jan. 23, 1856, but few changes were made in the Board. Messrs. William Appleton, Henry Andrews, and Marcus Morton, jun., were respectively re-elected as President, Treasurer, and Secretary. Mr. N. I. Bowditch was chosen Vice-President, in place of Mr. Robert Hooper. The Trustees on the part of the Commonwealth were the same as last year; and on the part of the Corporation they were Messrs. James B. Bradlee, W. W. Greenough, Robert M. Mason, Charles H. Mills, H. B. Rogers, J. T. Stevenson, Charles H. Warren, and Edward Wigglesworth.

At the first meeting of the Trustees, on Feb. 3, after this organization, Mr. Henry B. Rogers was elected Chairman. The same six Physicians and Surgeons as last year were re-chosen as the Board of Consultation. On the Board of Visiting Physicians, Dr. A. A. Gould took the place of Dr. Jacob Bigelow; that of Visiting Surgeons was the same. Dr. John Bacon, jun., was re-elected Chemist; Dr. Calvin Ellis, Curator of the Pathological Cabinet; Dr. S. L. Abbot Admitting Physician, and R. Girdler Superintendent, of the Hospital. The choice of Physician and Superintendent of the Asylum was postponed; Mr. and Mrs. Tyler being re-appointed Steward and Matron. The Standing Committees were designated, and the Visiting Committees arranged for the year. It was provided that two thousand copies of the annual report be printed. This report estimates the amount of the property of the Corporation yielding income to be $173,179.27, that income having been for the last year $45,525, of which $18,000 had been an extra dividend from the Massachusetts Hospital Life Insurance Company. There had been admitted into the Hospital 915 patients, of which 414 were wholly free, and 147 more paid for board only a part of the time. The average length of time of the stay of free patients, which in 1853 had been seven weeks, had grown, in 1855, to eleven weeks and four days. The Committee think the causes of this increase should be investigated. The whole expense of conducting the Hospital for the year was $43,252.51, of which

$8,889.17 was repaid by the patients. The average weekly expense of each was $5.64. The rate of board had been slightly raised, and there had been an increase in the number of paying patients. The new wards, constructed during the year, had proved very satisfactory; and thanks are regarded as due to Mr. H. B. Rogers for his superintendence of the changes. During the year, 280 out-door medical and 356 out-door surgical patients had been prescribed and cared for. The munificent bequest of Miss Pratt is noticed. The resignation of Dr. Jacob Bigelow calls forth a renewed tribute to his abilities, services, and virtues; while the Committee say, "No panegyric of ours could add to the esteem which he has won by a long course of honorable labor." Extraordinary outlays at the Asylum for gas-fixtures, bowling-alleys, billiard-tables, and piano-fortes, had increased the expenses there to $60,867.26, while the receipts had been $57,115.38. The cost of each patient a week was $5.50. There had been admitted 318 patients: of these, 192 remained.

Dr. Bell, having tendered his resignation, as before noticed, to take effect at this time, offers in his report some general and some personal suggestions. He refers to the accessories gathered at the institution by the liberality of friends and the co-operation of the Trustees, to secure there a well-ordered and a well-furnished home, in order to keep up the character of the establishment in its provisions for the comfort, interest, and restoration of the inmates. The erection of a beautiful, well-warmed bowling-alley, the fitting up of two new billiard-tables, and the purchase of three new pianos for the female side, and the provision of a third billiard-table for the male side, have added to the means of healthful amusement. The introduction of gas, and of Cochituate water, and the improved ventilating apparatus, have added largely to the comfort of the inmates. The first attempt in this country to warm institutions for the insane, by the medium of steam or hot water, had been successfully made here. It has secured an almost fixity of heat, and at a moderate outlay. The partitions under the dome of the male wing having been removed, a spacious and beautiful apartment had been secured as a dormitory for ten or twelve persons. The farm-buildings had been largely added to. The two noble edifices for the Appleton wards had been occupied, and had proved of eminent advantage.

Dr. Bell then refers to his own withdrawal as a candidate for re-election. With a clinging of heart to the place and scenes of such devoted service as he has rendered, he says that he has made his —

"Arrangements to retire to a spot not far distant where

I shall have the happiness of opening my eyes each morning on this blessed institution, and feeling that my own happiness will be intimately connected with witnessing its continued prosperity. I hope hereafter to be no stranger within its walls; hence I feel that no melancholy valedictory is required or would be in keeping with the occasion of my handing over this charge to another. I will only say that, as far as I know, I leave this asylum prosperous in its own affairs, and amply possessed of the confidence of the community. I leave it with a heart grateful to that Superintending Providence which shielded me for so many years from those bereavements and that ill-health which have of late overwhelmed me, so that I have been enabled to do something for those placed under my care, as well as for the general cause of the insane over our country. Grateful for the uniform support, the indulgent forbearance, the kind sympathy in my many trials, of the members of your Board, present and past; grateful to the medical profession, whose cheerful and ready confidence and uniform courtesy are and ever will be very dear to my memory; grateful to a community which has, in the various attacks to which this and all such institutions are ever liable from the mistaken, the ungratified, and the malignant, sprung promptly to our relief, rendering explanations and defences superfluous; grateful to a long line of recovered patients, of both sexes, whose kindly recognition of our efforts has inspired new activity and made labors pleasant, however in themselves anxious and exhausting; and, lastly, grateful to those associated with me in various capacities — most of them for many years, and some during my entire service — in the discharge of our holy functions; — I can mark the day of my leaving these walls, with a 'white stone,' and enter again the world without one feeling other than that of kindness and good-will to all mankind."

Dr. Bell was elected Superintendent of the Asylum in December, 1836. Having thus given nineteen years to its service, he refers to the fact that he had made no application for the office, and had not known even that he was thought of for it, being a stranger to every member of the Board and almost to the Commonwealth. Yet he trusts that the years have not passed for him without adding something to the common stock of knowledge of the treatment, moral and medical, of insanity. The Institution, almost the earliest of the curative hospitals of the land, had freely shared its experience with the successive institutions which had since been established from Maine to California. "Christianity," he says, "can hardly show a mightier triumph than the fact that the number of hospitals for the insane in the United States has increased from half-a-dozen to between forty and fifty." Each of the four larger British Provinces adjoining us has provided its large and well-furnished Institution, substantially on this model. Experience has led to a discriminating as well as an improved use of means of moral treatment trusted in for the care of the insane. Some fancied schemes have been abandoned, as has much reliance upon mechanical and agricultural labor, because of a change in the class of patients. For several years there was a disuse of all the forms of muscular restraint, but the experi-

EXPERIMENTS IN THE ASYLUM. 505

ment, very much vaunted, proved that no such exclusive system was, here at least, compatible with the true interests of all patients. A trial also was made of allowing very many patients to go abroad on parole. No accident occurred, and the pledge was rarely broken. But the patients were invariably found to be made by it less contented, and the conclusion was forced upon the officers " that almost every patient who was so far disordered in mind as to justify detention at all, was too much disordered for even a qualified liberty." The experiment of permitting the intermingling of the sexes in daily religious exercises and in occasions of festivity, though under the close supervision of officers and attendants, was thoroughly tested for several years, but its inconveniences long ago led to its abandonment. The interdiction of the visits and correspondence of friends, in so many cases, has always proved to be one of the severest trials of those in charge of such institutions, as well as one of the grounds of the distrust, impatience, and censorious criticism of outside observers. But the indispensable necessity of this restriction, as it was one of the earliest of the recorded facts of medical observation, so has it been confirmed in every day's experience of every asylum. On no point is the head of such an institution more tempted to yield or evade his convictions of duty than on this, pressed as he is by the solicitations, the importunities, and the teasings of those most interested in his patients, and subjected to the false reasonings, the caprices, and the murmurs of those influenced by only one set of their feelings, while jeopardizing the recovery of the sufferers who engage them. Dr. Bell expresses himself with earnestness and decision on this point; for he had had sore trials of his fidelity to a course on which his full experience and his intelligent and conscientious observation had given him fixed convictions. He was glad to have the love of those under his charge and of their friends, but he would not win that love by acting, as does a so-called indulgent physician, who allows his patient to have his own way as to diet and regimen. The friends of patients, however nature may sway them, should respect such convictions as these, and of such a man. Having devoted so much of his life to this specialty, he leaves it as his one full counsel to any one who may be called to like trust " to stand firm to his convictions on this greatest item of moral treatment." It is to be remembered, too, that this system of restriction of correspondence and visits is not a general rule applied to all patients, but only to those who are probably recoverable.

The whole number of patients admitted into the Asylum up to this time had been 4,006; Dr. Bell having had the care of 2,696 of them. The Committee in their report refer with much feeling to the services of Dr. Bell, and pay a most deserved tribute to his abilities and virtues. The number of patients had nearly trebled under his administration, and the Institution had gained a high and wide-spread reputation. The Committee declare, —

"It is unnecessary for us to say how much the Trustees regret to lose his services. His skill and kindness and care, his activity, decision, and fertility of resources, have been conspicuous in his management of the patients; his quick perception and uniform courtesy have given him that influence over their friends which is one of the first requisites for the successful treatment of the insane; while his weight of character has won the confidence of the community, and preserved the Asylum in a great measure from that suspicion and obloquy to which such institutions are peculiarly exposed."

It will be remembered that Mr. Bowditch has quoted, on a previous page, the explicit condition on which Dr. Bell, then a stranger to the Board, was put in charge of his responsible trust. It was that he should pledge himself to " pursue the course of moral and religious treatment of patients adopted by Dr. Lee." The occasion of his death, six years after this date, while giving his professional services to his country in her patriotic army, will call for a subsequent reference to him in these pages. But, in connection with the close of his devoted labors at the

Asylum, it is but proper to recognize here how he had so faithfully fulfilled his first pledge, not only in its terms, but in self-consecration to a most arduous work. In the touching farewell words which have just been copied from his report, it will be observed that he described the offices which he shared with his subordinates at the Asylum as " holy functions." No simpler, no more fitting terms could be chosen for defining his own devout, reverential, and lofty estimate of the nature of his duties, and of the character and spirit required in himself for their discharge. His tenderness, sympathy, refinement, and spirituality, his perfect self-command, his patience and earnestness, were combined with a vast intellectual power and with talents of philosophical and scientific breadth and vigor which are rarely bestowed on one man, and if possessed would be more rarely given and concentrated as they were by him on such an uninviting and limited sphere of service.

At the annual meeting of the Corporation, held Jan. 23, 1856, it was, —

" *Voted*, That the Corporation have heard with deep regret of the resignation of Dr. Luther V. Bell, the Physician and Superintendent of the M'Lean Asylum for the Insane ; and, in parting with him, they desire to record their grateful recognition of the profound knowledge, devoted zeal, and remarkable sagacity with which he has performed the delicate and responsible duties of the office he has so long honored."

CHAPTER XIV.

March 16, 1856, to Feb. 5, 1862.

Routine Business at the Meetings of the Trustees. — New Fence at the Hospital. — Dr. C. Booth elected Superintendent of the Asylum, and Dr. J. C. Smith an Assistant Physician. — Resignation of Dr. Perry. — Notice of the Death of Dr. J. C. Warren. — Proposal for a Sea-Wall on the Hospital Bounds. — Bequest of William Read. — Important Votes concerning the Asylum. — Annual Meeting. — Organization for 1857. — Report for 1856. — Illness of Dr. Booth. — Contribution to Dr. Morton. — Dr L. M. Sargent, Jun., chosen Artist of the Hospital. — Gift from Dr. J. M. Warren. — Death of Dr. Booth. — Temporary Service of Dr. Bell. — Annual Meeting. — Organization for 1858. — Report for 1857. — Bequests of M. P. Sawyer and W. Pickman. — Dr. J. E. Tyler, Superintendent of the Asylum. — Bequest of Dr. J. G. Treadwell. — Office of Resident Physician at the Hospital. — Resignation of Superintendent Girdler, and of the Secretary. — Malignant Fever at the Hospital. — Donation from Executors of Thomas Dowse. — T. B. Hall chosen Secretary. — Dr. B. S. Shaw chosen Resident Physician, and Dr. S. L. Abbot, Physician to Out-Patients, at the Hospital. — Application of a Female Student. — Mr. and Mrs. Gallison chosen Steward and Matron of the Hospital. — Thanks to Capt. Girdler. — Tribute to Dr. Storer. — Dr. F. Minot chosen a Visiting Physician. — Bequest of Mrs. A. Austin. — Establishment of the Treadwell Library. — Estate of M. P. Sawyer. — Filling of Flats. — Annual Meeting. — Organization for 1859. — Report for 1858. — Resignation of the Treasurer, and Election of Mr. Stevenson. — More Land at the Asylum. — Bequests of George Hills and of Mrs. S. B. Thompson. — Annual Meeting. — Organization for 1860. — Report for 1859. — Dr. Tyler's Report. — Important Votes. — Bequest of Jonathan Phillips. — Reduction of Expenses. — Annual Meeting. — Organization for 1861. — Report for 1860. — New Cottage at the Asylum. — Death of Mr. Bowditch. — Sketch of his Life and Character. — His Work on Suffolk Surnames. — The Civil War. — Preparations to receive Diseased and Wounded Soldiers. —

A New Form of Bond for Patients at the Asylum. — Absence of the Chairman. — Bounds of the Hospital Grounds. — Donation by Mr. W. Appleton.

In deriving the substance of the matter for the pages of this History from the records of the Trustees and from the annual reports made to the Corporation, many details of business and of discipline are necessarily omitted, as either trivial in the retrospect, or of mere routine, or such as are naturally to be inferred in the management and oversight of such a trust. The Trustees at their very frequent and never intermitted meetings, held once in a fortnight, inform themselves upon all the facts connected with the internal working and discipline of both the institutions under their charge; they direct the repairs and alterations of the buildings, and their furnishings; they give attention to all proposals for change, where change promises improvement; they listen to reports from the Visiting Committees as to the number, condition, and circumstances of the patients; they are informed as to the investments of their funds; they fix the number of free beds, the rates of board and the time, extended when necessary in special cases, during which invalids or convalescents may remain under care, and they elect from year to year the six House Pupils, with the aid of testimonials offered by applicants and of recommendations from the Surgical and Medical Boards. At regular quarterly meetings at the Hospital and Asylum, the Finance Committee examines the accounts of either institution. In these pages only matters apart from this routine are brought to notice.

At the meeting of the Trustees on March 16, 1856, Mr. G. H. Shaw, for the Committee on a new fence around the Hospital grounds, reported that he had procured subscriptions to the amount of $3,250 for that object, made on the condition that enough to cover the expense should yet be obtained. It was then " voted that the Chairman of the Board be authorized to subscribe, in behalf of the Trustees," the needful balance.

Dr. Chauncey Booth was, by ballot, elected Physician and Superintendent of the M'Lean Asylum. A Committee appointed upon the subject of the resignation of Dr. Bell were authorized to procure a bust or portrait of him to be placed in the Asylum. At the meeting on April 16, on the nomination of Dr. Booth, Dr. Jerome C. Smith was elected additional Assistant Physician at the Asylum, at a salary of $600. The salary of Dr. Ranney, the Assistant Physician, was fixed at $700.

At the meeting on May 4, a letter was received from Dr. M. S. Perry, resigning his office as one of the Visiting Physicians. Whereupon it was —

"*Voted*, That the Trustees accept with regret the resignation of Dr. M. S. Perry. His professional ability, his uniform courtesy to his colleagues, his kindness to the patients, and his faithfulness manifested in the discharge of the duties of his office, entitle him to the grateful remembrance of the Board."

The Secretary was instructed to communicate this vote to Dr. Perry.

The Chairman announced the death of Dr. John C. Warren, when it was voted that the Chairman and Mr. Wigglesworth be a Committee to prepare suitable resolutions expressive of the sense the Trustees entertain of this loss, to be reported at the next meeting, which was held on May 5. The following votes proposed by the Committee were then unanimously adopted: —

"*Voted*, That the death of John Collins Warren, though deferred by a kind Providence until the labors of a long life had come to a natural close, is an event that cannot be passed over by the Trustees of the Massachusetts General Hospital without a tribute of respect for his character, and of gratitude for the services which he has rendered to this Institution and the community at large.

"*Voted*, That Dr. Warren, in conjunction with his friend and contemporary, Dr. James Jackson, who still lives among us honored and beloved, was mainly instrumental in originating the General Hospital and M‘Lean Asylum by issuing in August, 1810, a circular letter to the public on the need of such an institution, and afterwards rendered valuable service in arranging and perfecting its organization. That for nearly thirty-six years, viz., from April 6, 1817, to Feb. 1853, he

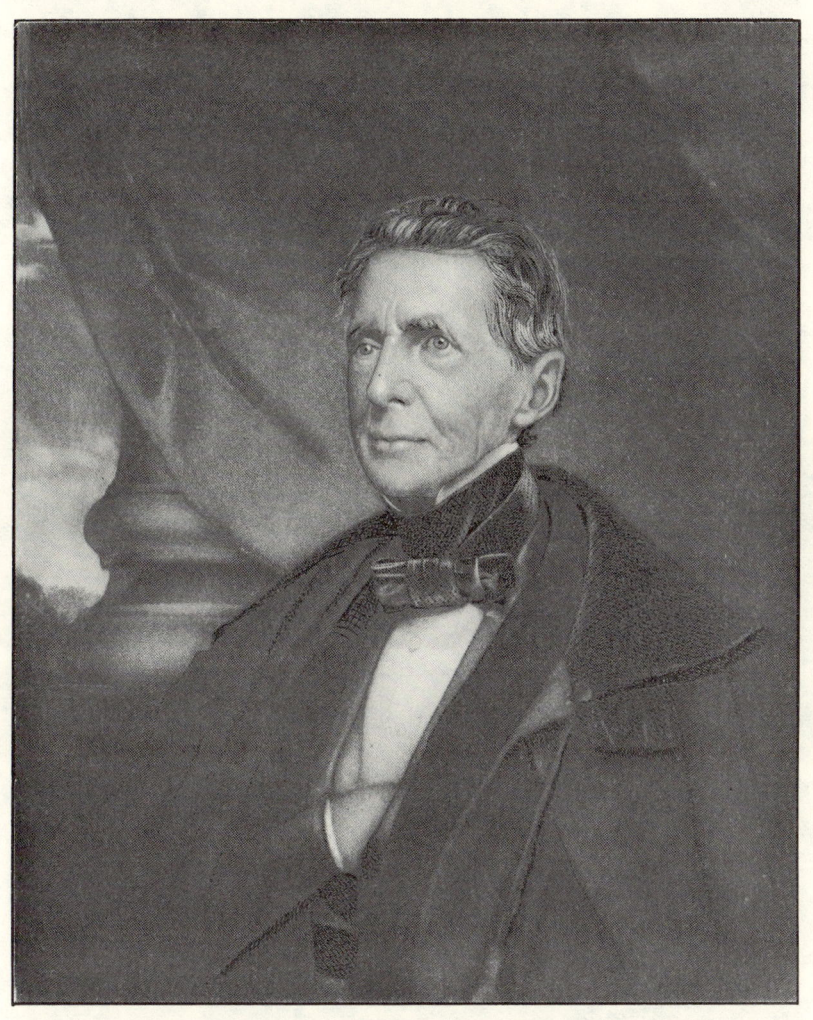

ENGRAVED BY T.B.WELCH, PHILA. FROM A DAGUERREOTYPE BY JOHN A. WHIPPLE, BOSTON.

JOHN C. WARREN.

John C Warren

& Professor of Anatomy & Surgery

IN THE UNIVERSITY OF CAMBRIDGE.

was at first the sole and subsequently the principal acting Surgeon, in daily attendance upon its wards, and by his eminent talents, knowledge, and practical skill, as well as by his fidelity, energy, and untiring devotion, in behalf of all the interests of the Institution, largely contributed to make it what it now is, an honor to the city and to the Commonwealth.

"*Voted*, That during his long life Dr. Warren spared neither labor nor expense in the pursuit of professional eminence and usefulness; maintained his position in the front rank of the surgeons of his time; did much by personal effort and liberal donations to promote the cause of natural science, and added to the lustre of the name which he inherited from a distinguished father, and transmits to a distinguished son.

"Notwithstanding a delicate and enfeebled constitution, his resolute spirit sustained his professional activity and interest to the last, and he found his reward in his own consciousness as well as in fortune and fame. The community in which he has been for so many years conspicuous will long hold his memory in honor.

"*Voted*, That the Trustees sympathize with the family of the late Dr. Warren in their bereavement, and in token of their respect for his memory will attend the funeral, if agreeable to them.

"*Voted*, That the Secretary be directed to enclose a copy of these votes to the family of the deceased."

At the meeting of the Trustees on May 18, Mr. Charles H. Warren communicated to the Board his resignation as a member of it.

Dr. Charles E. Ware, at the meeting of the Board on June 1, was chosen Visiting Physician, in the place of Dr. Perry, resigned. Mr. John Lowell was, on June 24, elected a Trustee, in the place of Mr. C. H. Warren, resigned. Proposed changes in the Rules and Regulations, reported by a Committee, were adopted by the Board.

The proposed extension of Charles Street, by the city authorities, over the flats belonging to this Corporation, was brought to a renewed notice by the Board, on Aug. 12, through a letter addressed to the Chairman, from the Chairman of the Committee on Streets, notifying the Board that that Committee " will report in favor of building a substantial seawall on the Commissioners' Line, in consideration of the Hospital's accepting the same, in liquidation of any and all damages in consequence of the laying out by the city of Boston a street over the flats belonging to the Corporation, provided said Corporation will give permission for and to the city to enter upon their flats for the purpose of building said wall." An early answer was desired, as the Committee added that, in case the offer was declined, they should forthwith make a contract for a pile bridge. The Board voted that it was not expedient to accept the proposition.

On Sept. 23, by election of the Board of Visitors, the Hon. John P. Bigelow again became a Trustee, filling the vacancy caused by the resignation of Mr. Henry M. Holbrook.

At the meeting of the Board on Oct. 10, a legacy of $2,000, left to the institution by the will of William Read of Marblehead, was accepted by the Trustees, on the conditions set forth by the testator. Messrs. Lowell and Bradlee were appointed, on Dec. 14, a Committee to examine the Treasurer's accounts, and to prepare the annual report.

The following very important votes were passed by the Trustees, at their meeting on Jan. 21, 1857: —

"*Voted*, That the Physician and Superintendent of the M'Lean Asylum be requested to communicate by letter to the Chairman of the Trustees the death of any patient under his charge, as soon as may be after the happening of the same, together with all the important facts and circumstances relating thereto. Also, that he cause all occurrences of any importance, which transpire within the Asylum, to be reported to him by all persons under his authority, as soon as practicable after they take place."

"*Voted*, That he cause a night-watch to be organized in both the male and female wards, which shall pass through each gallery as often as once in each half hour during each night, from ten to six o'clock. Also, that in case of any violent death, he cause a coroner to be summoned. Also, that at no time, excepting during the night-watch, shall any gallery, in either ward, be without a person actually present there as an attendant; and that such arrangements be made as shall effectually carry this object into operation."

The annual meeting of the Corporation was held on Jan. 28, 1857, when the annual report of the

Committee, with accompanying documents, which had been accepted by the Trustees, were laid before it. At the next meeting of the Trustees on Feb. 8, it appeared that the Corporation had elected the following officers for the ensuing year: William Appleton, President; N. I. Bowditch, Vice-President; Henry Andrews, Treasurer; Marcus Morton, jun., Secretary; with Messrs. J. B. Bradlee, W. W. Greenough, John Lowell, R. M. Mason, C. H. Mills, H. B. Rogers, J. T. Stevenson, and Edward Wigglesworth, Trustees on the part of the Corporation; and Messrs. J. P. Bigelow, W. S. Bullard, W. J. Dale, and Thomas Lamb, Trustees on the part of the Commonwealth.

The Board elected Mr. Rogers as its Chairman for the ensuing year. Drs. James Jackson, John Jeffries, Edward Reynolds, George Hayward, John Homans, and Winslow Lewis, were chosen as the Board of Consultation; Drs. D. H. Storer, J. B. S. Jackson, H. I. Bowditch, G. C. Shattuck, A. A. Gould, and C. E. Ware, the Board of Visiting Physicians; Drs. S. D. Townsend, J. M. Warren, H. J. Bigelow, H. G. Clark, Samuel Cabot, jun., and G. H. Gay, the Board of Visiting Surgeons. Dr. John Bacon, jun., was chosen Chemist; Dr. Calvin Ellis, Microscopist and Curator of the Pathological Cabinet; Dr. Samuel L. Abbot, Admitting Physician; and Richard Girdler,

Superintendent of the Hospital; Dr. Chauncey Booth, Physician and Superintendent of the M'Lean Asylum; and Mr. and Mrs. Tyler, as Steward and Matron. The Standing Committees were appointed, and the Visiting Committees were arranged for the year.

It was voted that two thousand copies of the annual report be printed. This report states that the expenses of the institution have considerably exceeded its receipts from all sources, — a state of things which calls for the serious consideration of its Trustees and friends. The income has been $24,719.53; the expenses have been $40,986.77, — the excess being largely accounted for by repairs and permanent improvements, especially the brick and iron fence around the grounds of the Hospital. But a deficiency has existed for many years. There had been 976 patients in the Hospital, at an average weekly expense for each of $5.49½. The resignation of Dr. Perry and the death of Dr. Warren are noticed. The receipt of legacies, of $2,000 from the Hon. William Read of Marblehead, and of $40,000 from the late John Bromfield, Esq., is acknowledged. At the Asylum, 149 patients had been admitted, and 196 remained at the end of the year. The average weekly cost for each patient had been $6.11. Dr. Chauncey Booth, having for thirteen years filled with great acceptance the post of Assistant Physician, had entered upon the higher position left vacant by the resignation of Dr. Bell. The hope and confidence of the Trustees in this appointment were saddened and thwarted by the early death of this excellent and accomplished gentleman, in the very vigor of his years. The report which he made — and Providence disposed that it should be his only official return — is long, elaborate, and full of interest. It proves with what devotion of heart and mind, and with what pains-taking inquiries of observation and research, he had given himself to the specialty of his profession. He reviews the working of the system known as *Moral Treatment*, introduced into the institution by its first medical director, Dr. Wyman, and now accepted " throughout the civilized world," — "not an arbitrary, but a progressive system." He discusses the question of the increase of insanity, with a cursory examination of its causes, in the manners and habits of the people, the mode of educating the young, the neglect of physical training, and hereditary transmission. He calls attention to the jurisprudence of his subject and the need of a more thorough investigation of the relations between insanity and crime. The earnest and intelligent spirit which Dr. Booth thus manifested in magnifying the high and responsible office to which he had given his youth and early manhood is a token of the work which he would have effected had his life been prolonged. Before the close of the year he was prostrated in a decline, from which he was not to find restoration.

At the meeting of the Board on Feb. 22, on the nomination of Dr. Booth, the Trustees chose Drs. Mark Ranney and Jerome C. Smith Assistant Physicians, and George C. Lincoln and Miss Relief R. Barber male and female Supervisors, of the Asylum.

At this meeting action was taken on the report of a Committee, Messrs. Stevenson and Lowell, to whom, at a previous meeting, had been referred a proposition that the Trustees, in behalf of the Hospital, should subscribe $1,000 to the fund then solicited from the public at large in behalf of Dr. W. T. G. Morton, for his discovery and use of an anæsthetic. The Committee remark that no ordinary circumstance would justify the Trustees, should they apply any portion of the funds under their control to any object other than the direct relief of the sick under their care. But the relations between Dr. Morton and the Hospital, in regard to the great discovery which prompts the proposed memorial, are peculiar. "He is known to have been chiefly instrumental in conferring a great good upon his race." He has received no pecuniary compensation for his agency in a discovery of so beneficent a character, but, on the contrary, has borne many sacrifices. While by justice he is entitled to a remuneration, the government of the country having omitted to provide a proper reward, the only mode in which it seems probable that it can be furnished is by a voluntary contribution. As to the question whether the Trustees may properly give any thing to it from the funds of the institution, the Committee decide in the affirmative on the following grounds: " The first important surgical operation to which that discovery was applied was performed within its walls, at his instance;" he gave the Hospital the privilege of a free use of his discovery at a time when he expected pecuniary advantage from it from other quarters; the Hospital has continued to receive benefit from it, which no reasonable amount of money could compensate; the refusal of a subscription by the Hospital might with reason prevent the foundation of the fund; and such a subscription finds precedents in the appropriations which the Trustees have made in procuring memorials of their benefactors.

The Committee therefore recommended the following vote, which, with the report, was unanimously approved by the Trustees: —

"*Voted*, That the Chairman of this Board be requested to subscribe, on behalf of the Massachusetts General Hospital, one thousand dollars towards the fund which it is proposed to establish for the benefit of Dr. W. T. G. Morton, as a memorial of the great service which that gentleman has rendered to science and humanity, in connection with the discovery of the uses of ether."

At the meeting of the Trustees on March 8, Messrs. Rogers and Stevenson were appointed a Committee to procure a bust or portrait of Dr. George Hayward for the Hospital.

At the meeting of the Board on April 10, the Trustees, on the report of a Committee to whom the subject had been referred, —

"*Voted*, That the Rules and Regulations be amended so that the title of the Admitting Physician shall hereafter be 'Admitting Physician and Physician to Out-Patients.'"

The same Committee recommended the establishment of the office of Artist of the Hospital. The Board approving, it was —

"*Voted*, That the said office be hereby established, and the following rules and regulations be adopted : —

"'Artist of the Hospital.

"'Art. 1. He shall, under the direction and at the discretion of the Physicians and Surgeons, make accurate drawings of such anomalous and rare cases of disease as shall be useful for future reference and examination.

"'Art. 2. He shall be present and assist the Physicians and Surgeons whenever his services may be desirable.

"'ART. 3. All copies and drawings shall be carefully preserved in a portfolio provided for the purpose, and shall be placed in the Pathological Cabinet, under the care of the Curator; and they shall not be taken from the Hospital without the consent of the Visiting Committee.'"

Upon the recommendation of the same Committee, Dr. L. M. Sargent, jun., was then elected Artist of the Hospital.

On the nomination of Dr. Booth, at the meeting Oct. 16, the Trustees appointed Mr. Henry H. Benson male Supervisor of the Asylum for the remainder of the year.

At the meeting of the Board on Nov. 22, a donation was announced from Dr. J. Mason Warren of a case of surgical knives, a large chair to be used in cases of lameness, and eighteen volumes of the Edinburgh Medical and Surgical Journal. The Secretary was instructed to return the thanks of the Board to Dr. Warren for this acceptable and valuable gift.

An application having been received at the meeting on Nov. 8, and then laid on the table, from Sarah W. Salisbury, "a graduate of the Female Medical College, to be admitted to the Hospital for the purpose of obtaining practical knowledge in some of the branches of Medical Science,"— it was at this meeting taken from the table, when it was —

DEATH OF DR. BOOTH.

"*Voted*, That the Secretary communicate to Miss Salisbury a copy of the rules and regulations of the Hospital, and inform her that the Trustees deem any departure from the rules and regulations to be inexpedient."

At the meeting of the Board on Dec. 20, Messrs. Greenough and Mason were appointed a Committee to examine the Treasurer's accounts, and to prepare the annual report. The illness of Dr. Booth having disabled him from the performance of his duties, the Visiting Committee reported that they had engaged Dr. Bell, then residing in Charlestown, to take temporary charge of the Asylum. The Board approved of this action.

At the meeting of the Trustees on Jan. 15, the death of Dr. Chauncey Booth was announced, whereupon it was —

"*Voted*, That this Board have heard with much sorrow of the death of Dr. Chauncey Booth, late Superintendent of the M'Lean Asylum, a man of sterling worth, and most esteemed by those who knew him best. His connection with the Asylum has been long and useful and honorable. He was quiet and modest, but resolute and self-possessed. He sustained himself well amid the arduous duties of his office, the weakness of disease, and the certainty of approaching dissolution. His services, both as Assistant and Principal Physician of the Asylum, have been highly appreciated by the Trustees, and are held in grateful remembrance by hundreds who have experienced his skill and kindness and care. He lived without reproach, and died with the calmness which comes from the consciousness of duty done.

"*Voted*, That in token of our respect for the memory of the deceased we will attend his funeral at the Asylum to-morrow.

"*Voted*, That a copy of the above votes be sent to the family of Dr. Booth."

The annual meeting of the Corporation was held at the Hospital, on Jan. 27, 1858, when the annual reports were presented and acted upon. No change was made in the officers of the Corporation from last year, except that Mr. Abbott Lawrence was elected a Trustee on the part of the Commonwealth, in the place of Hon. John P. Bigelow, who had declined a re-election. The Board subsequently voted its thanks to Mr. Bigelow for his long and valuable services.

At the next following meeting of the Trustees, on Feb. 7, 1858, Mr. Rogers was again elected Chairman. The Boards of Consultation and of Visiting Physicians and Surgeons remained unchanged; and the same gentlemen that were in the other offices of the Hospital during the last year were re-elected thereto respectively. The election of a Physician and Superintendent of the Asylum was postponed, Mr. and Mrs. Tyler being re-appointed Steward and Matron. The Standing Committees were chosen, and Visiting Committees were arranged for the year. It was directed that two thousand copies of the annual report be printed.

In this report the Committee state that the property yielding an income applicable to the general purposes of the Corporation is $171,603.55. The expenses of the Hospital and the Asylum for the past year have been $105,663.23; the receipts, $95,731.95. This excess of expenditure, steadily diminishing the property of the Institution which is exempted from special trusts, demands earnest attention. There had been admitted into the Hospital 920 patients, at an average weekly expense for each patient of $5.90, or, including repairs, of $6.45. There had been treated during the year 1,574 out-patients. There had been admitted into the Asylum 141 patients, and there remained at the close of the year 178. A very brief report comes from Dr. Bell, who, as has been noticed, a few weeks before the close of the year was put in charge of the Asylum temporarily, on account of the illness of Dr. Booth. The Committee refer with sadness to the death of this useful, beloved, and excellent man, and pay another warm tribute to his virtues, his amiability, and fidelity, and to the qualities, experience, and acquisitions which so eminently fitted him for his exacting and responsible trust.

A new brick stable and a mechanics' shop had been built at the Asylum, and new fences had been put up. Early in the spring the Board had received notice from Charles W. Storey, Esq., executor, that the Hospital had received a bequest by the will of the late Matthew P. Sawyer, Esq., of $7,000, and that it was also the residuary legatee of the estate. This donation — the amount not being as yet known — promised to be large. There had been paid to the Corporation during the year the bequest of William Pickman, Esq., of $4,000, to be apportioned equally to the Hospital and the Asylum.

A special meeting of the Board was held on Feb. 12, at which Dr. John E. Tyler was unanimously elected Physician and Superintendent of the Asylum, — Messrs. Rogers, Stevenson, and Mason being appointed a Committee to notify him of his election, and to make arrangements for his entrance upon his duties at as early a day as practicable. Thanks and compensation were voted to Dr. Bell for his valuable services during the illness and since the death of Dr. Booth. Oliver W. Webber was chosen Apothecary of the Hospital.

The Board voted, on Feb. 21, " that the Admitting Physician be instructed to receive patients with acute diseases into the Hospital to the full capacity of the wards, if applications of a suitable kind are made, until otherwise ordered by the Board."

A communication had been made to the Trustees at their meeting on March 7, relative to the interest of the Corporation in the will of the late Dr. John G. Treadwell, of Salem. The Committee to whom the matter had been referred reported at the meeting on March 21 as follows, the Board concurring in the report and votes : —

"Whereas the President and Fellows of Harvard College, by a vote passed at a stated meeting, on Feb. 27 last, have declined to receive or accept the bequest made to them in the will of the late John G. Treadwell, and renounced all benefit and interest under said will, as by an attested copy thereof hereby ordered to be placed on our records will more fully appear : therefore it is —

"*Voted*, That this Corporation doth hereby receive and accept the devises and bequests made to them in trust in the will of the late John G. Treadwell, subject to the conditions and limitations therein contained respecting the same ; and that Messrs. Rogers, Lamb, and Mason be, and they are hereby directed and empowered, in behalf of this Corporation, to take possession of the real estate, and receive and obtain from the executors proper transfers of the personal property, with full power to make such arrangements and settlements, execute such instruments, receipts, and discharges, and do and perform such acts and things as may be necessary and proper in the premises."

Another vote instructed the Treasurer to keep two accounts of the property thus received : one account to be credited with the sum of five thousand dollars, to be designated " The Treadwell Library Fund, in trust ; " and the other account, credited with the balance, to be designated " The Treadwell Fund, in trust." It was also voted that Messrs. Rogers, Lamb, and Mason "be a Committee to take charge of the Medical Library bequeathed to the Corporation by the late John G. Treadwell, and make such arrangements for its safe keeping, conveyance to Boston, and temporary reception in the Hospital, as may to them seem proper and advisable; and that said Committee consider and report what ultimate and permanent provision will be necessary and appropriate for the accommodation of the same."

The College had declined the bequest proffered to them in the will of Dr. Treadwell, because of "unusual and embarrassing conditions attached to it."

At the meeting of the Board on March 31, on the report and recommendation of a Committee appointed on Dec. 20, 1857, to examine into the internal affairs of the Hospital, it was "voted that in the opinion of this Board it is expedient to establish the office of Resident Physician at the Hospital, with powers and duties hereafter to be prescribed." The same Committee were requested to report to the Board such new Rules and Regulations, and such changes in those now in force, as would be necessary to define the powers and duties of the new officer and applicable to the change in the existing system; and also to report a suitable candidate for the said office. Dr. Dale was added to this Committee, which consisted of Messrs. Rogers, Bullard, Greenough, Lowell, and Mason.

Capt. Girdler on April 21 offered his resignation as Superintendent of the Hospital, and Mr. Morton his as Secretary of the Corporation. At the meeting on April 27, the Board directed the Committee on the Treadwell bequest to adapt the room then occupied by the Physicians and Surgeons to the reception of the Treadwell Library. Great anxiety was felt at this meeting on account of the existence of fever of a very malignant character in the Hospital. The Physicians and Surgeons were authorized to employ such additional assistance as the emergency required. The Committee, to whom had been referred the resignation of the Secretary, reported resolutions, which were unanimously adopted, expressing their regret therefor, and tendering their thanks for the fidelity, accuracy, punctuality, and promptitude with which he had discharged his arduous and responsible duties for sixteen years, courteously affording the Board the aid of his experience, knowledge, and ability. The salary of his successor, to be chosen, was fixed at $300.

A communication from Mr. George Livermore, in behalf of the executors of the late Mr. Thomas Dowse, of Cambridge, was received by the Board on May 9, enclosing a check of five thousand dollars, as a donation to the Hospital. The matter was referred to the Chairman, to consider and report.

Mr. Thomas B. Hall was by ballot elected Secretary, and was duly qualified. The Committee on the Treadwell estate were authorized to negotiate with the executors for a final settlement. The "Committee on the Internal Administration of the Hospital" reported on May 19 some Rules and Regulations defining the duties of the new office of Resident Physician, with certain changes in the duties of other offices. After certain amendments had been made in the draft, the report was accepted, and the changes were adopted, to take effect when either of the offices named therein shall be filled. It was voted that the salary of the Resident Physician be fixed at fifteen hundred dollars. The same Committee were empowered and requested to present candidates for the offices of Steward and Matron.

The Committee on the donation through the trustees under the will of Thomas Dowse reported on May 23, recommending that the Board accept it on the condition accompanying it; viz., that the income of it be appropriated to the support of free beds in the Hospital. The report was accepted, and it was —

"*Voted*, That this Board accept the donation on the above condition; and that in acknowledgment of the services rendered by the trustees of Mr. Dowse in this behalf, and of the favorable sentiments towards the Institution entertained by him, a free bed be, and the same hereby is, appropriated to the use of George Livermore and Eben Dale, Esquires, during the joint lives and the life of the survivor of them, subject to the rules and regulations from time to time made in relation to free beds."

It was also voted that this donation and all reinvestments of its proceeds be kept distinct, as "the Dowse Fund in trust," the income to be for the support of free beds; and that the Secretary send a certified copy of these votes to the trustees above-named.

At this meeting Dr. Benjamin Shurtleff Shaw was by ballot elected Resident Physician, and Dr. Samuel L. Abbot Physician to out-door patients at the Hospital, in conformity with the new arrangement of offices and distribution of duties which had been approved by recommendation of the Committee on the Internal Administration of the Hospital. In communicating his election to Dr. Abbot, the Secretary was directed to assure him —

"That the Trustees desire to avail of this opportunity to express to him their satisfaction with the manner in which he has performed the responsible duties of Admitting Physician for the past nine years, and to bear testimony to the faithfulness and zeal which have characterized all his relations with this Institution."

The Board, at its meeting on June 6, granted the request of Dr. John E. Tyler, to attend the annual gathering of the " Medical Superintendents of Institutions for the Insane," to be holden this year at Quebec; and, in consideration of the advantage resulting from such conventions, voted to pay his expenses on the errand. At the meeting of June 16, Miss Sarah W. Salisbury, by letter, renewed her urgent application for admission to the Hospital for the purpose before stated. The Trustees directed the Secretary to inform her that there had been no change in the views of the Trustees since the reply to her former application. Several candidates having been presented for the offices of Steward and Matron at the Hospital, on the ballots being taken, William B. Gallison was unanimously elected Steward. On the nomination of Dr. Shaw, in accordance with the rules, Mrs. Gallison was proposed as Matron, and was unanimously elected. The united salary of the Steward and Matron was fixed at $1,000. The previous resignation of Capt. Girdler was then acted upon and accepted, and it was " voted that the thanks of the Board be tendered to Capt. Girdler for his long and faithful services as Superintendent of the Hospital, and that in consideration thereof the Treasurer be directed to pay him his regular salary to October next."

RESIGNATION OF DR. STORER.

The Trustees, at their meeting on June 22, voted that the Committee on Accounts, by the new rule that had been adopted, should consist of two members of the Board, and that Messrs. Stevenson and Mason constitute that Committee.

Mr. Rogers, as Chairman of the Committee on the Treadwell property, read a report, which was accepted and placed on file. He also, as chairman of a Committee to whom had been referred the resignation of Dr. D. H. Storer as Visiting Physician, which had been offered at the meeting on July 6, recommended that the same be accepted, with the following vote, in which the Board concurred: —

"*Voted*, That although the term of service of Dr. D. Humphreys Storer has not been of so long duration as that of some of his predecessors in office, it has been, like theirs, distinguished for high professional knowledge and skill, and for promptness and exactitude in the discharge of duty. And this Board, in token of their appreciation of his valuable labors, self-sacrificing spirit, and independent and manly bearing, tender to him their sincere thanks, accompanied by their best wishes for his future happiness and success."

Dr. Francis Minot was, on July 20, elected a Visiting Physician to the Hospital, in the vacancy caused by the resignation of Dr. Storer.

The Board, at its meeting on Sept. 14, authorized the Superintendent of the Asylum to expend one hundred dollars for books for the use of patients, and to make such arrangements for amusements for them as he may deem expedient, all under the supervision of the Chairman of the Board.

At the meeting of the Board on Sept. 28, Dr. Shaw found it necessary to announce the resignation of Mr. Gallison, so recently elected Steward of the Hospital, on account of ill health. The Board accepted the resignation, and appointed Messrs. Stevenson and Lowell, with the Chairman, a Committee to nominate a candidate for the office, with authority to make all needful temporary arrangements. A communication was read from R. H. Eddy, Esq., executor of the will of the late Mrs. Agnes Austin, stating a bequest to this Corporation of two estates in Salem, and five thousand dollars to the Asylum. The same was referred to the Finance Committee. The salary of the Physician to out-door patients was fixed, on Nov. 7, at $300. The interest of the Corporation in the estate of the late M. P. Sawyer engaged the attention of the Board at its meeting on Nov. 21, and the matter was put in charge of two committees, and was in part disposed of at the meeting of the Board on Dec. 5. At this meeting, Mr. Rogers, in behalf of a Committee to whom had been referred the subject of the Treadwell Library, presented a report, with accompanying votes, and proposed rules and regulations

ESTATE OF M. P. SAWYER. 535

for its use. These were accepted, providing for the preservation, the careful oversight, and the annual examination of the books, and for the faithful performance of the requisitions contained in the will of the late Dr. Treadwell, respecting the care and use of said library, and providing also for additions to the same.

At the meeting of the Board on Dec. 19, communications were received from Messrs. J. B. Bradlee and C. H. Mills, resigning their places as Trustees. A claim had been advanced by Mrs. Lydia N. Raymond to an interest in the house No. 26 Beacon Street, then in possession of the Hospital, under the will of the late M. P. Sawyer. Mr. Rogers, in behalf of a Committee to which the matter had been referred, submitted a report upon it, with votes, which were accepted by the Board, as follows : —

"*Voted*, That in consideration of the doubt which exists as to the testamentary intentions of Matthias P. Sawyer, deceased, respecting the estate numbered 26 Beacon Street, now in the lawful possession of this Corporation, by virtue of the residuary clause of his will, and of the handsome sums of money which they have received, and still expect to receive from his benevolent disposition towards them, this Corporation hereby surrenders their legal rights in this estate, and relinquishes the same to Mrs. Raymond."

The Secretary and Treasurer were authorized and directed to prepare and execute a proper quitclaim deed of this estate, in conformity with the terms of this vote.

Messrs. Lawrence and Wigglesworth were appointed a Committee to prepare the annual report.

At its meeting on Jan. 14, 1859, the Board fixed the salary of the office of Steward at the Hospital at $1,000, and that of the Matron at $250; the present incumbents of those offices to be remunerated at those rates for their services since the resignation of Mr. Gallison. At the meeting on Jan. 19, authority was given to the Chairman of the Board to execute an indenture in behalf of the Corporation with the City of Boston, providing for the filling up of the flats lying between the Hospital grounds and the Harbor Commissioners' line.

The annual meeting of the Corporation was held at the Hospital on Jan. 26, 1859, when the annual report, including those of the Treasurer and of the officers of the Hospital and Asylum, was presented. At the first subsequent meeting of the Trustees on Feb. 13, it appeared that the election of officers for the year had been as follows: William Appleton, President; N. I. Bowditch, Vice-President; Henry Andrews, Treasurer, and T. B. Hall, Secretary; Messrs. N. H. Emmons, W. W. Greenough, George Higginson, John Lowell, R. M. Mason, H. B. Rogers, J. T. Stevenson, and Edward Wigglesworth, Trustees on the part of the Corporation; and Messrs. W. S. Bullard, W. J. Dale, Thomas Lamb, and Abbott Lawrence, Trustees on the part of the Commonwealth. Mr. Rogers was re-elected Chairman of the Board. The same gentlemen were chosen on the Board of Consultation as had served last year. The only change on the Board of Visiting Physicians was that Dr. Francis Minot took the place of Dr. D. H. Storer. The Board of Visiting Surgeons remained unchanged. Dr. J. Bacon, jun., was also re-elected Chemist; Dr. C Ellis, Microscopist and Curator of the Pathological Cabinet; Dr. B. S. Shaw, Resident Physician; Dr. S. L. Abbot, Physician to out-door patients. Lucius M. Sargent, jun., was elected Artist; Mr. Harvey Howard, Steward; and Mrs. Sarah L. Gallison, Matron of the Hospital. Dr. John E. Tyler was re-elected Physician and Superintendent of the Asylum; Columbus Tyler, Steward; and Mrs. M. E. Tyler, Matron. The Standing Committees were appointed, and the Visiting Committees were arranged. It was ordered that two thousand copies of the annual report be printed.

This report states the amount of the property of the Corporation yielding income to be $168,489.75. The income had been $97,422.25; the expenses, $110,477.96. There had been admitted to the Hospital 1,015 patients, at an average weekly expense for each of $6.53, including, and of 5.67\frac{1}{2}$ excluding, repairs. There had been treated during the year 2,223 out-door patients. The Trustees had made material changes in the Rules and Regulations for the Hospital, the most important of which was the establishment of the offices of Resident Physician and Steward, in place of a Superintendent. There had been admitted to the Asylum 155 patients, and there remained at the end of the year 186. Dr. John E. Tyler had succeeded Dr. Booth in charge. The respect and distinction which he had won while he had under his care the New Hampshire State Asylum, and his own eminent qualifications, were assurances that he would maintain and increase the high reputation of this institution. The sum of $7,000 had been received from the estate of the late M. P. Sawyer, for free beds at the Hospital, besides property in real estate estimated at $18,000, to accrue at some distant period. The reversionary bequest from D. J. G. Treadwell amounted to about $40,000, besides his valuable library, which had been suitably disposed in the Hospital. The donation of $5,000 through the trustees of Mr. Dowse, and the legacy of $15,000, received under the will of the late Mrs. Agnes Austin of Cambridge, consisting of real estate valued at $10,000 to the Hospital, and $5,000 to the Asylum, had been gratefully acknowledged. Both institutions were in a satisfactory condition, and were faithfully directed.

Dr. Shaw, in making his first report as Resident Physician of the Hospital, says that the ability to receive and treat an increased number of proper and curable patients has been secured by refusing, as a general rule, to receive such as did not admit of cure or of very decided relief, and by limiting the stay of patients to the period in which they actually needed medical or hygienic treatment. There had been in the Hospital at one time during the year 120 free patients. As the principal article of house diet, a nutritious soup had been introduced.

Dr. Tyler, in making his first report, states the fact that, while during the year the male wards of the Asylum had been seldom crowded, nearly as many female patients had been declined as had been received, which were seventy-nine; from which he infers that "it will hold true of this vicinity for the year past, that more females than males have been reached by mental disease." The year had been one remarkable for extraordinary religious excitement and interest, and for commercial disturbance and disaster, affecting deeply both sexes and all classes of society, and acting severely upon their intellectual and emotional faculties. Dr. Tyler discusses this subject in a very instructive and judicious way. He mentions the benefit found in the Asylum in the use of sulphuric ether, in a careful and discriminating way, for the tranquillization of the nervous system. He asks for an addition to the library at the Asylum. By request of the Trustees, he offers some suggestions as to improvement in heating and ventilating apparatus, and the reconstructing of apartments for excited patients. He promises an entire self-devotion to his sacred trust.

Dr. Tyler's request for an increase of the library at the Asylum was referred to the Visiting Committee for consideration and report. A communication was read from Henry Andrews, resigning the office of Treasurer of the Corporation, when it was "voted that the resignation be accepted." Also, on motion of Mr. Wigglesworth, it was "voted that the thanks of the Board be presented to our late Treasurer for his valuable services to this Corporation during the long period of twenty-four years, in which his uniform fidelity has gained for him the respect of all the Boards of Trustees with which he has been connected." At a special meeting of the Board, held on Feb. 18, Mr. T. J. Stevenson sent a communication resigning his office as a Trustee, and a vote of thanks was passed to him "for his long and faithful services." Mr. Stevenson was then elected, by ballot, Treasurer of the Corporation for the ensuing year. Thus began the term of service, which at this present writing still continues, of an officer of this Corporation, who has given to a most exacting and responsible trust signal abilities, the highest financial skill and judgment, with a warm interest in the cause of humanity which the institution represents. The complicated accounts which he administers form a lucid record even for those, not experts, who annually audit them.

Marcus Morton, jun., was elected a Trustee for the ensuing year, in the vacancy caused by the resignation of Mr. Stevenson.

On Feb. 27, the Board voted, after a report from the Committee on the library of the Asylum, to whom the request of Dr. Tyler had been referred, " that three hundred dollars per annum be placed at the disposal of the Superintendent and Physician of the Asylum to be used in the purchase of books for the permanent increase of the library."

At the meeting of the Board on March 27, measures were adopted for the settlement of the interest of the Corporation in the estate of the late M. P. Sawyer. At the meeting on April 20, similar steps were taken in reference to the bequests from the Treadwell property. A final report upon the latter subject was made and accepted at a meeting of the Board on May 8, and the selection was then approved of Dr. Shaw, as Guardian and Librarian of the Treadwell Library, at a salary of one hundred dollars. Mr. Morton resigned his seat on the Board, as a Trustee, on June 5, and the resignation was accepted. A Committee, of which Mr. Rogers was Chairman, reported on July 14 on the proposed purchase of "the Woodward Lot and Joy Farm," near the Asylum; and it was "voted that the Treasurer be authorized to purchase the 'Woodward Lot,' so called, next the Asylum, at Somerville, at a rate not exceeding twenty-five cents per square foot." The Treasurer reported on Aug. 9 that he had effected the purchase. G. Howland Shaw was, on Sept. 20, elected a Trustee in the vacancy caused by the resignation of Mr. Morton; but, in a communication received by the Board on Oct. 14, he declined the office.

The Board voted, at its meeting on Nov. 6, an amendment of a rule of the Hospital, so that it should read, "Any individual on the payment of one hundred dollars shall be entitled to a free bed at the Hospital for one year." Mr. Rogers, in behalf of a Committee to whom had been referred the question of the expediency of receiving inebriates as patients at the Asylum, raised by Dr. Tyler's last quarterly report, made a brief report, which was accepted: whereupon it was "voted that this Board deem the practice of admitting inebriates into the Asylum to be highly prejudicial to its best interests, and that hereafter no such persons be admitted as patients without the express order of the Board in each case." At the meeting of the Trustees on Nov. 20, Mr. N. I. Bowditch received the thanks of the Board for a newly bound copy of his "History of the Massachusetts General Hospital." The Board referred to Mr. Lowell, with full powers, the matter of building a sea-wall on the boundary of the Hospital grounds. Mr. Rogers, for the Committee on improvements at the Asylum, reported a proposition in writing from M. C. U. Cotting, agent for Miss Joy, for the sale of a strip of land one hundred and fifty feet wide, on the north-east side of the Asylum grounds, and the surrender of certain rights of way and restrictions on the south-east and south-west. This proposition coming before the Board on the next day, Nov. 21, at an adjournment, the following resolutions and vote were unanimously passed: —

"*Resolved*, That the extinguishment of all rights now held by any persons whatever other than this Corporation, in Asylum and Essex Streets, and of the restrictions upon building easterly of Essex Street, is desirable."

"*Resolved*, That the purchase of a strip of land one hundred and fifty feet wide, on the north-east side of the Asylum premises, is also desirable. Therefore, *Voted*, That the Committee on improvements at the Asylum be authorized, at their discretion, to effect these objects, at an expense not exceeding $33,000."

At the next meeting, held Dec. 4, the same Committee reported progress in negotiations to effect this object, and received further authority from the Board.

Grateful acknowledgments were made by the Board, on Dec. 18, to Mr. O. W. Bird, executor, for the receipt, through him, of a legacy of $1,000, bequeathed to the institution by his grandfather, the late George Hills; and thanks were voted to Dr. J. Mason Warren for the gift of a copy of the "Life" of his late father, Dr. J. C. Warren. A communication from Dr. H. J. Bigelow announced the bequest to him, by the late Mrs. S. Benton Thompson, of $492.40, for the benefit of the patients of the Hospital, with the request —

"That the income accruing shall be added to the principal, until the latter shall reach the sum of $500; after which the income shall be made payable annually to Henry J. Bigelow during his life, to be distributed at his pleasure, for the benefit of the patients in the Hospital, and after his death the income to be devoted to the support of free beds."

"*Voted*, That the Trustees accept the donation from Dr. Bigelow, on the conditions named, and that the same be called the 'Thompson Fund;' and that the grateful acknowledgments of the Board be presented through Dr. Bigelow to the executors of the will of the late Mrs. Thompson."

Messrs. Emmons and Higginson were appointed by the Board, on Jan. 1, 1860, to prepare the annual report for the last year. Henry H. Benson commu-

ORGANIZATION FOR 1860. 545

nicated to the Board, on Jan. 13, his resignation of the office of male Supervisor at the Asylum. The resignation was accepted; and the Board confirmed the nomination, by Dr. Tyler, of George A. Goodell, as his successor. The usual reports of the Treasurer and the other officers of the institution were presented at this and the next meeting, on Jan. 18, and referred to the Committee on the annual report. Appropriations were made for repairs at the Asylum, and for furniture for a Lecture-room there. The thanks of the Board were voted, on Jan. 25, to Messrs. Maynard & Noyes, of Boston, for their long-continued kindness in allowing the accommodation of their premises as a place for receiving packages for the Asylum; also, to the family of the late Dr. Perry for a photograph likeness of him, received from the hands of Dr. Bowditch.

The Committee on the annual report presented their report for the year 1859, which was read, accepted, and with the accompanying papers ordered to be laid before the Corporation at its annual meeting on this day.

At the first meeting of the Trustees, on Feb. 5, 1860, after the annual meeting of the Corporation, it appeared that the following gentlemen had been elected officers for the ensuing year: William Appleton, President; N. I. Bowditch, Vice-President; J. T.

Stevenson, Treasurer; T. B. Hall, Secretary; Messrs. J. M. Beebe, N. H. Emmons, W. W. Greenough, George Higginson, John Lowell, R. M. Mason, H. B. Rogers, and Edward Wigglesworth, Trustees on the part of the Corporation; and Messrs. Martin Brimmer, W. S. Bullard, W. J. Dale, and Thomas Lamb, Trustees on the part of the Commonwealth. On the organization of the Board of Trustees, Mr. H. B. Rogers was re-elected Chairman. No change was made in the last year's Boards of Consultation of Visiting Physicians and Surgeons, nor among the officers of the Hospital, except that Oliver H. Webber was chosen Apothecary, and there was no choice of an Artist, Dr. Sargent having declined a re-election. Dr. J. E. Tyler was re-appointed Physician and Superintendent of the Asylum, and Mr. and Mrs. Columbus Tyler Steward and Matron. The Standing Committees on Finance, on Accounts, on Free Beds, on the Warren Fund and Library, and on the Book of Donations, were appointed, and the Visiting Committees were arranged for the year. It was directed that two thousand copies of the annual report be printed.

The Committee, in this report, estimate the amount of the property of the institution, from nearly all of which income is derived, at $258,558.67. The expenses of the Hospital and the Asylum for the year

LEGACIES RECEIVED.

had been $98,789.64, and the receipts $94,076.47. The cost to the Corporation for the maintenance of 934 *free* patients had been $31,910.47; the income of funds specially appropriated to that purpose having been $14,816.06, leaving $17,094.41 chargeable to the general funds. There had been admitted to the Hospital 1,240 patients, at an average weekly expense for each of $5.75½, including, and of $5.33, excluding, repairs. Though there had been such an increase in the number of patients, yet at no time were all the beds occupied, nor was any proper applicant refused admission. Thus the new system adopted by the Trustees as to the discharge of convalescents had worked satisfactorily. The Committee commend the order and efficiency of the administration of Dr. Shaw. The Physician to out-door patients had treated 3,165 cases. There had been admitted to the Asylum 131 patients, and 175 remained at the end of the year, 317 patients having received its benefits during the year, at an average weekly cost for each of $6.16½. Several of the wards had been greatly improved and refurnished. The Committee express a high appreciation of the services of Dr. Tyler. Recognition is made of the legacy of $1,000 from the late Mr. George Hills, of Boston; of the donation of $3,857.22 from Dr. Rufus Kittredge, the income of which is to be applied to " Asylum " purposes ; and of the donation of $492.40 from Mrs. Thompson, for the " Hospital." Both Hospital and Asylum are reported to be in a satisfactory condition under the efficient and devoted management of their officers and attendants. Dr. Shaw reports that, besides the out-door patients, about five hundred persons had had the aid of dentistry in the extraction of teeth. The object of the Hospital being to afford substantial relief to the largest possible number of persons, it is not consistent with it to use even beds temporarily unoccupied for patients with incurable diseases. It is more in conformity with the design of the institution that eight or ten sufferers by acute disease should be successively relieved, than that the bed which they might occupy should be used, it may be for a year, by a chronic incurable. One half of those who during the year had been refused admission, being of foreign birth, had been referred to the State institutions provided for them. Beds must be reserved for urgent cases. Much relief is afforded to out-patients by the loan of Hospital furniture, surgical apparatus, fracture-beds, &c. A very complete catalogue had been made of the Treadwell Medical Library, which may be consulted by any proper applicant in the profession. By a new plan of administration there had been a reduction of the internal expenses of the Hospital, without any loss in good diet, or nursing and medical care.

Dr. Tyler, in his report, gives a condensed but most striking and classified statement of the individual and the classes of cases which in the course of the year come under his care, with the various forms of mental disease, — wild and destructive mania, frenzy, deep depression, suicidal tendency, delusion, and exhaustion, — all needing, and through their friends finding, the merciful refuge of the Asylum. The relief to those friends from manifold and painful anxieties, and the increase of comfort and safe liberty to the patients, are blessings hardly measurable. The number of perfect recoveries, and the restoring of useful and valued persons to their homes, families, and duties, call for gratitude. Recent improvements have added much to the convenience and elegance of the house arrangements. A great variety of amusements and means of recreation — billiard-tables, bowling-alleys, saddle-ponies, carriages, sleigh-rides, chess, cards, backgammon, bagatelle, the library, sewing-circles, and music — offer their resources. Many patients have attended concerts and lectures in Boston, and public worship on Sunday in various churches. Every Sunday evening a sermon is read, with singing, in one of the wings. Holiday parties, with dancing, and stereopticon, ventriloquism, &c.,

were held on Christmas, New Year's, February 22, July 4, and other occasions. The unremitting vigilance of attendants has prevented accidents and secured safety.

Dr. Tyler proceeds, at some length, to make one of those admirable contributions to the science and practical wisdom of his specialty, which give such high character and value to the series of reports offered by the heads of the Asylum. He pronounces insanity a disease, curable under conditions, like other diseases, and more hopeful of cure the earlier it is brought under specific treatment. He sets aside the absurdity of its being a disgrace. He opposes the fancy or theory that it can ever exist, without a derangement of the brain as an organ, or in its functions; yet he distinctly recognizes it as a secondary effect of diseases, like dyspepsia, not originating in the brain. Even hereditary victims of insanity are not to be considered incurable any more than if the disease were fever or rheumatism. Dr. Tyler then points at some of the causes which are influential in producing insanity, as warnings for those who would avert it for themselves or for others. An enlightened supervision of the training of childhood and youth, proper exercise and furnishing of the intellect, the recognition of moral laws and facts, self-control; the restraining of personal caprices, and of all appetites;

a regard for the intellectual, moral, and physical powers in their due relations and proportions; relaxation from too assiduous devotion to a special work or calling; the rational treatment of bodily ailments; and, above all, strict temperance, — are the safeguards which science and experience commend to all.

The Trustees instructed the Secretary to inform the Treasurer that it would be agreeable to them to have him participate freely in their discussions whenever he should attend the meetings. At the next meeting, Feb. 19, it was —

"*Voted*, That the Treasurer keep a separate and distinct account of all income received from, and all expenditures incurred on account of, each of the funds which have been or may be hereafter received for account of the Asylum, in respect to the use and application of which there are any special provisions; and that all unexpended balances of said accounts remaining at the close of the year be carried to the debit of the new account for the succeeding year."

It was also voted that the Superintendent of the Asylum, at each quarterly meeting of the Board, should present separate lists of such beneficiary patients as in his judgment should receive aid from the special trusts and funds for the ensuing quarter, that the Board might act on each case by a distinct vote. The Chairman from a Committee reported, recommending the appointing a " Standing Committee on Alterations and Repairs" at the Hospital and Asylum, with full powers in all cases in which the expense would not exceed one hundred dollars, the consent of the Board being requisite for any proposed outlay beyond that amount. The report and its recommendations were approved. The rules and regulations were amended according to these new provisions, and the new Committee was appointed for the current year.

An ice-closet was provided for the Hospital, by vote, April 1. A nuisance, caused by the city in filling the flats west of the Hospital, called for the action and protest of the Board, on May 6. Provision was made for proper diplomas for House Pupils at the Hospital. Mrs. George G. Lee subscribed $1,000 for a life free bed at the Hospital. Dr. Tyler received permission, on May 20, to be absent from the Asylum for attendance on the Convention to be held at Philadelphia, of Superintendents of Institutions for the Insane. The Treasurer was afterwards authorized to pay the travelling expenses of this visit, as for the benefit of the Asylum. On June 19, permission was granted to the House Pupils to sleep and take their breakfasts at the Hospital until otherwise ordered. During a contemplated absence of Mr. Rogers, Mr. Wigglesworth was, on July 3, chosen temporary Chairman of the Board. A communication to the Trustees, from Dr. Tyler, on Sept. 12, announced the resignation of Dr. Jerome C. Smith as Second Assistant Physician at the Asylum, and the nomination of Dr. J. Blackmer as his successor. The resignation was accepted, and the nominee was elected. The Board voted, on Oct. 12, "that in consideration of the advanced age of Miss Taylor, and her long and faithful services as nurse, which are held in grateful remembrance by the Trustees, she be relieved from all duties to the Hospital, and that her wages be continued till further order of the Board." A bequest made to the Corporation by the late Jonathan Phillips, Esq., to be appropriated to purposes designated by him, was gratefully acknowledged by the Trustees. The Committee on Accounts proposed on Oct. 23 the following vote, with its preamble, which were passed by the Board: "Whereas the expenses of the Hospital have increased largely during the past two years, voted that the Physicians and Surgeons of the Institution be requested to consider and to report to this Board, whether patients cannot be treated under its present system of administration at a less expense, and with equally satisfactory results." Prompted by this vote, Dr. Shaw communicated to the Trustees, on Dec. 9, a report of a sub-committee of the Medical Board as an answer to certain inquiries concerning the economy of the institution. This report was referred to the Committee on Accounts. Messrs. Rogers and Greenough, as a Committee, were instructed to consider and report whether any and what changes are desirable in the rules and regulations of the Hospital and Asylum. Messrs. Bullard and Beebe were appointed a Committee to prepare the annual report of the Board; the several reports of the respective physicians and officers of the institution, which were presented on Jan. 11 and Jan. 16, 1861, being referred to them. A report was made by the Committee and accepted by the Board, that, under existing circumstances, no change should at present be made in the terms of admission to the Hospital. The Committee on the rules and regulations asked for and received further time.

The annual report of the Board for 1860, with the accompanying documents, was laid before the Corporation at its annual meeting, on Jan. 23, 1861. All the officers of the Corporation during the last year were re-elected for the year ensuing, except that Dr. Samuel G. Howe was appointed, in place of Mr. Thomas Lamb, as one of the Trustees on the part of the Commonwealth. In the organization of the Board of Trustees, at its first meeting, on Feb. 10, Mr. Rogers was re-elected Chairman. Mr. Greenough, for the Committee of the old Board, on the revisal of the rules and regulations for the Hospital and the Asylum, reported, recommending certain changes and additions. The Board accepted the report, and adopted its recommendations. Mr. N. H. Emmons communicated to the Board his resignation as a Trustee. The same was accepted, and thanks were returned to him for his valuable services in that capacity. Mr. J. Amory Davis was then elected, by ballot, to fill the vacancy in the Board. The Boards of Consultation, of Visiting Physicians and Surgeons, and all the officers of the Asylum and Hospital, were unchanged, save that Mrs. Sarah L. Gallison having resigned the office of Matron of the Hospital, her resignation was accepted, with a continuance of her salary through the current quarter. Dr. Shaw was requested to consult with the Chairman relative to a proper person for Matron. The Standing Committees were appointed, and the Visiting Committees were arranged for the year.

The report for the previous year, 1860, is very elaborate, and contains matter of much interest. The expenses of both departments for the year had been $110,329.16; while the receipts had been $91,550.66, accruing from the ordinary sources. In addition to other general funds, there had been an extra dividend of $15,000 from the Hospital Life Insurance Company, without which there would have been a great deficiency of means. The Corporation had, up to this time, received from that insurance company since its establishment, according to the provisions of its charter, $231,687.50, being "the most munificent of all its munificent benefactors." The cost of the maintenance of 1,137 free patients at the Hospital, for an aggregate of 5,685 weeks, had been $36,148.06; of which amount, after deducting the income from endowments and subscriptions for free beds, there remained $18,955.69 to be charged to the general funds of the Corporation. The average cost per week of a patient at the Asylum, $6.58; at the Hospital, $6.42. The unproductive property of the institution in land and buildings is estimated at $607,209.99, the productive property being $258,330.36. A legacy had been received during the year of $10,000, for the support of free beds at the Hospital, by the will of the late Hon. Jonathan Phillips, who had been connected with the institution as a Trustee and Vice-President for more than a quarter of a century.

Mr. William I. Bowditch had made a donation of $274.25, being the amount of his bill for valuable professional services. The purchase of five acres of land adjoining the Asylum estate secures the premises from intrusion and extends the facilities for the out-door exercise of patients. Plans were in preparation for a *Cottage*, a suitable building, felt to be now very necessary, for imbecile female patients. The Committee express in high terms their sense of the fidelity and value of the services of the heads and of the subordinate officers of the Asylum and the Hospital, and acknowledge thankfully the labors of Dr. S. L. Abbot, who, as Physician to out-patients, had administered to 4,271 persons during the year. The resignation of Miss Rebecca Taylor, " who has efficiently and faithfully performed the duties of nurse in the Hospital for thirty-four years, and to more than four thousand persons," is noticed, with the remark that " she has won the gratitude and affection of the patients, and the cordial regard of all who know her, by her gentle manners and truly Christian life." The provision made for this excellent woman has been already noticed. The Treadwell Library, for consultation, contained 2,534 volumes. There had been in the Hospital since it was opened 23,351 patients, and in the Asylum 4,702. Nearly half of these in each department had been discharged *well*.

By Dr. Shaw's report it appeared that the whole number of patients in the Hospital for the year had been 1,394, of whom 1,240 had been admitted during that time : 1,137 had been wholly free. Of the patients, 555 were from Ireland. No applicant whose case was suitable for treatment had been rejected, and no one had been refused admission on account of inability to pay board.

Dr. Tyler reports that 121 new patients had been received into the Asylum during the year, and that 187 remained at its close. Holding in the reserve of a sacred confidence many of the experiences and incidents of his professional duties, he gives expression to some general and useful suggestions. Recognizing the fact that insanity, in any given case, is a sad experience, and brings a crushing sorrow upon the family of the afflicted one, he says it by no means follows that all the experience of an Asylum is of a gloomy character. The necessity and expediency of a separation from home and friends having been deliberately admitted, in spite of all the yearnings, reproaches, misgivings, and imaginary apprehensions that come with the effecting it, there is still another side to the experience. A glimmer of something like light comes where all has been darkness. Removal from the scenes and associations of the origin of the disease, the regularity and method of Asylum life, diversion of thought, the sense of being cared for wisely and kindly, gradually work their blessed influence. When restoration in its processes and its results is realized, it brings with it a clear comfort and an intensity of happiness. There are resources of peace, relief, and enjoyment also, for those for whom there is no reasonable hope of recovery. They appreciate the method, the comfort, the amenities of the house, its system and routine; they are observant of their dress and appearance, and the furnishings of their rooms; they enjoy their walks, drives, and amusements, and the interchange from solitude to companionship. Many of these regard the Asylum almost with reverence, and are alway on the side of order in a time of murmuring. Such patients are more than an offset to their antipodes in faith and feeling, and so are sources of benefit to others. Those who are under strong and grotesque delusions, in their own fixed belief, — kings, prophets, the world's benefactors, inventors, deities even, — if not seriously disputed, enjoy themselves and amuse their fellows, in the complacency of their fancies and plans. If imagination can invest with wealth and power, the Asylum has nabobs whose wealth and possessions are unmatched by any of the princes or potentates of the earth. All the passing trains of cars are carrying their goods, and the ships on all oceans are doing their traffic. The pitiable victims of hallucination who torture themselves into despair, of course, must not be forgotten; nor is it wise to dwell upon their miseries. The querulous and the perverse are to be borne with, neither encouraged nor roughly withstood. What the officers and attendants of an Asylum must be to meet the demands of a charge covering all these and many other workings of disease, it needs no full rehearsal of qualities to be set before an intelligent mind. Fidelity and kindness are the laws of the house. Patients taken away *uncured*, and employés discharged for unfitness, are the sources of all the malign reports about a well-ordered Asylum. Those who are *thoroughly recovered* are always enthusiasts in their praise and gratitude. An *early* resort to the Asylum in *every* case of insanity, and a patient delay till the cure is thorough and confirmed, before removal, are the prime conditions of benefit.

Dr. Dio Lewis had spent much time during the year in introducing his new system of gymnastics for classes in both sides of the Asylum, with great delight for the practitioners and the by-standers. Among the ladies there is an enthusiastic interest in "fancy-work." They contribute many valuable articles to charity-fairs. A generous friend had sent them two hundred dollars for the purchase of materials. Dr. Tyler, after stating that the political and social excitements of a most disturbed and startling year of time had all received attention in the Asylum, slyly adds that they "had been commented upon with as much interest and perhaps as wisely as in the great world outside of us." Many of the patients had attended entertainments in the city, and more still had been gratified by concerts, games, and lectures within the walls. Regattas and sleigh-rides yielded their delights.

Provision was made by the Trustees, at their meeting on Feb. 20, for the printing of five hundred copies of the Rules and Regulations in their amended form. At the meeting on March 31, the Board received a donation of $500 for the purchase of books for the patients in both branches of the institution. Grateful thanks were returned for the gift, and its proper use was referred to the consideration of a Committee. Plans, specifications, and an estimate of cost for a new cottage for female patients at the Asylum, were laid before this meeting by a Committee. The Board approved and adopted the same, and appointed Messrs. Rogers, Bullard, and Greenough a Building Committee, with full powers, up to the limit of an outlay of $32,000.

At the quarterly meeting of the whole Board, held at the Asylum on April 17, the death of Mr. Nathaniel I. Bowditch, Vice-President of the Corporation, was announced. The following resolutions offered by Mr. Rogers were unanimously adopted : —

"*Resolved*, That the Board of Trustees of the Massachusetts General Hospital have heard with unfeigned sorrow of the decease, on yesterday evening, of Nathaniel Ingersoll Bowditch, Esquire, its respected Vice-President.

"*Resolved*, That his long connection with this institution, as Secretary, Trustee, Chairman of the Board, and Vice-President, extending through a period of thirty-five years; the untiring devotion of all the faculties of his mind and heart to the promotion of its interests; his fidelity, intelligence, ability, patience, and firmness in the discharge of duty; his gentle, joyous, and modest demeanor, at all times and under all circumstances, so peculiarly remarkable in him; his sympathy with suffering and his many noble and generous acts for its alleviation, so characteristically performed, and so beneficial and grateful to those who were the subjects of them, — in short, his whole character, moral and intellectual, constantly developing and maturing, and his whole life always growing wiser and better and more useful to the last, have won for him the respect, admiration, and love of all the members of the successive Boards of Trustees of this Corporation, and of the Physicians and Surgeons and other officers who, from time to time, have been connected with it, and demand from us this tribute of regard for his memory.

"*Resolved*, That this Board, as a mark of respect for the character and services of its late Vice-President, will attend his funeral in a body, provided the same be in accordance with the feelings of the family.

"*Resolved*, That we sympathize deeply with the family of our deceased friend in the severe dispensation of Providence which has fallen upon them, and respectfully tender to them this token of our sorrow and regard.

"These resolutions to be entered on the records, and a certified copy of them to be transmitted to the family of the deceased."

In a volume of which this truly excellent and much loved man was the author, and the present reproduction of which was provided for by a liberal bequest in his last will, it is but right that he himself should find a special commemoration. The preceding pages from his pen will be evidence enough to a thoughtful reader of the love which he bore this institution; of his painstaking in dealing with its history; of his grateful estimate of every service which it received, from its origin to its maturity, from the professional skill and fidelity of its officers, and from the generosity and munificence of its benefactors. He labored to trace out and authenticate every fact which formed its annals. He acquainted himself with all the incidental matters which marked its development. He was jealously watchful for its good repute, and resolved that it should have no other repute. He kept its claims for the supply and enlargement of its resources before a community whose respect for him was an additional motive for listening to the cause which he pleaded. He directly solicited the gifts of others, and tried to conceal his own. And this, it might almost be said, was but the lesser part of what Mr. Bowditch did for the Massachusetts General Hospital; for he might have done it all outside of the walls of its spacious edifices. It may be added, without risking any extravagance in the statement, that during most of the thirty-five years of his official connection with the institution no officer within or without its walls was more heartily, laboriously, and effectively engaged than he was in promoting its objects, or was more thoroughly and minutely acquainted with all that occurred in it. The nurses and the patients came to know him best through his sympathies and his tender solicitude, and through a thousand kindly offices of thoughtful ministration, by gentle words, by the toy put into the hand of the little wondering child, crippled or languishing on its bed; by the rosebud, the nosegay, or the luscious garden fruit offered to a sufferer, in whom gratitude created the appreciation of the unwonted luxury.

Mr. Bowditch was born in Salem, June 17, 1805, a son of the eminent Nathaniel Bowditch, LL.D., whose genius in mathematical and nautical science, while it gave him a world-wide fame, places him among the greatest men of our Continent. The son graduated with high rank at Harvard College in 1822, and at once entered upon the study of the law in the office of the late Benjamin R. Nichols, Esq., — then residing in Salem, and himself a generous benefactor of this institution. The family having removed to Boston, Mr. Bowditch entered the law-office of the late Hon. William Prescott and Franklin Dexter, Esq., with the latter of whom Mr. Bowditch was for a short time a partner in business. He was very soon drawn into that specialty of his profession, "conveyancing," for which he had a peculiar taste and aptitude, and in the pursuit and practice of which he obtained a distinction in Boston which made him the supreme authority in tracing, verifying, and transferring the titles of parcels of real estate. No careful man who proposed to buy or to take a mortgage on such property thought he had done his full duty to himself unless he had the warrant of Mr. Bowditch. He was thoroughly acquainted with the voluminous contents of the Registry of Deeds for the county, and his own iron safe was crowded with fifty-five autograph folios, of five hundred pages each, of abstracts of titles, of copied instruments and carefully drawn plans of original and subdivided estates under their successive owners. As parcels of land became of enhanced value in the city, inches became of importance in the measurement; and the owner of an estate was inclined to great precision or over-precision in his claims in fractions. The writer of these lines heard Mr. Bowditch once pleasantly remark, in reference to some of these elastic measurements, that he should be satisfied with the fortune which would accrue from the actual sale of the supposititious inches of territory specified in deeds, *beyond* the actual surface of the soil in the city. His fame as an accurate investigator and conveyancer came to the knowledge of

Lord Chancellor Lyndhurst, and drew from him a high certification. His special acquisitions in connection with his legal training were drawn upon in very important cases, in which he was summoned for testimony or an opinion by the Legislature and the City Council.

A volume which bears the name of Mr. Bowditch as its compiler, and which appeared in three editions, successively increasing in size, — so that the third edition contains seven times as many pages as the first, — is unique in our literature. It involved incredible labor and research, and is a marvellous witness to the thoroughness and fidelity of his devotion to his special profession. The volume was not put on sale, the copies of it being given by the author privately to his friends as a pleasant token of his personal regard, and to public libraries and institutions. I copy from the third edition, now before me, containing nearly eight hundred octavo pages, and printed in 1861 : the title and motto are as follows : —

"Suffolk Surnames. By N. I. Bowditch.

"A Name! If the party had a voice,
What mortal would be a Bugg by choice?" — Hood.

The dedication is "To the Memory of A. Shurt, 'The Father of American Conveyancing,' whose name is associated alike with my daily toilet and my daily occupation."

The work is a direct result of his investigations in the Suffolk Registry of Deeds. The first edition appeared in 1857; the second, enlarged, in 1858. The prefaces contain much interesting historical matter relating to the Records of Suffolk County, and much curious information on the general subject of names, and the bibliographical sources on which the author drew, in the expansion of his work far beyond its original design. There is a vast deal of instruction and humor to be found in the volume, more than any one would imagine could come from an arrangement of the classification and derivation of names. It needed, however, the compiler's own charming fancy and subtile wit to make so much of his theme and materials.

The reader will peruse, with full appreciation and sympathy, this closing portion of Mr. Bowditch's preface: —

"I will conclude with a few words of 'personal explanation.' I was born in 1805. Of a vigorous frame and active habits, I enjoyed for fifty years almost uninterrupted health. During the summer months, I seldom omitted a daily swim in Charles River; and the coldest weather of winter rarely induced me to resort to an outside garment. In 1835, on a bridal tour, I visited Niagara, and swam across that river, below the Falls, on two successive days; and once, when the thermometer was at zero, the gentlemen who had gathered around the fire in an insurance office in

Boston proposed, as I entered the room, to subscribe to buy me an overcoat, because, as they said, it made them cold to look at me. At fifty, however, I ceased to be a young man; and my dress was no longer such as to exert a chilling influence over my friends. In February, 1859, I slipped upon the ice, but did not fall; and I supposed that I had escaped with merely a slight sprain, and the laugh of the bystanders. I had, however, injured the head of the thigh bone; and the result was a gradually increasing lameness. In June I removed to my summer residence in Brookline. Here, in an apartment curtained by forest trees, I sat, day after day, week after week, a prisoner; my sole occupation being the collection and arrangement of the materials for the present edition, and the laborious preparation of the Index. On Aug. 2, a visit was made by my attending surgeons. I arose to receive them; and in the effort to open the drawer of a small writing-table, which was partly behind me, I pulled it out so that it fell upon the floor. From this slight cause, a severe fracture of the thigh occurred while I was standing up. I have been thenceforth condemned to a state of horizontal meditation, which must last as long as I live. Twice already have I here seen the foliage of summer give place to the snows of winter. My misfortune has received every alleviation which science could suggest, or the kindness of family and friends bestow; but my bodily pain and weariness soon made some fixed employment almost indispensable. I accordingly commenced the printing of this work in the autumn of 1859; and it has enabled me to attain a state of cheerful discomfort.

Until my confinement, I had never permitted my mustache and beard to grow: they are now of a truly patriarchal length and whiteness. Had my book been a grave, philosophical treatise, my head, with these hairy appendages of

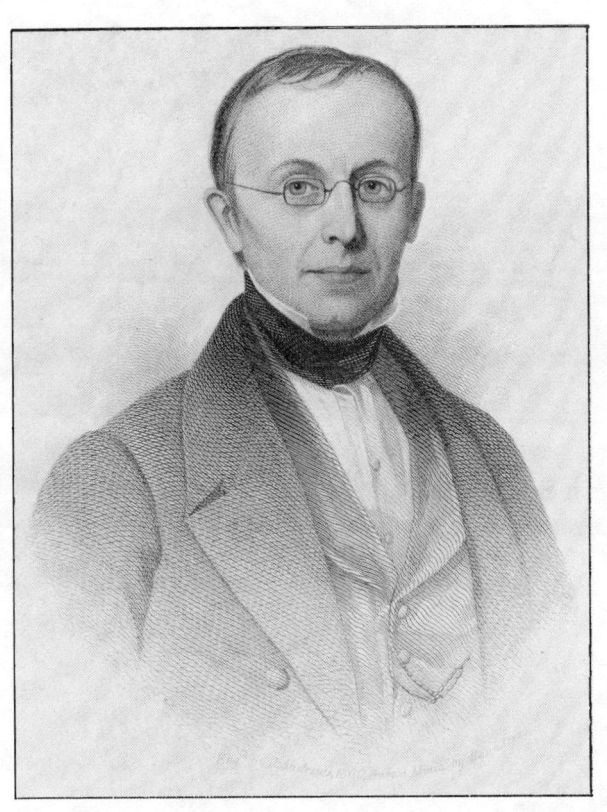

wisdom, would have made for it a most appropriate frontispiece. But, considering its light and lively character, I have preferred a *retrospective* view of my face. The engraving is from a miniature painted by a British artist, while on a professional visit to this country, about twenty years ago. Truth compels me to admit that no one recognizes me through this disguise of youth.*

"If my volume shall sometimes dispel the cloud of care or thought from the brow of manhood, or call forth a smile upon the face of youth and beauty, I may perhaps hope, if not for the sympathy, at least for the indulgence, of my readers."

This preface bears date, " Brookline, Mass., February, 1861." The writer, who had borne his severe and protracted sufferings with Christian patience, sustained by Christian hope, was released on the 16th of April following. Those who were privileged to visit him in his cheerful chamber will always remember his sweet smile of welcome, the resignation of his spirit, and his lively interest in the nobler concerns of the world without. There was a curious satisfaction — associated with his long series of visits to other sufferers in the Hospital — with which he drew the attention of his visitors to the ingenious devices and

* There is an excellent likeness, in photograph, of Mr. Bowditch, in the Trustees' room at the Hospital, the gift of Mrs. Bowditch. This, as having "the appendages of wisdom," would have been given by preference in this volume, had not the subject of it made his own choice.

mechanism of the couch on which he lay, for raising him and affording slight changes of position. He had another resource on that bed of pain besides the revising of his book of Names. He bore in remembrance very many who were poor, in sorrow, or under trial; loving to be told of any new ones on the Bethesda list who were strangers to him, that he might send to them regularly the tokens of his sympathy and bounty. His philanthropy was of the widest, his humanity was of the purest and the fullest.

In accordance of purpose with his wife, Mr. Bowditch, in 1860, gave to Harvard College the sum of seventy thousand dollars, for the establishment of sixteen scholarships, four for each class, of an annual value of two hundred and fifty dollars each.

At the meeting of the Trustees on April 17, the Committee on Repairs were instructed to procure plans for laying out and improving the grounds, and for the better drainage of the Asylum. It is interesting now to note how the alarming condition and prospects of the country at the opening of the civil war are recognized by an entry on the records at the meeting of the Trustees on April 24. The Committee appointed to contract for the new "Cottage" at the Asylum reported that the proposals in their hands for the work were within the estimates. But they hesitated, without further conference with the Board, to proceed with the work " under the circumstances now existing in the country." " After a full discussion of the subject," the Board, in strong faith, gave the Committee authority to go on with the work.

The Board, at its meeting on May 5, were informed by the Treasurer that the late Mr. Bowditch had in his will bequeathed to the Hospital $5,000 to constitute a " Wooden-leg Fund," and $2,000 as a fund for the republication of the History of the Hospital. The Treasurer was directed to establish the two funds accordingly. At the same meeting, the Secretary was directed to communicate to His Excellency Governor Andrew the following vote, passed in view of the pending civil war : —

"That the Trustees of the Massachusetts General Hospital assure the Executive of the Commonwealth that, in the event of any diseased or wounded soldiers being returned to this city, they shall consider it their duty and privilege to extend to them all the succor and relief that may be within their power."

A communication from Governor Andrew acknowledging this vote was received by the Board on May 19; and by a second, subsequent letter to Dr. Shaw, on Aug. 27, he expressed his high appreciation of the attentions rendered by the Hospital to returned soldiers.

The House Pupils having petitioned for leave to board in the Hospital, the Trustees, by vote on Aug. 27, granted permission until further order. A new form of bond, with reference to sureties, for the admission of patients to the Asylum, having been found desirable, Mr. Lowell, to whom the subject had been committed, reported a form at this meeting, which was adopted. Mr. R. M. Mason, on Sept. 10, resigned his place on the Board, on account of intended absence abroad. The Secretary was directed to communicate to him the thanks of his associates for his long and valuable services. The Treasurer was authorized to borrow the money needed for the construction of the new "Cottage" at the Asylum. On Nov. 17, the Chairman, Mr. Rogers, having previously announced to the Board that he would be unavoidably absent from Boston during much of the coming season, in attendance at Washington as a member of the National Sanitary Commission, the Board elected Mr. Bullard as Chairman *pro tem.* while Mr. Rogers should be absent. Measures were instituted by the Board, on Dec. 15, for disposing the boundary line between the flats belonging to the Corporation and those belonging to the heirs of the late Dr. Parkman. Messrs. Wigglesworth and Davis were appointed the Committee, on Dec. 29, to prepare the annual report of the Board; and the annual reports of the Treasurer and other officers, as presented on Jan. 10, and Jan. 15, 1862, were referred to them. At the meeting on Jan. 10, the Treasurer read a communication from the Hon. William Appleton announcing his donation of $10,000 to be added to the "Appleton Fund," for the assistance and support of needy curable patients at the Asylum. A suitable acknowledgment was made of this munificent gift.

CHAPTER XV.

FEB. 5, 1862, TO FEB. 22, 1867.

ANNUAL MEETING AND ORGANIZATION FOR 1862. — REPORT FOR 1861. — DEATH OF THE PRESIDENT, MR. APPLETON, AND TRIBUTE TO HIM. — INVALID SOLDIERS AT THE HOSPITAL. — BEQUEST FROM MISS TOWNSEND. — UNITED STATES SANITARY COMMISSION ASK THE SERVICES OF DR. SHAW AND DR. TYLER. — RESIGNATION OF THE STEWARD AND MATRON OF THE ASYLUM. — SERVICES OF DR. MORRILL WYMAN. — LEGISLATION ON ASYLUMS. — ANNUAL MEETING. — ORGANIZATION FOR 1863. — REPORT FOR 1862. — RESIGNATION OF DR. TOWNSEND. — DR. TYLER'S TRIBUTE TO DR. BELL. — SKETCH OF HIM. — NEW COTTAGE FOR MALES AT THE ASYLUM. — RESIGNATION OF DR. BACON AS CHEMIST. — HOUSE PUPILS TO BOARD AT THE HOSPITAL. — DR. J. C. WHITE ELECTED CHEMIST. — BEQUEST OF JOHN PICKENS. — DEATH OF DR. HAYWARD. — DR. TOWNSEND ELECTED CONSULTING PHYSICIAN. — ADDITIONAL SURGICAL HOUSE PUPILS. — LITIGATION CONCERNING BEQUEST OF MISS LORING. — BEQUEST OF DR. B. D. GREENE. — HOURS FOR THE VISITS OF SURGEONS AND PHYSICIANS. — A SURGEON TO OUT-PATIENTS. — ANNUAL MEETING. — ORGANIZATION FOR 1864. — REPORT FOR 1863. — HISTORICAL PAMPHLETS PRESENTED BY DR. SHAW. — LEGACY OF WILLIAM OLIVER. — RESIGNATION OF SECRETARY HALL. — ELECTION OF MR. W. S. DEXTER. — RESIGNATION OF DR. BOWDITCH AND CHOICE OF DR. C. ELLIS AS A VISITING PHYSICIAN. — OTHER CHANGES AMONG THE OFFICERS. — TRIBUTE TO DR. J. B. S. JACKSON. — BEQUEST OF MISS SEVER. — ANNUAL MEETING. — ORGANIZATION FOR 1865. — REPORT FOR 1864. — DEATH OF J. AMORY DAVIS. — RESIGNATION AND APPOINTMENTS AT THE ASYLUM. — OTHER RESIGNATIONS. — ANNUAL MEETING. — ORGANIZATION FOR 1866. — REPORT FOR 1865. — IMPORTANT REPORT ON THE FINANCES AND CIRCULAR. — CHANGES OF OFFICERS AT ASYLUM. — BEQUEST OF DR. WORCESTER. — A NEW OPERATING THEATRE. — LEAVE OF ABSENCE TO DR. TYLER. — GIFT FROM REV. J. SPAULDING. — LEGACY FROM MISS S. PRATT. — ANNUAL MEETING. — ORGANIZATION FOR 1867. — REPORT FOR 1866. — GENEROUS SUBSCRIPTION. — DEBT PAID. — DR. TYLER'S REPORT.

THE annual meeting of the Corporation was held at the Hospital on Feb. 5, 1862. The following gentlemen were elected officers for the ensuing year, William Appleton, President; Robert Hooper, Vice-President; J. T. Stevenson, Treasurer; T. B. Hall, Secretary; Messrs. J. M. Beebe, J. Amory Davis, W. W. Greenough, George Higginson, John Lowell, H. B. Rogers, J. C. Wild, and Edward Wigglesworth, Trustees on the part of the Corporation; and Messrs. W. S. Bullard, W. J. Dale, Martin Brimmer, and S. G. Howe, Trustees on the part of the Commonwealth.

The annual report for 1861 estimates the productive property of the Corporation at $307,166.05. The value of the property at Somerville is fixed at $332,712.27; that of the Hospital estate in Boston at $289,347.64. The expenses of the Hospital have been $38,954.30; and of the Asylum $63,311.87, the income of the Corporation having been $95,996.44; showing an excess of expenses of $6,269.73. An appeal to our citizens is recommended for the purpose of increasing the fund for free beds at the Hospital. There had been admitted to the Hospital 1,416 patients; whole number under treatment 1,552; the average cost of each, per week, being $5.35. Testimony is borne to the efficiency of the Resident Physician and other officers. No case suitable for treatment had been rejected. The Hospital had ministered to the comfort of many of our volunteer soldiers who had become disabled. The Physician to out-patients had treated 4,775 during the year. The Treadwell Library contained 2,577 volumes. The Superintendent of the Asylum reports 298 patients under treatment during the year, 188 remaining at its close; the average weekly cost of each being $6.07. The Asylum has maintained its high reputation for the fidelity of its officers, and the merciful efficiency of their work. The new building for highly excited female patients is in a state of forwardness. The gifts of J. Bowdoin Bradlee and of William Appleton, and the bequests of N. I. Bowditch, are gratefully mentioned; and the tribute of warm regard to the last-named gentleman is renewed.

Dr. Shaw repeats his suggestions as to the intent of the Hospital for the treatment of curable patients, rather than for an Infirmary, and refers to the proposed City Hospital as designed to receive contagious and incurable cases.

Dr. Tyler, in his report, congratulating himself on the progress of the new building on the Asylum grounds, and giving a general summary of the year's duties, and gratefully referring to all the means of amusement and relaxation enjoyed by his large household, devotes the rest of his pages to a most admirably condensed and eloquent statement of the experiences of the country under the terrible discipline of war, with especial reference to the effect of its exciting events upon his patients. We can recall no more adequate or striking picture and summing up, than that which he has here drawn of those days and scenes of woe. His devoted predecessor, Dr. Bell, was at the time in the field as a minister of mercy to the patriot army.

The President of the Corporation and the generous benefactor of the institution, Hon. William Appleton, having died on Feb. 15, at Longwood, a special meeting of the Corporation of the Massachusetts General Hospital, which had been duly notified, was held at the Hospital in Boston, on Monday Feb. 24, 1862, at $3\frac{1}{2}$ o'clock P.M.

Robert Hooper, Esq., the Vice-President, called the meeting to order, and took the chair.

The death of the Hon. William Appleton, late President of the Corporation, being announced, the following resolutions offered by the Treasurer, J. Thomas Stevenson, were unanimously adopted: —

"*Resolved*, That in the death of the Hon. William Appleton this Corporation has met with a great loss. He was connected with the management of its affairs for twenty-five years, always with a lively interest in the promotion of its charitable purposes. The institution is greatly indebted to his prudent counsels, as well as to his well-directed benevolence. His munificent donations have enabled the Trustees to do much for the comfort, as well as for the cure of those insane, whose limited means might otherwise have deprived them of the full advantages of a residence at the Asylum. The fund which he established for the assistance of the curable insane has abounded in rich fruits. The buildings bearing his name at Somerville, which were erected at his suggestion and chiefly by his bounty, are honorable monuments both of his sagacity and of his benevolence.

"*Resolved*, That a copy of these proceedings be communicated to the family of Mr. Appleton, with assurances of the sympathy of the members of this Corporation with them in their bereavement, and of their appreciation of the honorable and Christian character of the deceased."

A communication from Edward Wigglesworth, Esq., was read, declining to accept his re-election to the office of Trustee, and it was voted that the same be referred to the Board of Trustees.

The meeting was then dissolved.

Attest: T. B. HALL, *Secretary*.

At the first subsequent meeting of the Board of Trustees, on Feb. 24, 1862, Mr. H. B. Rogers, then absent at Washington, was re-elected Chairman, Mr. Bullard being chosen to fill the place temporarily. A communication from Mr. Wigglesworth, resigning his place as Trustee, having been referred to the Board by the Corporation, the Trustees voted to him their thanks " for his long, faithful, and efficient services." The following professional gentlemen were then elected by ballot for the ensuing year: as the Board of Consultation at the Hospital, Drs. J. Jackson, J. Jeffries, E. Reynolds, G. Hayward, J. Homans, and W. Lewis; as Visiting Physicians, Drs. J. B. S. Jackson, H. I. Bowditch, G. C. Shattuck, A. A. Gould, C. E. Ware, and F. Minot; as Visiting Surgeons, Drs. S. D. Townsend, J. Mason Warren, H. J. Bigelow, H. G. Clark, S. Cabot, jun., and G. H. Gay; Dr. B. S. Shaw, Resident Physician; Dr. S. L. Abbot, Physician to Out-patients; Dr. J. Bacon, Chemist; Dr. C. Ellis, Microscopist and Curator of the Pathological Cabinet; O. H. Webber, Apothecary; Harvey Howard, Steward; Mrs. Mary Wiggin, Matron. Dr. J. E. Tyler was chosen Physician and Superintendent of the Asylum, and Mr. and Mrs. C. Tyler Steward and Matron. The Standing Committees of the Board were appointed, and the Visiting Committees were arranged for the year. The thanks of the Board were voted to Mrs. N. I. Bowditch for the gift of a photograph likeness of her late husband, " whose services and benefactions are gratefully remembered by this Corporation." It was —

" *Voted*, That the subject of proper accommodations in this Hospital for the sick and wounded of the United States army be referred to Drs. Dale and Howe, to consider and report to this Board at an early meeting; and in the mean time that Dr. Dale shall have authority to place for treatment in the

Hospital any invalid soldier for whom there is suitable room, the rate of their board being $4.50 per week."

Dr. Dale reported at the next meeting, March 23, —

"That, unless some extraordinary exigency should occur, the accommodations now afforded by this Institution are ample for the present."

A communication from the Custom-house Collector of Boston was received, enclosing a copy of an inquiry from the Treasury Department at Washington, relative to obtaining contract proposals from public and private hospitals, for the accommodation of sick seamen. Whereupon it was —

"*Voted*, That the Resident Physician be directed to reply to the Collector, that, whilst the Trustees would be glad to receive all patients for whom there is room in the Hospital, the organization and rules of the Institution and its relation to the City and State are such as to prevent any contract-undertaking of the kind desired."

On May 4, Miss Susan L. Kilborn made a communication to the Trustees, asking leave to visit the Hospital. The communication was laid on the table. Mr. Henry A. Whitney was elected a Trustee, on May 18, to fill the vacancy in the Board caused by the resignation of Mr. Wigglesworth. Mr. Lowell, at the meeting of the Board, on June 3, offered a new

Form of Admission of patients to the Asylum, made in accordance with recent legislation. It was adopted by the Board. He also submitted a document relative to the use of land of the Parkman heirs adjoining the Hospital grounds. This document disclaimed all rights and easements being acquired to the Hospital by the enclosure of land of the Parkman heirs, and the opening of a gate upon the same. The document was approved, and the Treasurer was authorized to execute it in behalf of the Corporation. The Committee on improvements of the Asylum grounds were authorized, on June 3, to remove the old cottage as soon as the excited patients were transferred to the new building. Dr. Tyler received permission to attend the approaching annual convention of " the Association of Superintendents of Institutions for the Insane," at Providence, — his expenses to be met by the Board.

At the meeting of the Board on July 15, the Chairman, Mr. Rogers, took his seat, having returned from service at Washington, on the Sanitary Commission.

The Trustees, at their meeting on Aug. 26, received the following letter, of that date, addressed to them: —

"The late Miss Mary P. Townsend, by her last will, authorized us, as her executors, to dispose of the residue and remainder of her estate to such charitable and public institutions as her executors may think meritorious.

"In such residue and remainder is a parcel of real estate in Hanover Street, in this city, which was appraised at $7,500, after her decease, and is now under lease to a good tenant, for three years from the first day of July last, at a rent of $450 for the first year, and $500 a year for the last two years. The tenant pays the taxes and keeps the estate in repair at his own cost.

"We think we cannot more exactly fulfil the benevolent intentions of Miss Townsend in giving us the power to dispose of the residue of her estate, than by presenting the house in Hanover Street to the Massachusetts General Hospital, as her gift. Accordingly, we send you a deed of it, and an assignment of the lease.

"We have thought it best that the deed should be absolute and without limitation; but we wish and earnestly hope that the income of the estate may hereafter and always be appropriated for the support of free beds in the Hospital." Signed by the executors, William Minot, and William Minot, jun.

This benevolent donation was accepted; the Secretary being directed to communicate to the executors the sincere thanks of the Board, and the Treasurer to establish the "Townsend Free Bed Fund," from the estate and its income. A communication was received from the Surgeon-general of the United States army relative to the termination of any contract for board of United States soldiers at the Hospital, and their future removal. Dr. Tyler, on Sept. 9, communicated to the Board his appointment of Dr. James H. Whittemore as Assistant Physician at the Asylum, in place of Dr. John Blackmer, who, after two years of faithful service, had left, on his appointment as surgeon of the 47th Massachusetts Regiment. The nomination was confirmed.

A communication from Dr. Shaw was laid before the Trustees, on Oct. 10, relative to a request of the United States Sanitary Commission that he would act on a Board of Special Inspection of General Hospitals of the army, requiring a service for two terms, of two weeks each, during the next six months. It was then " voted that leave of absence be granted to Dr. Shaw for the time and purpose named, provided he makes such arrangement for supplying his place during his absence as shall be satisfactory to the Chairman of this Board."

The same leave was granted by the Board to Dr. Tyler, on Oct. 15, for the same purpose and on the same conditions.

Dr. Bacon, Chemist at the Hospital, was authorized to employ an assistant in the performance of his duties, in such way and at such time as he cannot attend to them himself, at an expense not exceeding $250 annually.

Mr. Bullard, for a Committee, reported on Nov. 2 that a marble bust of the late William Appleton had been procured and placed in the Trustees' Room at the Asylum.

The resignations of Mr. and Mrs. Tyler, as Steward and Matron of the Asylum, were received by the Board on Nov. 16, and were accepted, with the understanding that the incumbents would remain in office until suitable successors could be found.

Messrs. Howe and Wild were appointed on Dec. 28 to prepare the annual report of the Board to the Corporation. Mr. Higginson was afterwards added to this Committee, to whom the reports of the Treasurer and of the officers of the Hospital and Asylum, as they were regularly submitted, were referred. At the meeting on Jan. 21, 1863, the Trustees passed a vote of thanks to Dr. Morrill Wyman, of Cambridge, "for his careful examination of the plans of ventilation for the new Cottage for females at the Asylum; for his valuable suggestions thereon; and for the cordial interest manifested by him in the welfare of the institution."

Dr Howe and Mr. Lowell were appointed a Committee, on Feb. 4, "to look after the interests of this institution in the proposed legislation on the subject of Asylums for the Insane, now pending before the Legislature of this State."

The annual meeting of the Corporation was held at the Hospital on Feb. 4, 1863, at which the report of the Trustees was presented. Mr. Robert Hooper, who had been Vice-President, was chosen President, in place of the late William Appleton; Edward Wigglesworth was chosen Vice-President; J. T. Stevenson, Treasurer; and T. B. Hall, Secretary. Only two changes were made in the Board of Trustees, Mr. Henry A. Whitney taking the place of Mr. Wigglesworth, on the part of the Corporation; and Mr. Harrison Ritchie taking that of W. J. Dale, on the part of the Commonwealth.

At the first meeting of the Board, on Feb. 15, it was organized by the choice of Mr. H. B. Rogers as Chairman. A communication was read from Dr. Solomon D. Townsend, declining to be re-elected one of the Visiting Surgeons of the Hospital. The following resolves were thereupon unanimously adopted: —

"*Resolved*, That in accepting the resignation now tendered to them, by Dr. Solomon D. Townsend, the Trustees, in justice to him and to themselves, feel bound to express their high appreciation of his long, faithful, and valuable services in behalf of this Institution. 'Consulting Surgeon' of the Hospital from the year 1835 to 1839, and 'Acting Surgeon' from that time to this, a period of nearly a quarter of a century, he has daily, without fee or pecuniary reward, given a full share of his time and professional skill to the patients committed to his charge; and by his ability, sound judgment, assiduity, kindness, and consistent and gentlemanly conduct, has, at all times during this long term of years, won the respect and esteem of his professional associates and of all the various Boards of Trustees. In parting from him, the Trustees therefore would offer to Dr. Townsend their hearty thanks for all the good he has done to them and the public in the past, and their most sincere wishes for his welfare and happiness in the future.

"*Resolved*, That Dr. Townsend be requested to sit for his portrait or bust, and that Messrs. Rogers, Bullard, and Stevenson be a Committee to carry this resolve into effect."

A communication having been received from Dr. W. J. Dale, announcing that he had declined re-election as one of the "State Trustees," it was thereupon —

"*Voted*, That the thanks of the Board be presented to Dr. Dale for his long, faithful, and efficient services as a member of the Board from which he has now retired."

The elections for Boards of Consultation, of Visiting Physicians, and Visiting Surgeons resulted in the choice of all the members of those Boards during the previous year, save that upon the last named Dr. Richard M. Hodges was chosen to supply the place of Dr. Townsend. Dr. Shaw was chosen Resident Physician of the Hospital; Dr. Abbot, Physician to out-patients; Dr. Bacon, Chemist; Dr. C. Ellis, Microscopist and Curator of the Pathological Cabinet; George T. Sears, Apothecary; and Mrs. Mary Wiggin, Matron. Dr. Tyler was chosen Superintendent of the Asylum. The Chairman then appointed the Standing Committees, and the Visiting Committees were arranged for the year. The Chairman and Mr. Lowell were made a Committee to consider and report upon the duties of the Steward of the Hospital, with power to make such temporary arrangements relative to that office as may be necessary.

The annual report of the Trustees, of which two thousand copies were printed, contains references to many matters of interest. The pressure of the times had not caused any anxiety in diminishing the income, in increasing the number of patients, or abating the earnestness of the friends and officers of the institution. There had been received and treated within the Hospital during the year 1,611 patients, in addition to the 140 who were there at its beginning. There remained at its close 145. There had been treated 4,800 out-patients. There had been received and treated at the Asylum 270 patients, of whom there remained at the close of the year 176. This whole summing up presents to us a ministration of mercy in an impressive form, especially when we contemplate the accumulative results gathering in the lengthening course of years. The gift through the executors of the late Miss Townsend is a recognition of a continued liberality which is expected to constitute an item in every report. The expenses of the Hospital were $42,114.81; the average weekly cost of each patient, $6.04. The expenses of the Asylum were $71,823.46, the average for each patient being $7.27, though this covers some extraordinary outlays on the grounds, &c. The value of the productive property is set at $318,397.96; that of the real estate, — the Asylum, $348,441.93, the Hospital, $280,347.64. The outstanding debt is $78,164.81, incurred by the purchase of the Joy and Woodworth estates, and by the building of the new cottage for female patients. An appeal is suggested for aid in removing this debt, without diminishing the beneficent work of the Institution.

Dr. Shaw reports that, though 277 applicants had been refused as unfit at the Hospital, no case suitable for treatment had been rejected for inability to pay board. The capacity of the Hospital is 180 beds. It had sent home well, during the year, 843 patients. There had been received and treated 212 United States soldiers, besides a large number as outpatients. Before the establishment of a government military hospital in Boston, such patients had been paid for at the rate of $4.50 a week. Since that time they had been free.

Dr. Tyler's report is written in a grateful spirit for the large additions which have been made to the comforts and curative agencies of the Asylum. The new edifice for patients under the most demonstrative forms of mental disorder, with its spacious and cheerful apartments, and the enlarged and beautiful grounds improved by Mr. Cleveland, are realized as blessings already. The war, the distractions and miseries of which are more and more daily felt, has not yet caused any appreciable increase of insanity. Seventeen of the attendants of the Asylum had enlisted in the army, and Dr. Blackmer had gone into service as surgeon. Dr. Tyler repeats, as with the force of his increased experience, that insanity in almost all its forms is curable, and generally is so according to the promptness with which it is put under treatment; in its incipient stages its subtle approaches and vague manifestations being too often slighted till the mischief is confirmed. The decease during the year of the Hon. William Appleton and Dr. Luther V. Bell is regarded by Dr. Tyler as properly calling forth from him a tender reference to their services and virtues. They had been so long and harmoniously associated as officers in this Institution, — the one, by his sympathy and large pecuniary gifts and administrative skill, contributing so munificently and wisely to its means and its government; the other, by his humane and gentle spirit, his profound knowledge, and his enriched experience, presiding within its walls over the dependent subjects of his skill, — that death, coming to them after protracted feebleness, seemed to make one more bond of union between them. The "Appleton Wards," with their elegant and convenient apartments, are to some extent a compensation to a socially favored class of patients for their removal from luxurious homes. The "Appleton Fund," for the assistance and support of needy curable patients, is a form of benevolence already blessed by many of the recovered among its grateful receivers. Thus the rich and the poor were alike embraced in Mr. Appleton's considerate kindness. It is but right that Dr. Tyler's just and beautiful tribute to his predecessor and associate should be transferred to these pages: —

"For nearly twenty years Dr. Bell held the position of Superintendent of the Asylum, identifying himself with all its interests, and directing its daily management, with a comprehensive skill, sagacity, and forecast, a purity and elevation of purpose, and a scrupulous faithfulness to every relation involved, which secured for him, for those intrusted to his care, and for the Institution, the happiest and the most abundant results. The accuracy and variety of his knowledge, the soundness of his judgment, and his remarkable faculty of adapting means to ends, meet one here at every step; while the recognized method of treatment, the traditionary usages and rules of the house, bear the indelible stamp of his thorough and exact comprehension of the needs of the insane, and his wonderful tact in providing for them. His active and commanding intellect, his extraordinary attainments as a scholar, philosopher, and psychologist; his extensive knowledge of every thing pertaining to the phenomena, management, and history of insanity; his able and long-continued efforts and success in diffusing and establishing correct views of the nature and treatment of the disease, — have justly caused him to be regarded as one of the most distinguished of the many great men who have ever adorned the medical profession. His inbred sense of honor, his entire removal from all meanness and duplicity, his sterling integrity and inflexible moral courage, his keen sense and ardent love of right, leading him to its defence, in utter disregard of any personal consideration, and in the face of any obstacle, and qualifying and inspiring all his every-day life, and yet with no touch of pharisaical exactness or pretension, commanded the admiration and respect of all who knew him, and gave him an uncommon power of personal influence, while it made him of inestimable worth as a friend. His courteous and dignified bearing, his gentle manner and quiet humor, his inexhaustible store of anecdote and useful information, gave him a wonderful charm as a companion. Strong, though not demonstrative in his feelings, warm in his attachments, he loved his home, his friends, and his daily associations, and devoted himself to their welfare. He loved his country, and felt the severity of her fiery trial; and, faithful as always to his convictions of right and personal obligation, he gave her as his last offering the rich accumulation of his experience, and his life, — a brilliant example of lofty Christian patriotism."

The reference made in the last sentence of Dr. Tyler's affectionate tribute to his predecessor may justify a few words of explanation. It was the privilege of the writer, in another associate relation, to be charged with the office of a biographer of Dr. Bell.* Dr. Bell came of an honored ancestry of the Scotch-Irish settlers in New Hampshire. His father was governor, one of his brothers senator in Congress, and another the chief-justice of that State. He had predilections for and would have won eminent distinction in political life, had not his chosen profession first drawn and then engrossed the faculties of his mind. The last years of his connection with the Asylum were saddened by repeated and severe afflictions. He was there bereaved of three children and of his wife. On the resignation of his office, he retired to a dwelling which he had built for himself in Charlestown, that he might be near to the scene of his long-continued service, which he hoped frequently to visit. Here he suffered much from the symptoms of pulmonary disease. On the opening of the civil war, by letter dated April 19, 1861, and addressed to the adjutant-general of the State, beginning with the words, " We are at that point where every man who can devote himself to his country's service should come forward," he asks to have put on file his application for any position in the

---

* Memoir of Luther V. Bell, M.D., LL.D. Prepared by vote of the Massachusetts Historical Society. Printed in the " Proceedings," &c., for 1863.

medical service of the Commonwealth in which he could be useful. He says that he had been originally educated for a surgeon in the New York hospitals. Governor Andrew at once gladly commissioned him, June 10, 1861, as Surgeon of the 11th Regiment of Massachusetts Volunteers. This office he resigned on being appointed by General Hooker, the commander of his division, "Acting Brigade Surgeon." He was soon after promoted to be " Medical Director " of the division, having under him twenty-two medical officers, in charge of fifteen thousand men. He performed devoted service in the camp, on the field, and in the hospital, and was a witness of some of the most direful horrors of the war. In January, 1862, Congress proposed the appointment of a corps of " Inspectors of Hospitals." To all persons to whom his character and qualifications were known, it would be obvious that he would be considered as among the first of those to whom such a responsible trust should be offered. As there was something characteristic of the nobleness and dignity of the man in the course which he pursued in reference to the matter, and as he made the writer the medium for the accomplishment of his wishes, I will venture to transcribe a portion of one of his letters to me which relates to the subject.

"HEADQUARTERS, HOOKER'S DIVISION,
LOWER POTOMAC, Jan. 13, 1862.

"A bill now on its way through Congress reorganizes the Medical Department of the army. The Brigade Surgeons, in which class I stand as No. 10, are merged with the surgeons of the regular army, and certain 'Inspectors' are provided for, with rank and emoluments a little higher than we now enjoy. Their duties are to exercise a supervision over the hospitals, the hygienic regulations, &c.

"I propose applying for one of these places, feeling confident that my pursuits and studies hitherto will make me more useful in such a position than in the ordinary line of duty. Of course one's expectations of success depend entirely on the influence which friends can bring to bear on the appointing power."

He then refers to the exhaustive professional testimonials which were already on file in his favor, and to the friendly relations existing between him and the incumbents of national and State offices; and yet, looking outside of the usual means employed for political patronage, he adds: —

"It seems to me that for an office requiring capacity for such duties and trusts as those suggested, if offices are ever bestowed because of fitness, the appointing power should have the testimonials of some other than political names. I should be glad at least to offer something different, and my thoughts have turned towards our associates in the distinguished societies," &c.

His wish was to have gathered to a petition in

his favor the names of some prominent gentlemen, Fellows of the American Academy of Arts and Sciences, and Members of the Massachusetts Historical Society. The paper which I obtained and transmitted to him in answer bears the following signatures: Robert C. Winthrop, William Appleton, Governors Everett and Washburn, Presidents Sparks and Walker, Professors Parsons, Parker, and Pierce, J. G. Palfrey, David Sears, and Josiah Quincy. To his own signature Mr. Appleton added these words: —

"I am not satisfied with simply signing the annexed; but will add that I for many years was intimately acquainted with Dr. Bell while I was acting as President and Trustee of the M'Lean Asylum. I do not nor did I ever know the man I could so highly recommend for the office asked for."

A special testimonial in his behalf, addressed to the President of the United States and to the Secretary of War, went from members of the Massachusetts Medical Society and from the Medical Faculty of Harvard University. Dr. Bell was informed that his friends with cheerful alacrity were preparing these papers, and warmly expressed his thanks in a letter. But the papers did not reach his tent till the day before his final illness. They are now before me bearing his indorsement. It is soothing to think of him as in his last hours enjoying in this form the sympathetic pleasure of communion with distant friends. After a severe attack on Feb. 5, he died under his canvas shelter at Camp Baker, near Budd's Ferry, on Feb. 11, of metastasis.

At the meeting of the Board on March 1, Messrs. Bullard, Beebe, and Brimmer were appointed a Committee to raise by subscription a sum of money sufficient to pay the cost of building and furnishing a new cottage for male patients at the Asylum; and they were instructed, after securing the amount, to consult with Dr. Tyler, and to cause to be built on the grounds an edifice conformed in general arrangements and for a corresponding class of male patients to that built last year for females. On March 15 the Committee on the subject reported to the Board that temporary experimental arrangements had been made relative to the office of Steward at the Hospital. The report was accompanied by a communication from Harvey Howard, resigning that office: his resignation was accepted. Leave was granted to Dr. Shaw to accept the appointment of Commissioner, or Examining Surgeon, under the authority of the United States Pension Office, — his services to be rendered at the Hospital. This office was to be held by him in accordance with documents communicated to the Board relative thereto. The Committee on the Warren Fund and Library were authorized to expend a sum not exceeding fifty dollars for the supply of illustrated papers at the Hospital. On March 29, by request of the Visiting Physicians, the Board made a change in the regulations, which allowed Dr. Ellis, the Microscopist and Curator of the Pathological Cabinet, to perform their duties in case of their necessary absence. On April 10, the Committee on that subject reported that a sum sufficient for building and furnishing a new cottage for excited male patients at the Asylum had been subscribed. Thanks were voted to each of the subscribers. On April 15, Dr. Tyler received permission, at the expense of the Corporation, to attend the annual meeting of the Association of Superintendents of Institutions for the Insane, to be held in New York on May 19. Dr. Tyler having recommended Mr. and Mrs. George W. Whittle as persons suitable to fill the positions of Steward and Matron at the Asylum, and a Committee having reported in approval of the nomination, they were elected by ballot to those offices. Permission was granted by the Board, on May 3, to Messrs. C. Tyler and J. M. Pinkerton, executors of the late Dr. Bell, to take his portrait from the Asylum that an engraving might be made from it. In terminating the connection which Mr. and Mrs. Columbus Tyler had so long held, as Steward and Matron at the M'Lean Asylum, the Trustees " desire to express their entire satisfaction with the manner in which they have discharged their respective duties, their regret at their departure, and their sincere wishes for their future welfare and happiness." It was voted that their salaries should be paid to the 1st of July ensuing, and that a copy of these votes be transmitted to them by the Secretary. Mr. Tyler had entered the Asylum as attendant, on July 29, 1827; was made Supervisor in 1830, and Steward, Feb. 1, 1835, making thirty-six years of service. He had found his future wife a patient in the Asylum, of which, on her recovery, she was made Supervisor in the autumn of 1830, and Matron in 1835, making twenty-eight years of service.

A nuisance existing on the water border of the Hospital grounds, Messrs. Lowell and Beebe, with the Treasurer, were appointed a Committee to wait upon the mayor of the city to urge the immediate filling of the flats.

On May 17 Dr. John Bacon resigned his office as Chemist at the Hospital. His resignation was accepted, the thanks of the Board were voted to him " for his long and valuable services," and the Physicians and Surgeons were requested to nominate a

BEQUEST OF MR. PICKENS. 599

suitable candidate to fill the vacancy. Mr. Rogers, for a Committee that had been appointed to endeavor to obtain a reduction of the charge for water, reported that they had had a full hearing before the Board of Aldermen, who had rejected the petition for a reduction of the rates, upon legal grounds, stated in City Document No. 47, for 1863.

By recommendation of Dr. Shaw, it was voted, on May 31, that the present House Pupils be permitted to board in the Hospital until further order of the Trustees.

A communication having been received from the Medical Board recommending Dr. James C. White as a candidate for the office of Chemist of the Hospital, he was, by ballot thereupon taken, declared elected. The rules regarding the House Pupils of the Hospital were amended. Mr. Lowell, on June 16, made a report on the use of the John Redmond bequest, which was accepted and placed on file. Dr. Tyler was authorized, on July 14, to engage the services of a landscape gardener, for the proper ornamenting of the Asylum grounds. On Aug. 25, a bequest of $950.00 to the Corporation from the late John Pickens was announced to the Board by the Treasurer, which was gratefully acknowledged.

At the meeting of the Board on Oct. 21, Mr. Wild, for a Committee, reported the following resolution, which was unanimously adopted:—

"In view of the recent death of Dr. George Hayward, which occurred suddenly on the 7th instant, at the advanced age of seventy-two, the Trustees of the Massachusetts General Hospital would express their sympathetic interest in this sad event, and their regret for the departure of one so long and intimately connected with this Institution. Dr. Hayward was first chosen Assistant Surgeon in 1826, then junior Surgeon in 1830, and chief in 1838, which post he resigned in 1851, after twenty-five years of active service; still, however, continuing to the day of his death as an efficient member of its Board of Consultation. The history and records of the Hospital bear enduring testimony to his faithful and devoted labors in all these relations, and of the high appreciation in which they were held by our predecessors in office; and now that his life of varied usefulness on earth is closed the present Board of Trustees desire to offer this last and grateful tribute of respect to his memory.

"*Voted*, That the foregoing resolution be entered upon the records, and a copy of the same be communicated to the family of the deceased."

Dr. Solomon D. Townsend was then elected by ballot to fill the vacancy in the Board of Consultation caused by the death of Dr. Hayward.

On Nov. 22, in consideration of additional services rendered by the Resident Physician and the Matron of the Hospital, the salary of the former was increased to $2,000, and of the latter to $650. On Dec. 20, Messrs. Whitney and Lowell were appointed a Committee to prepare the annual report of the

Trustees to the Corporation. At this meeting a recommendation, made at a previous meeting by Dr. Shaw, of the election of two additional Surgical House Pupils, was adopted; and the Secretary was instructed to report the changes necessary to be made in the rules and regulations conformably thereto, which he did at the meeting on Jan. 3, 1864, his report being approved by the Board. A question having arisen as to the use of the surplus income of Mr. Bowditch's Wooden-leg Fund, a Committee appointed for that purpose reported, on Jan. 20, that the representatives of the family of the donor objected to any diversion of the income from the object specified by him. On Feb. 3, an appropriation of $200 was made for enlarging and improving the greenhouse at the Asylum. An increase was voted to the salaries of the Superintendent, the Assistants, the male Supervisor, and the Clerk, at the Asylum. The annual report of the Board was read to the Trustees, and accepted, and ordered with the accompanying documents to be laid before the annual meeting of the Corporation to be held this day.

A special meeting of the Board was held on Feb. 28, at which information was given and action taken upon a matter of great interest. It appeared that the late Mrs. Abigail Loring, of Boston, had ordered that the residue of her estate, amounting to more than $71,000, should be distributed among incorporated Charitable Institutions of this city, according to the decision and direction of three persons to be appointed for that purpose by her executor. Such distribution having been made, the sum of $30,000 was assigned to this Institution for the support of free beds. It also appeared that the provision of the will under which such distribution had been made was claimed by the heirs-at-law to be illegal and void; and that one or more suits at law had been commenced to test its validity. The Board thereupon resolved that it gratefully received the assignment to it in the order of distribution, and that the Treasurer and Mr. Lowell be a Committee with full power, in behalf of this Corporation, to employ counsel, sign and execute instruments and papers, and do every thing in their judgment proper and desirable for facilitating and securing to this Corporation the payment of the above amount. Further reference to this subject will be found under the year 1868. The Treasurer, for the Committee on the bequest of the late Dr. B. D. Greene, reported that the executors of his will were prepared to pay over the sum of $5,000, for the purpose of establishing a free bed at the Hospital. It was voted that the bequest be gratefully accepted for the purpose indicated, and that the Treasurer invest the sum as the " Greene

Fund," the income to be for the support of free beds in the Hospital.

A Committee, to whom had been referred the subject of the hours of visiting of the Surgeons and Physicians, reported that they had called a meeting of those officers, and, having fully impressed them with the desirability of the greatest possible regularity in their visits, had presented the subject in all its relations. The Committee after deliberation had adopted the following resolution: —

"That the hour for the daily visits to the patients shall be ten o'clock, A.M., or as near that time, between the hours of ten and one, as possible. The faithful performance of the letter and spirit of this rule is, in the opinion of the Committee, compatible with the best care of the patients and the good internal management of the Hospital."

Upon the report and recommendation of the same Committee, the following preamble and vote were adopted: —

"Whereas the interests of the out-surgical patients will be promoted, the convenience of the Visiting Surgeons be subserved, and the benefits of the Institution increased, by the appointment of a Surgeon to this class of patients, —

"*Voted*, That a Surgeon to out-patients be and hereby is established, whose duties shall correspond generally with those of the Physician to the same department."

The Rules and Regulations were altered in adjustment to the provision in this vote. Dr. Algernon Coolidge was then by ballot elected Surgeon to out-patients.

The first regular meeting of the new Board of Trustees for the current year was held on March 13. The officers of the Corporation were the same as in the previous year, save that Dr. William J. Dale took the place of Martin Brimmer among the four Trustees on the part of the Commonwealth.

At the organization of the Board, Mr. H. B. Rogers was re-elected as its Chairman for the ensuing year. In the election of the members of the various Boards, and of the officers both of the Asylum and the Hospital, all who had filled those places during the previous year were again chosen to them respectively. The Chairman appointed the Standing Committees, and arranged the Visiting Committees for the year.

The annual report for 1863 takes notice that a variety of causes had made the year one of marked interest for the institution. The great rise in the prices of the commodities of life, with no corresponding increase of receipts, had caused anxiety. There had been a generous response to the appeal for funds for erecting the new building at Somerville, and several valuable bequests had been received, still the Treasurer has to report an increasing debt. The new City Hospital, now about ready to be occupied, — in the construction, arrangement, and preparation of which the experience of our own institution has furnished valuable aid, — will hardly diminish, to any practical extent, the draft upon our resources. The increasing population, and the accommodation of classes of patients, lying-in women and sufferers by cutaneous diseases, for which we have no provision, will probably require all its added space and means. The report notices the resignations, the changes, and the elections in the official staff of the institution, which have been already referred to as they severally occurred. During the year, 1,793 patients had been treated in the Hospital. The assumption of the general superintendence of the Hospital by the Resident Physician, Dr. Shaw, has been found to be an improvement on the old system. The applicants for treatment as out-patients have numbered 5,214, all but 227 of whom were cared for: 1,590 prescriptions had been furnished without charge.

The Committee congratulate the Trustees on the appointment by the Governor of an able Board of Commissioners, — Hon. Josiah Quincy, jun., and Drs. Alfred Hitchcock, and Horatio Storer, — to examine into and report upon the subject of Insane Asylums in this State. The sum of $44,450.00 had been munificently subscribed for the erection of a cottage for excited male patients, corresponding to that which was built two years ago for female patients, and which has proved so beneficent in its advantages. The legacies made to the institution for the year are, — from the estate of John Redman, to be added to the Redman Fund, $7,500; from the late Captain Percival, $1,000; from the late John Pickens, $1,000; and from the late Miss Elizabeth Hill, $250; the last three sums being subject to the legal United States tax. The productive property of the institution is estimated at $287,528.95; the income was $102,877.05; the value of the estates at the Hospital and Asylum is $651,189.57. The debt of the Corporation amounts to $73,559.50. The expenses of the Asylum were $69,300.63; of the Hospital, $47,421.71. The weekly cost of each patient was, at the Asylum, $6.98; at the Hospital, $6.66. There had been admitted to the Asylum, as Dr. Tyler reports, during the year 94 new patients; and there remained at its close 201. There had been perfect recovery in many severe cases, and in several of very long standing. The new cottage of the ladies' wing, with the fine gardens, have proved of incalculable benefit. It had been a busy, and, so to speak, a cheerful year, among the inmates, working for the great " Sanitary Fair." The amusements and festivities of the year have been varied and much enjoyed. The subscription of $45,000, raised in four weeks, for the designed new building, and the kind payment by a friend, Mr. W. S. Bullard, of a sum of $800 to purchase an enlargement of the grounds, are warmly recognized. The whole household parted with Mr. and Mrs. Columbus Tyler with deep regret, and follow them with gratitude and good wishes.

Dr. Tyler then, at considerable length, with a view to inform and to meet the prejudices and misstatements which prevail among some classes of the community, defines the conditions and safeguards which regulate the admission and detention of the patients at the Asylum. These are presented by him with specific and minute detail, and to an intelligent and candid mind will prove in every respect satisfactory.

At the meeting of the Board on April 15, Dr. Shaw presented to the Trustees six volumes of pamphlets relating to the institution, which he had collected and had caused to be bound. This gift was highly appreciated and gratefully recognized by the Board, and the volumes were ordered to be placed under the special charge of the Resident Physician. The collection has proved very serviceable in the preparation of these pages. At this meeting, Mr. S. P. Loud, executor of the will of the late William Oliver, informed the Board that a legacy of

$37,580.00, under said will, had fallen in to this Corporation, by the recent death of Miss Nancy Oliver. The matter was referred, for proper action, to the Treasurer. On account of the enhanced cost of the necessaries of life, it was found requisite to raise the rates of board for patients at the Asylum. Their sureties were to be informed of this, the Visiting Committee for the time being receiving full power to dispose of all questions which might arise in any case from this needful measure. On April 20, the Committee on repairs received full powers to make all necessary arrangements for taking the supply of water for the Asylum from the Charlestown Water-works, instead of from the Cochituate.

At the meeting of the Board on May 8, Mr. Wild was appointed Secretary *pro tem.*, in the absence of Mr. Hall, from whom a communication was received, resigning that office held by him. His resignation was accepted, and the thanks of the Board were voted to him for his faithful and valuable services. Messrs. Davis and Lowell were made a Committee to nominate at the next meeting a candidate or candidates for the office of Secretary, and the latter was requested and authorized to act as such till the vacancy should be filled. Dr. Tyler received permission to attend, at the expense of the institution, the annual meeting at Washington, of Medical

Superintendents of the Insane. On the nomination of the Committee, at the meeting of the Board on May 24, Mr. William S. Dexter was unanimously elected Secretary, and was duly qualified as such on June 7. On May 24, Dr. H. I. Bowditch resigned his office as one of the Visiting Physicians. The Board accepted his resignation with great regret, and expressed to him " their gratitude for his long, faithful, and laborious services, and for his constant and deep interest in the welfare of the Hospital." Dr. Calvin Ellis was, on June 7, unanimously chosen to fill this vacancy. A change in the Rules was made by which the Board of Consultation was increased to eight members. Drs. H. I. Bowditch and C. E. Brown-Séquard were then elected members of that Board. An increase of salaries and wages was voted to employés at the Asylum on July 15, and on July 19 the salary of the Steward and Matron was increased $300 *per annum*. The thanks of the Trustees were voted, on Aug. 16, to the Directors of the Public Institutions of Boston, for their kindness in giving the use of the city boat to the Asylum patients on three occasions during the present summer. It was voted, on Oct. 19, to hold the regular meetings of the Board henceforward on Friday, instead of, as heretofore, on Sunday. Dr. Algernon Coolidge, on Nov. 4, resigned his position as Surgeon to out-patients. His resignation was accepted, and a Committee charged with the selection of a gentleman to be proposed for that office. The thanks of the Board were voted to Dr. Coolidge for his faithful and valuable services. Messrs. Greenough and Higginson were appointed, on Dec. 16, a Committee to examine the Treasurer's accounts, and to prepare the annual report of the Board to the Corporation. On Dec. 30, Dr. J. B. S. Jackson communicated his resignation as a Visiting Physician. The Board, on accepting it, resolved, —

"That the official services of Dr. Jackson, as House Apothecary, Assistant and Admitting Physician, and Visiting Physician in this Hospital, extending as they do through a period of thirty-one years, twenty-five of which have been devoted to the important duties of the last office, deserve, and should receive the grateful acknowledgments of the Board and of this community; and, in accepting the resignation of his present official position, the Trustees desire to bear their testimony to the punctuality, precision, skill, and thorough fidelity with which all its requirements have been discharged, and to extend to him their best wishes for his future health and welfare."

The Treasurer reported on Jan. 18, 1865, a bequest from Miss Martha Sever, of Kingston, of five shares in the Western Railroad Company for the support of free beds. The annual report of the Trustees, having been presented and accepted by the Board, was, with the accompanying documents, laid before the Corporation at its annual meeting on Feb. 1. The Committee necessarily have much to say about the pecuniary affairs of the Corporation. This is the fifty-first annual report. The expenses are still steadily exceeding the income. The numerous personal changes in the administration and conduct of the institution, already noticed in the order of their occurrence, are referred to. Leading practitioners have within a few years devoted themselves to the special investigation of a certain obscure class of diseases, and the Board of Consultation has been enlarged by the addition of the two distinguished practitioners, Drs. Bowditch and Brown-Séquard. There had been admitted to the Hospital 1,599 patients, of whom $55\frac{1}{2}$ per cent were discharged cured. The Physician to out-patients had treated 3,761 medical cases; and 1,858 surgical out-patients had been cared for. There had been 302 patients at the Asylum, 195 remaining there. The property of the Corporation, other than the real estate in use by it, is $337,395.02. The debt amounts to $83,414.50; and the excess of expenses over income for the year had been $26,704.12. The Treasurer's accounts go into full details on all these matters, and prepared the way for the measures of relief which were soon to be munificently afforded. Dr.

Tyler, in his report from the Asylum, also refers to these financial perplexities, and to the slight increase in the charge of board for patients, — though, he adds, these have known no abridgment of care, convenience, comfort, or recreation, however the managers have been embarrassed. The entertainments have been numerous and much enjoyed. The improvements in the grounds and buildings are highly appreciated. Dr. Tyler then devotes eight pages of his report to a very instructive statement of one of those lessons of a full and enriched experience as to the uses of an Asylum, and its benefits and its modes of soothing patients, for which this series of reports is so valuable.

The first meeting of the Trustees for the current year was held at the Hospital on Feb. 24. The officers of the previous year had all been re-elected, save that in the place of Mr. J. C. Wild, Mr. George B. Emerson had been chosen a Trustee on the part of the Corporation. He, however, declined to serve. Mr. Rogers was re-elected Chairman of the Board. Drs. H. I. Bowditch and D. H. Storer were joined to the previous Board of Consultation; Drs. G. C. Shattuck, A. A. Gould, C. E. Ware, F. Minot, C. Ellis, and S. L. Abbot, were chosen Visiting Physicians; the Visiting Surgeons were the same as before, as were the other officers and employés of the

Hospital and Asylum. The Chairman appointed the Standing Committees, and arranged the Visiting Committees for the year. The Board at several successive meetings gave much attention to measures for increasing the funds of the institution. A Committee had been appointed; and a circular prepared by its Chairman, Mr. Rogers, was considered at the meeting on April 20, and approved, with a vote that three thousand copies of it be printed. To this circular and its results subsequent reference will be made. Dr. Tyler made a short visit to Charleston, S.C., this spring, for the benefit of his health.

The death of Mr. J. Amory Davis, one of the Trustees, was communicated to the Board at its meeting on May 5; and the Trustees gave expression to the great sorrow with which they heard of the removal of their late associate, and resolved, —

"That this institution, in common with the whole community, has sustained great loss in the death of Mr. Davis, whose comprehensive spirit of humanity, perfect fidelity, and sound judgment, united with most conscientious devotion to the duties of his office, had rendered his services of great value to this institution and to all connected with it."

This tribute was communicated to the widow of Mr. Davis, and the Board attended his funeral.

Dr. Alexander D. Sinclair was, on May 19, chosen to serve for the remainder of the year as associate to the Physician to out-patients. On June 2, leave of absence was given to Dr. Tyler to attend at Pittsburg the Convention of Medical Superintendents of American Institutions for the Insane. On July 20, it was voted " that the Physicians and Surgeons to out-patients be authorized to charge such fees for their first visits as they may think proper, whenever they are satisfied of the ability of patients to pay the same." Donations of large amounts were received by the Board at this, and on subsequent meetings, which will be mentioned at the close of the year. A communication was received from Dr. Tyler on Sept. 5, announcing the resignation of Dr. Ranney, and relating to the appointment of a successor. This was acted upon at the meeting of the Trustees on Oct. 2. Dr. Ranney's resignation was accepted, and the thanks and good wishes of the Board were voted to him. Dr. Whittemore was then appointed Assistant Physician at the Asylum, and Dr. Isaac H. Hazelton was appointed in Dr. Whittemore's former place. It was voted that the quarterly meetings of the Board at the Asylum be henceforth held on the Fridays after the third Wednesdays of January, April, July, and October. Mr. Greenough, on Nov. 3, resigned his place as a Trustee. Messrs. Storrow and Rogers were appointed, on Dec. 15, to prepare the annual report of the Board. To this Committee

ORGANIZATION FOR 1866.

were referred in order the various reports of the officers and of the Treasurer as they were presented.

At the meeting of the Board on Jan. 19, 1866, Mr. Bullard communicated the offer of Mr. Nathaniel Thayer of a donation of the sum of twenty-five thousand dollars to the Corporation, provided that seventy-five thousand more were raised. Messrs. Bullard, Beebe, Higginson, and Rogers were appointed a Committee to obtain subscriptions for the same. The Secretary, Mr. W. S. Dexter, resigned that office on Feb. 7; his resignation was accepted, with thanks for his faithful and efficient services. Mr. Thomas B. Hall was then elected Secretary *pro tem*. Dr. Tyler's salary was fixed at $3,000, commencing from January first. The annual report, which had been offered to the Board and accepted, was, with the accompanying documents, laid before the annual meeting of the Corporation held on Feb. 7, 1866.

The Corporation re-elected Messrs. Hooper, Wigglesworth, and Stevenson, respectively, as their President, Vice-President, and Treasurer, and chose Mr. Thomas B. Hall Secretary; with Messrs. Beebe, C. H. Dalton, S. Eliot, G. Higginson, J. Lowell, H. B. Rogers, C. S. Storrow, and H. A. Whitney, Trustees. Messrs. W. S. Bullard, S. G. Howe, James L. Little, and Harrison Ritchie had been appointed Trustees on the part of the Commonwealth. The Trustees, on their organization, Feb. 23, unanimously chose Mr. Rogers as their Chairman, notwithstanding he had declined to be a candidate for re-election. No change was made in the old Boards of Consultation, of Visiting Physicians and Surgeons, or in the officers of the Hospital or Asylum. Dr. J. Theodore Heard was chosen Surgeon to out-patients. The Chairman appointed the Standing Committees and designated the terms of the Visiting Committees for the year. The Special Committees of the last year, who had not reported, were re-appointed on their respective subjects.

The report of the Trustees for 1865, with the documents accompanying it, are of especial interest. An anxious solicitude had steadily increased with the successive statements of the Treasurer as to the excess of expenditures over income, and the accumulating debt. The Asylum might be regarded as self-supporting, from the board of patients and the income of special funds. The Hospital was the great absorbent and the occasion of the debt. The special report and the circular, soon to be referred to, indicate the measures taken to relieve the embarrassment. The donations and legacies for the year amount to $22,920; viz., a bequest of $500 from Miss Martha Sever; from the estate of M. P. Sawyer, $1,000; from the Redman estate, $6,500; donations from William Minot, $100; from Mrs. H. F. Lee,

$1,000; from Stephen Salisbury, $5,000; from Edward Whitney, $5,000; from Edward Wigglesworth, $1,000; bequest by E. A. Raymond, $2,820.

The death of their associate, J. Amory Davis, is appropriately noticed by the Committee. Dr. Shaw reports that there had been admitted to the Hospital 1,199 patients, 140 of whom were on account of accidents. The average number had been 113. There had been treated as out-patients 5,356 persons. The weekly cost of a patient in the Hospital had been $9.86; in the Asylum, $12.50. There were remaining in the Asylum 192 patients; 277 having been under treatment during the year. The list of resources for the diversion, amusement, instruction, and excursions of the patients, as presented by Dr. Tyler, exhibits an amount of kindness and sympathy exercised towards them which makes by itself an impressive lesson. In May, the new building for gentlemen, called the "Bowditch Ward," was occupied; and its excellent adaptations have afforded the most solid satisfaction. Another of those instructive contributions to the science of his theme, with pregnant suggestions as to the causes, the workings, and the "moral treatment" of mental disease, will be found in this report of Dr. Tyler's. Where but to the keen and intelligent observation, the discriminating judgment, and the carefully matured experience of such well-tried officials as himself, are we to look for wise counsel? Dr. Mark Ranney, his senior assistant, having assumed the superintendence of the Iowa Asylum, Dr. Whittemore fills his place, Dr. I. H. Hazelton being Dr. Whittemore's successor.

To this annual report is attached the " Report of a Committee on the Financial Condition of the Hospital," and a Circular. The Committee, after a most thorough and protracted investigation into the management, oversight, internal economy, and daily administration of the Hospital, had entirely satisfied themselves that there was no waste, no extravagance, no needless or unwarranted outlay. Relief from embarrassment was not to be sought in reducing the expenses, but was offered only by the alternative of an appeal to the public for generous gifts, or of increasing the number of paying patients. Considering the circumstances of the community, under the pressure of many burdens and the exaction of many claims, at the close of an exhausting war, a direct appeal for new gifts is to be made only from absolute necessity. The publication of a circular which shall set the wants and appeals of the institution before affluent and benevolent persons, so that they may be induced to remember it in the disposal of their estates, is strongly recommended. The Committee then give reasons to justify the effort for increasing the number of paying patients. The institution in its early years, received its patients chiefly from that industrious class of our native population, who, by paying a reasonable board, enabled it, with the help of its income from invested funds and donations, to meet its expenses. Immigrations from abroad, with a consequent change in the social and pecuniary condition of the laboring classes, have led to an extraordinary increase in the number of free patients humanely cared for in the Hospital. During the last five years, of 7,668 patients, only 1,601 have paid any thing; and of those who paid any thing very few met the actual cost of their board. Nearly 25,000 other patients had freely received medical or surgical advice or treatment. The excess of expenditures beyond income has thus, in five years, swelled to $60,827.04. The debt of the institution, after all the splendid endowments it has received, is now $86,698.47. The city, within the last year having provided a commodious hospital for the poorer classes, will justify this institution in diminishing the number of its free patients. The Committee therefore recommend measures to that end.

The Circular, of which three thousand copies were printed, under date of April 1, 1865, earnestly presents the claims of the institution. With the exception of a similar one at Philadelphia, it is the oldest in the country. Having received substantial aid from the State in its first year, it has ever since depended wholly on subscriptions, donations, bequests, and devises, in which it has had a truly munificent share. It has prompted the formation and endowment, and been the model for the management of many other hospitals. It has been an effective agent in the development and improvement of the medical and surgical professions. It has nobly ministered to suffering humanity. Apart from its property in the lands and buildings which it occupies, its invested funds, most of them restricted in their use, amount to $230,380.03, with a debt, arising from the sum of yearly deficits, of $86,698.47. Unless the institution receives further aid, its necessary course will be to reduce the average number of its free patients, which is now 114, to 50. Waiving for the present, for reasons assigned, a direct appeal for donations, the Circular asks that the claims of the Hospital may be remembered in testamentary bequests. The fruitful results effected by this Report and Circular will come under grateful recognition in the review of the current year. The thanks of the Trustees were voted, on March 23, to the contributors who had responded so generously to this appeal.

Dr. Tyler received leave of absence, on April 20, to attend the meeting of Superintendents of Asylums at Washington. On May 4, Miss Wiggin resigned her office as Matron of the Asylum. Her resignation was accepted. On May 18, Dr. Tyler communicated to the Board the resignation of Mr. G. A. Goodell, as Supervisor at the Asylum, and the nomination to the Board of Mr. Dexter Gray as his successor. The resignation was accepted, and the nomination was confirmed. Measures were adopted to provide for renovations in the surgical department of the Hospital, as desired by the Surgeons. A report and plans were submitted on June 29, for alterations and improvements in the surgical operating theatre; and Dr. H. J. Bigelow appeared to urge their adoption. The subject was recommitted for further details on July 13. On Aug. 31, an anonymous bequest of $1,500 from a friend of the institution was announced to the Board. This gift proved to be an offering of gratitude from the Rev. Dr. S. M. Worcester, whose wife had been a patient at the Asylum. On Oct. 19, Dr. Tyler having communicated to the Board the resignation of Miss Relief R. Barber, after a service of thirty years as female Supervisor at the Asylum, it was "voted that the Chairman be requested to communicate in writing to Miss Barber the high appreciation of her services held by the Board." Dr. Tyler having proposed as her successor Miss Georgiana W. Mills, the Board voted approval. Progress was announced, on Nov. 2, in the plans for a new surgical theatre. Messrs. Eliot and Little were appointed, on Dec. 28, the Committee to prepare the annual report. On Jan. 11, 1867, Dr. Tyler wrote to the Board stating his need of relaxation from his cares, and his desire for leave of absence for six months. The Board voted an expression of sympathy for him, and in consideration of the value of his services gave him leave of absence for a year, with a continuation of his salary. Thanks were voted to the Rev. J. Spaulding, of New York, for the donation of $500, made by him to the institution at the request of his wife. Mr. Ritchie, on Feb. 6, announced his intention to decline a re-appointment as a Trustee on the part of the Commonwealth. The Treasurer announced his reception of a legacy of $20,000 from the executor of the will of the late Miss Sarah Pratt, one half for the Hospital and one half for the Asylum.

The annual meeting of the Corporation was held on Feb. 6, 1867, at which the reports were submitted; and these were referred to the Trustees, by whose Committee they were to be prepared for print. The only change made in the Corporation was in the appointment, on the part of the Commonwealth, of Ezra Farnsworth as Trustee, in place of Harrison Ritchie, who had declined longer service. Mr. Rogers was again chosen Chairman of the Board; Dr. C. E. Brown-Séquard was added to the Board of Consultation of the previous year; Dr. James C. White took the place of Dr. A. A. Gould, as Visiting Physician; the Board of Visiting Surgeons was unchanged. Dr. Shaw was re-appointed Resident Physician of the Hospital; Drs. Sinclair and H. J. Oliver, jun., Physicians to out-patients; Dr. J. T Heard, Surgeon to out-patients; Dr. C. Ellis, Microscopist and Curator of the Pathological Cabinet; Dr. J. C. White, Chemist; D. G. Wilkins, Apothecary; Mrs. M. A. Colesworthy, Matron. Dr. J. E. Tyler was re-chosen Superintendent of the Asylum, and Mr. and Mrs. Whittle Steward and Matron. The Chairman, with the approval of the Board, appointed the Standing Committees, and arranged the Visiting Committees for the year.

The report for 1866 is in every particular a cheerful and a hopeful document. The income of the year had been $190,935.60; the expenses, $194,802.63; the excess of the latter being chargeable to the Hospital; while the Asylum, owing to the difference in the class of its patients, more than supports itself. The debt, which, after a previous reduction, had amounted to $68,369.97, has been paid during the year; the productive general fund has increased from $53,002.27 to $95,213.82, and the productive special funds from $308,056.01 to $331,782.51. These gratifying results are due chiefly to the liberal subscriptions in answer to the appeal in the Circular. Mr. Nathaniel Thayer had offered to give $25,000, on condition that $75,000 more were subscribed in the community. The sum was soon raised, with a surplus of eight hundred dollars, contributed by ninety-eight persons. The list of subscribers will be found near the close of this volume. Other donations and legacies received during the year amounted to $10,072.03, and new subscriptions for free beds to $4,100.00. Dr. Shaw reports that 1,224 patients had been under treatment during the year; 95 remaining. Of medical and surgical out-patients treated, there had been 5,608. The relief provided by the City Hospital is appreciated here. Very extensive renovations had been made in the Hospital during the year. A new operating theatre is now the greatest necessity. The death of Dr. A. A. Gould, " one of the most faithful and amiable of the medical staff," is tenderly referred to. The assets of the Corporation, exclusive of the Hospital and Asylum estates, amount to $426,996.33.

Dr. Tyler reports that there had been 103 new patients received at the Asylum during the year, and that 197 remained at its close. While great improvements have been made in the grounds, " several new and valuable items of purely medical treatment have been successfully tried;" the general management, or *moral treatment*, tested by long and varied trial, having remained the same. Holidays, amusements, excursions, lectures, games, &c., organ concerts at the Music Hall, and free access to the Museum given by Mr. Kimball, have continued to contribute their pleasures to the patients. The resignation of the Supervisor, Mr. Goodell, after twelve years of varied service, deprived the Asylum of a most faithful officer and a most trustworthy man. Miss Barber's retirement, after thirty years of the most devoted toil and sympathy given to the hundreds who had been under her charge, sets the seal of a cherished and affectionate remembrance upon her peculiar usefulness and her wonderful adaptation for her life's work.

Dr. Tyler devotes several pages of his report to a discussion of that form of insanity which is produced by inebriety. There is, he says, a large increase in the habits of intemperance, and in the class of sufferers from that vice who become thereby mentally diseased. His advice is sought constantly by the victims and by their friends. The latter, in very many cases, naturally seek to avail themselves of the retirement, discipline, and remedial processes of the Asylum. But it is not expedient — on the contrary, it is highly objectionable — to receive such a class of patients. It is not fitting that they should be domiciliated with the general insane. Very many and very serious practical embarrassments would arise from receiving them. This report may be profitably consulted by those interested in this special subject, either from their relation to any victim of inebriety, or from their concern for the establishment of an institution devoted to the care of inebriates.

CHAPTER XVI.

FEBRUARY 22, 1867, TO 1872.

DR. TYLER'S ABSENCE IN EUROPE. — GIFT THROUGH DR. J. M. WARREN. — NEW GROUNDS AT ASYLUM. — FEMALE STUDENTS AT HOSPITAL. — DEATH OF DR. J. M. WARREN. — DR. J. H. DENNY, ASSISTANT AT ASYLUM. — LEGACY FROM DR. J. M. WARREN. — DEATH OF DR. J. JACKSON. — BEQUEST FROM HIM. — RELIGIOUS SERVICES AT ASYLUM. — RESIGNATION OF MR. WHITNEY. — ANNUAL MEETING. — ORGANIZATION FOR 1868. — REPORT FOR 1867. — NEW OPERATING THEATRE. — DR. TYLER'S FOREIGN OBSERVATIONS. — DEATH OF THE PRESIDENT OF THE CORPORATION, MR. HOOPER. — FURTHER BEQUESTS. — CHANGES IN THE MEDICAL STAFF. — ANNUAL MEETING. — ORGANIZATION FOR 1869. — REPORT FOR 1868. — DR. TYLER'S REVIEW. — LADY VISITORS AT HOSPITAL. — NEW OFFICERS. — GIFT FROM JOHN C. GRAY. — WARREN PRIZE. — APPEAL FROM DR. MORTON'S FAMILY. — ANNUAL MEETING. — ORGANIZATION FOR 1870. — REPORT FOR 1869. — DEPARTMENT FOR SKIN DISEASES. — POST MORTEM REGISTER. — COMMITTEE ON AUTOPSIES. — DONATIONS FROM DR. H. J. BIGELOW. — FEMALE SUPERVISOR AT ASYLUM. — CHANGES OF OFFICERS. — NEW SURGICAL INSTRUMENTS. — LEGACY FROM REV. DR. WORCESTER. — EXPERIMENT OF A SKIN DISEASE WARD. — ANNUAL MEETING. — ORGANIZATION FOR 1871. — REPORT FOR 1870. — RESIGNATION OF DR. TYLER. — RESIGNATION OF DR. WHITTEMORE. — AN INCIDENT CONNECTED WITH THE ASYLUM. — AWARD OF THE WARREN PRIZE. — PROPOSALS FOR A NEW LOCATION FOR THE ASYLUM. — RESIGNATION OF MR. FARNSWORTH. — DONATIONS RECEIVED. — SUBJECT AND ADVERTISEMENT FOR THE NEXT WARREN PRIZE. — DR. RAY IN TEMPORARY CHARGE OF THE ASYLUM. — STATISTICS OF SURGICAL OPERATIONS. — DR. JELLY CHOSEN SUPERINTENDENT OF ASYLUM. — DR. H. P. QUINCY, ARTIST OF THE HOSPITAL. — S. D. WARREN, TRUSTEE. — DONATION OF JAMES MCGREGOR. — THE NABBY JOY FUND. — RESIGNATION OF DR. SHAW. — ELECTION OF DR. N. FOLSOM AS RESIDENT PHYSICIAN OF HOSPITAL. — REMARKS ON THE HOSPITAL AND ASYLUM. — CONCLUSION.

At the meeting of the Trustees on Feb. 22, 1867, Mr. Rogers, in behalf of a Committee appointed to consider what arrangements should be made at the Asylum during Dr. Tyler's proposed absence, *reported* " that they had instructed Dr. Whittemore, acting Superintendent, to consult Dr. Morrill Wyman, of Cambridge, and Dr. Bancroft, of Concord, N.H., and that those physicians had consented to serve the institution, as Visiting and Consulting Physicians, during Dr. Tyler's absence. The Committee also recommended the appointment of Dr. James H. Denny, as Assistant Physician at the Asylum, for the same period." The action of the Committee was confirmed, and Dr. Denny was elected.

On March 8, a Committee of the Trustees was appointed to inquire and report " whether the conduct of the officers, and the treatment of the patients, at the Asylum, are, in all respects, humane, considerate, and faithful." Mr. Rogers, for the Committee, on March 22, reported a plan, with estimates of cost, for the proposed new surgical theatre; and a special meeting was ordered for considering and acting thereon. At such a meeting, on March 27, the Board voted " that it is expedient to erect, on the Hospital grounds, a building for surgical operations, and for the accommodation of out-door patients ; and that the plans and estimates for such a building, presented to the Board, be adopted." Messrs. Rogers, Bullard, and Storrow were appointed a Building

Committee, with full power in the case, the expense not to exceed fifty thousand dollars. The Rules and Regulations for the Hospital were amended so as to provide for the annual election of six House Pupils, two for the medical, and four for the surgical department. On April 12, Dr. J. Mason Warren addressed a note to the Board enclosing $2,000 towards the cost of the new surgical theatre. Thanks were returned to him, and, through him, to the contributors of that gift. On April 19, Dr. Warren presented to the Board a copy of his new work, entitled " Surgical Observations, with Cases and Operations," dedicated to the officers of the Hospital Corporation. Thanks were voted for the gift, — the book to be deposited in the Treadwell Library. A proposition had been suggested to charge medical students a fee for admission to the lectures and operations at the Hospital. A report of a Committee, which thought it inexpedient to do this, was approved by the Board. The Committee "on the conduct of officers, and the treatment of patients at the Asylum," made a full report, which was accepted and placed on file, on May 3. On that date, Mr. Bullard, for a Committee, reported the purchase of the " Barrell Farm," adjoining the Asylum grounds, for $40,000. The purchase was approved and confirmed. Mr. Beebe was, on May 17, elected temporary Chairman of the Board during Mr. Rogers's proposed absence abroad. Mr Rogers had sought to resign that place, but, by request of the Board, had consented to withdraw his resignation. Mr. Beebe was added to the Building Committee of the Surgical Theatre. Messrs. Beebe, Bullard, and Eliot were instructed to consider and report upon the subject of religious services at the Asylum. At the meeting of the Board on May 17, a letter from Hon. Charles G. Loring had been read, recommending the admission of Miss Sophia Blake to "the medical visitations at the Hospital;" also a note from Miss Blake and Susan Dimmock, asking leave to share the educational advantages of the Hospital, especially in the female wards. The subject had been referred to the Visiting Committee, with the addition of Mr. Eliot, whose report, recommending the passage of the three following resolutions, was adopted by the Board, on June 28: —

1. "That Chap. III., Art. 3, of the Rules and Regulations for the Hospital, may be so interpreted as to include female, as well as male students. 2. That the admission of female students be left to the discretion of the Visiting Physicians and Surgeons, individually. 3. That female students, whenever admitted, shall be placed in classes separate from male students, and shall attend the clinical practice of the female wards exclusively."

At the meeting of the Board on Aug. 30, the

following preamble and resolutions, offered by Mr. Eliot, were unanimously adopted : —

" The Trustees of the Massachusetts General Hospital, at this their first meeting after the death of Dr. J. Mason Warren, in noticing an event so generally lamented by the community, and so particularly afflicting to the Hospital, resolve as follows : —

"1. That they bear their united testimony to the variety and excellence of the services which Dr. Warren has rendered to the Hospital for nearly twenty-one years as a member, and nearly five years as the head, of its professional staff. Fitted no less by nature, than by descent, for a high position in his profession, uniting great gifts with great acquirements, and using his scientific abilities with a vigor that commanded respect, and a kindliness that inspired attachment, he was remarkable even among the remarkable Physicians and Surgeons who have been connected with the Hospital.

" 2. That they dwell with peculiar feeling upon the last proofs of his interest in the institution : upon the dedication of his recent volume, describing the most eminent among his life-long labors, to the government of the Hospital; upon the subscription of $2,000, which he secured in aid of the operating theatre now building; yet more upon the fidelity with which he went through his last term of service, though suffering acutely from the development of the disease under which he died; all of these acts being not only consistent with his unbroken devotion to the Hospital, but likewise characteristic of the science, the liberality, and the conscientiousness which distinguished his whole career.

" 3. That, speaking for other interests as well as for those of the Hospital, they lament the early close of a life from which, though it had already done its full share, even more might have been expected, had it continued but a few years longer in ministrations to the sick and the poor, in the relief of suffering, in the promotion of medical science, and in the furtherance of public and private designs for the improvement of society. Yet, while lamenting that the life on earth has closed, they rejoice that the memory of their departed associate will not fail to live among those who knew him, and those who are to come after him.

"*Voted*, That the Secretary be requested to communicate the resolutions to the family of the deceased, and to furnish a copy to the public press.

" *Voted*, That Messrs. Lowell and Eliot be a Committee to prepare, and report at the next quarterly meeting, such resolutions as they may think proper to express the feelings of the Board upon the decease of the last survivor of the earliest founders and officers of this institution, the venerable Dr. James Jackson."

The Massachusetts Board of State Charities, having required a report from this Corporation, under chapter 243 of the Acts of 1867, the Secretary, on Sept. 27, stated " that he had in reply informed the Board of State Charities that this Corporation would make no report unless further called upon, on the ground that this Corporation is not a State Charity within the meaning of the statute." On Oct. 18, the nomination by Dr. Tyler of Dr. James H. Denny, as second Assistant Physician and Apothecary at the Asylum, in place of Dr. Hazelton resigned, was confirmed. Dr. J. Collins Warren, in a letter acknowl-

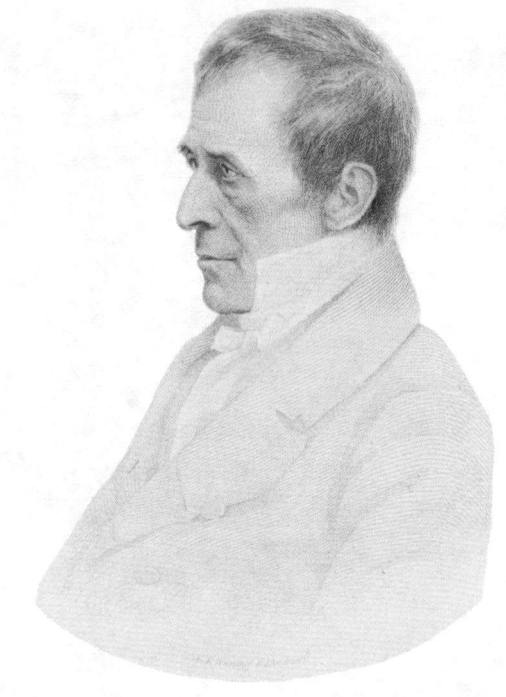

edging the receipt of the resolutions passed by the Board on the death of his late father, informed the Board of a legacy under his father's will, to the Trustees, of $2,000, to be called the "Warren Prize Fund." The communication was referred for future consideration. On Oct. 18, Mr. Eliot, for a Committee, offered the following preamble and resolutions: —

"The death of Dr. James Jackson, one of the founders of the Massachusetts General Hospital and its first Physician, whose active service extended from April 6, 1817, to Oct. 13, 1837, and who, as Consulting Physician, was connected with the Institution to the close of his earthly life, Aug. 27, 1867, is an event of so singular and so affecting an interest to the Hospital, that the Trustees have delayed noticing it officially until a quarterly meeting should draw them together in full numbers. They can add nothing to his well-deserved reputation, but they perform an act of simple duty in offering a sincere and grateful tribute to his honored memory.

"*Resolved*, That the Trustees of the Massachusetts General Hospital recall, with deep sensibility, Dr. Jackson's long connection with the Institution, which he was prominent in founding and extending, and to which, while he retained his powers, he gave the great benefit of his name, his science, his advice, and his influence.

"*Resolved*, That his remarkable traits as a Physician, well-known and appreciated before the Hospital was founded, and fully acknowledged during the half-century of its existence, have been of inestimable value to its administration not only during the term of his attendance in our wards, but in the subsequent period, during which his counsel and support, while he could give them, have never failed our predecessors or ourselves.

"*Resolved*, That his personal as well as his professional qualities, his activity without imprudence, his decision without dogmatism, his dignity that never wounded, his conscientiousness that never provoked, his exhaustless sympathies, which made him the brother or the father, as well as the physician of those to whom he ministered, bearing their troubles as his own, and alleviating by the charm of his presence the pains which he could not remove by his skill, his unwearied study, his fruitful knowledge, his contributions to the science and literature of medicine, and his relations to the elder and younger members of the profession, gave him a position at the Hospital as exclusively his own as that which he held in the community.

"*Resolved*, That his labors, as efficient as they were devoted, and his counsels, as wise as they were earnest, rendering him both the ornament and the safeguard of the Hospital, are among its most precious traditions, and that they are to be cherished for the sake not merely of its past history, which they had so large a share in forming, but of its future course, to which, if they are faithfully preserved, they will be the helpful guides.

"*Resolved*, That the Trustees remove his name from the list of their living associates, only to place it, where it belongs, at the head of the departed benefactors of the Hospital. And to the end that his memory may continue among us, as we think he would have best preferred it to continue, the free bed which was placed in 1837 at his disposal for life shall remain the Jackson Free Bed, perpetuating his attachment to the Hospital, and his benevolence to humanity."

These resolutions having been unanimously adopted, the Secretary was directed to communicate them to the family, and to furnish a copy to the public press.

Mr. F. H. Jackson, son of Dr. Jackson, communicated to the Board a bequest from his late father to the Hospital, of a portrait of M. Louis, of Paris. The same was gratefully accepted, and placed upon the walls of the Hospital. It was voted that the nomination to the Jackson Free Bed be vested in the oldest daughter of the deceased.

On Nov. 15, Mr. Beebe, for a Committee that had been appointed in May, upon the subject of religious services at the Asylum, made a report, on which the Board resolved that it is expedient to establish such services; that they should be wholly free from a sectarian character; that the Committee procure plans and estimates for a chapel at the Asylum, the present hall to be in the mean while used for the purpose; and that the Committee consult with the Superintendent with regard to a chaplain *pro tem.*, and for a suitable incumbent of the office. Mr. Whitney having resigned his place on the Board, and being unwilling when solicited to remain, his resignation was accepted with much regret on Nov. 29, and with thanks for his long and useful services.

Messrs. Beebe and Dalton were appointed on Dec.

27, a Committee to prepare the annual report. The nomination by the Committee of Rev. David G. Haskins to the office of Chaplain, *pro tem.*, at the Asylum, was confirmed on Jan. 17, 1868. Dr. Charles E. Ware declined to be a candidate for re-election as a Visiting Physician, and could not be induced, by a Committee appointed for the purpose, to withdraw his letter of resignation.

The annual meeting of the Corporation was held on Feb. 5, 1868, and the first subsequent meeting of the Trustees was on Feb. 21. The only change in the officers of the Corporation was in the election of Mr. Edmund Dwight in place of Mr. H. A. Whitney as a Trustee.

The annual report of the Trustees for 1867, it being the fifty-fourth of the series, is a document of much interest in its contents. The death of Dr. J. Mason Warren, and that of the venerated Dr. James Jackson, are properly the first subjects of respectful notice. The former, besides his active efforts in aid of the new operating theatre, now in progress, left a bequest of $2,000 as a fund for a prize to be called the Warren prize, in memory of his father, the interest of which, every three years, is to be awarded for the best dissertation considered worthy of a premium, on some subject in physiology, surgery, or pathological anatomy. The bequest by Dr. Jackson of the portrait of M. Louis has been already mentioned. The portrait was a gift from M. Louis, in 1833, to a son of Dr. Jackson, who had died in early manhood. Dr. Jackson " valued this picture more highly than any thing that he owned." When M. Louis heard what disposition had been made of it " he expressed himself as highly pleased." The new operating theatre is said to be nearly completed. A safe and commodious elevator has been constructed by which patients can be taken from any story of the building and along covered galleries to the new room. The structure contains in addition convenient apartments for receiving patients before and after operations, rooms for etherization, for sulphur and other baths, rooms for out-patients, a private operating room, and offices for the surgeons and physicians. Science and humanity will find the most efficient aids in the new arrangements, beyond what had been afforded in the old operating room under the dome of the Hospital. The income for the year had been $204,059.56; the expenditures, $194,843.36. The property, real and productive, is valued at $1,154,836.14. Still the expenses of the Hospital department had exceeded its income by $15,664.97. The additional subscriptions for the year to the Free-bed Fund were $3,900; but the cost of them had exceeded all the income for them by nearly twenty per cent.

The donations and legacies during the year had amounted to $43,312.75. There had been 1,301 patients in the Hospital. Of surgical out-patients there had been 2,569; of medical, 2,957. More than one half of all the cases received at the Hospital had been cured. At the Asylum, 89 new patients had been admitted; 178 remained. Dr. Tyler had been abroad from February to October, and expresses his gratitude to the Trustees for affording him the privilege, and for making such admirable and efficient arrangements for the oversight of his charge during his absence. Though the great object of his vacation was to lose sight for a season of hospital life, yet his inclination and his opportunity led him to make many visits with extended investigations in the Asylums of Great Britain and the continent. He had been received everywhere courteously and fraternally. As the result of his wide and inquisitive investigations, so fully and intelligently directed by his own private experience and official professional authority, we have in his report a document of permanent value as a contribution to the highest department of the literature of his theme. Any one who shall for years to come assume to discuss, as from a point of advantage or influence, the comparative views of insanity, and of the methods of treating it, cannot wisely neglect to read this report. With a generous catholicity of spirit, an admirable candor of judgment, and a most discriminating allowance for differences of opinion in details, where there is a general harmony on the part of qualified judges in the case, Dr. Tyler presents his observations and conclusions with an emphasis of personal assurance, and a freedom from dogmatism, that alike give a charm and a warrant to his expressed convictions.

Mr. Rogers was re-elected Chairman of the Board of Trustees. On the Board of Consultation, Dr. J. B. S. Jackson was chosen to fill the vacancy caused by the death of Dr. James Jackson; the Visiting Physicians of last year were continued in office, with the exception of Dr. C. E. Ware, who had declined; and the only change among the Visiting Surgeons was in the election of Dr. Algernon Coolidge in place of the late Dr. J. Mason Warren. Dr. Charles B. Porter was chosen an additional Surgeon to Out-patients; all the other officers of the Hospital and Asylum being again elected. The Chairman, with the approbation of the Board, designated the Standing Committees and the Visiting Committees for the year. Thanks were voted to Dr. Charles E. Ware " for his faithful, efficient, and sympathetic service of ten years, as Visiting Physician, and for the unfailing interest he has always shown in all matters affecting the usefulness of the Hospital." The Treasurer was instructed to establish a permanent fund for the Warren prize, conformed to the conditions in the bequest. The salary of the Treasurer was increased to $1,000. The death of Mr. Robert Hooper, President of the Corporation, was announced to the Board on March 6; and at the meeting on March 20, Mr. Bullard, for a Committee appointed for the purpose, reported the following resolution, which was unanimously adopted: —

"That while we acknowledge the mercy of God in the tender manner in which He released from the weariness and infirmities of his earthly life Robert Hooper, the President of this institution, the event cannot fail to affect our sensibilities and recall his long and useful services. Of uncommon individuality of character and manner, of singular probity of mind and independence of thought, of large and cultivated capacities, he was faithful and sagacious in all his trusts, most honorable in the conduct of affairs, affectionate and tender in all his social relations.

"Mr. Hooper was elected a Trustee in 1837, Chairman of the Board in 1842, Vice-President in 1850, and President in 1863, serving in these several offices over thirty years. And we desire to record our grateful sense of the fidelity, ability, and sympathetic interest with which he performed these services, and to bear witness to the deep concern he felt in all that affected the welfare and usefulness of this institution.

"*Voted*, That a copy of the foregoing resolve be sent by the Secretary to the family of the deceased."

Official notice was received, on April 3, from the

Trustees under the will of Mrs. Abigail Loring, of their readiness to pay the amount, $35,000, awarded to this Corporation. The award was received with gratitude, and the Treasurer was authorized to receipt for it. Messrs. C. H. Parker and W. P. Mason, executors of the will of the late W. P. Mason, having paid over to the Corporation $10,000, being the amount of a bequest provided for in said will, less United States revenue tax, it was —

"*Voted*, That this Corporation gratefully accepts the same upon the conditions of said will; and that the Treasurer be directed to establish a special fund, to be called the 'Mason Free-bed Fund,' the income of which shall be annually appropriated to the support of free beds in this Institution; and that he be further directed, in conformity with said conditions, to confer upon Mr. W. P. Mason and Mrs. Walter C. Cabot each the rights of life free-bed subscribers."

On April 17, permission was granted, on request, to the Massachusetts Medical Society to hold their annual meeting in June in the operating theatre of the Hospital. Measures were adopted by the Trustees, on April 24, to co-operate with Dr. Tyler in extending proper civilities to the Association of Superintendents of American Institutions for the Insane at their coming meeting in Boston, in June. The salary of the Chaplain at the Asylum was fixed at $1,000. On May 8, Dr. A. D. Sinclair resigned his office of Physician to out-patients. His resignation was accepted, and thanks were voted for his faithful services. Two free beds at the Hospital were placed at the disposal of St. Stephen's Chapel, Boston, on the payment of $2,000. Dr. Charles E. Ware was elected on the Board of Consultation in the vacancy caused by the death of Dr. Homans. On May 22, Dr. Henry K. Oliver, jun., was elected a Visiting Physician for the remainder of the year; and Drs. Hall Curtis and George G. Tarbell were elected Physicians to out-patients. Miss Sturtevant was appointed, on July 31, as Matron of the Hospital, in the vacancy caused by the recent decease of Mary A. Colesworthy. The Trustees had voted the sum of two hundred dollars to Dr. Morrill Wyman, for his kind services at the Asylum during the absence of Dr. Tyler; and, in grateful recognition of the bounty, Dr. Wyman sent a gift of the same amount for the aid of needy patients there. A faithful attendant on the kitchen of the Asylum, on leaving after twenty-five years of service, received a present of one hundred dollars, with an appreciative letter of thanks. On Dec. 18, acknowledgments were returned to Miss M. Louisa Shaw for the donation of $500, " for the Free Bed and Ward for Incurables." Messrs. Dwight and Bullard were, on Jan. 6,

1869, appointed a Committee to prepare the annual report, and to them were referred the Treasurer's and the other reports as successively presented. On the report and advice of a Committee, on Feb. 3, authority was given to sell all the land lying east of the Eastern Railroad at the Asylum.

The annual meeting of the Corporation was held on Feb. 3, 1869, and the first subsequent meeting of the Trustees on Feb. 19. Mr. Edward Wigglesworth, who had been Vice-President, was chosen President; Mr. Nathaniel Thayer, Vice-President; and Messrs. Stevenson and Hall were respectively re-elected Treasurer and Secretary, and the Board of Trustees remained unchanged. The Board, on its organization, re-elected Mr. Rogers as Chairman. The Board of Consultation bears the name of Dr. C. E. Ware in place of that of the late Dr. Homans. The only changes made in the staff of officers at the Hospital and Asylum were such as have been noted during the last year, except in the choice of Mr. David J. Dearborn as male Supervisor at the Asylum, in place of Mr. Dexter Gray, deceased.

The report for 1868 states the expenses of the Hospital to have been $67,564.47, of which only $14,671.45 had been received from patients. The expenses of the Asylum had been $142,535.36; the net deficit of income below expenses had been

$17,124.50. There had been 1,265 patients in the Hospital, of which 771 were wholly free. The average weekly cost of each was $12.74. As out-patients, 5,264 persons had been treated. A Dental Service had been added during the year, in connection with the Dental School of Harvard College, 1,078 persons having received its services. The Treadwell Library has a constant increase by the addition of costly works not to be found in private medical libraries. The Trustees are increasingly solicitous for the prosperity and advancement of their institution. They stand between the bounty of a rich and liberal community and a body of professional men of great skill and self-devotion, and they desire to be the medium of a great benevolence for the good of their fellowmen. They are now considering whether they may be able to afford accommodations for the treatment of special diseases. The death of the President, and of the Matron of the Hospital, is properly noticed.

The legacies and donations received during the year amount to $77,939.79. The receipts for annual subscriptions for free beds had been $4,300. The Treasurer's statement gives a full and lucid account of all the classified and restricted and general funds, with an exhaustive exhibition of the economy of the institution. Dr. Shaw, the Resident Physician, presents the statistics of the patients with the usual details and specifications. He refers to religious services held for convalescents, and to the visits of kindly friends to the patients with books and other offerings. Dr. Tyler reports that 270 persons had been under treatment at the Asylum, and 176 remained. About a third of the patients have attended religious services in the hall on Sunday afternoons, receiving thus an influence evidently soothing and beneficial. The late Supervisor, Mr. Dexter Gray, is spoken of with warm respect and affection for his virtues and his services. He had intermitted his relation to the Asylum to serve his country in the war, and returned with a wound which was one of the causes of his lamented decease. The Asylum had a history now of fifty completed years. Its first patient — whose case the Trustees spent three hours in examining — was a young man whom his father believed to be one of those spoken of in the Bible as possessed with a devil. The father said the remedial measure which he had employed was *whipping*. This patient completely recovered. There are now about seventy like institutions in the American States and the Provinces. Dr. Tyler makes his report chiefly a condensed and concise, but still a very adequate, sketch of the history of the Asylum; which, as a whole, is a profoundly instructive illustration of the application of the resources of Christian benevolence, munificence, and science to one of the most grievous of all human woes. The Association of Medical Superintendents of American Institutions for the Insane, having met this year at Somerville, had made a thorough examination of the Asylum, and of its methods and conduct. After a prolonged discussion of the "legal relations of the insane," they unanimously agreed upon a "project of a law" which would aid to assure the prompt care of a patient, the protection of his personal liberty, and the safety of the public. This document appears with Dr. Tyler's report.

The Trustees, on March 19, voted that the Resident Physician be requested to prepare for publication a simple statement, that children have long been, and will continue to be, received and properly cared for at the Hospital. After the Board had for some time had under consideration the appointment of two or more ladies to serve as visitors to the female wards of the Hospital, on June 4 the measure was approved. Four ladies were elected by ballot to that service, and a Committee was appointed to confer with them on their proposed duties. It was voted that all Hospital out-patients affected with diseases of the skin be placed under the special care and treatment of Dr. J. C. White. In answer to a suggestion in a letter from Dr. Calvin Ellis, then in Paris, relative to the purchase of improved electrical apparatus for the

Hospital, the Visiting Physicians, who had been consulted on the subject, reported in favor of the proposition; and the Board, on June 18, appropriated two hundred dollars in gold for that object. The sum of £300 was put at the disposal of Dr. Henry J. Bigelow, for the purchase in Paris of surgical instruments for the Hospital. On Aug. 20, Dr. Tyler communicated to the Board the resignation by Dr. James H. Denny of the office of Second Assistant Physician and Apothecary at the Asylum, and the nomination of Dr. George F. Jelly as his successor. The resignation was accepted, and the nomination confirmed. On Oct. 1, the Board found it necessary to increase the number of physicians to out-patients, and chose Drs. John Collins Warren and Robert Willard as additional officers. On Oct. 22, Mr. John C. Gray received the thanks of the Board for the donation of $1,000 for the support of free beds. Messrs. Farnsworth and Lowell were designated, on Dec. 17, a Committee to prepare the annual report. On Jan. 14, 1870, Mr. Bullard, for a Committee on the "Warren Prize," reported a form of advertisement, which was accepted, as follows: —

"MASSACHUSETTS GENERAL HOSPITAL. — The Warren Prize, founded by the late J. Mason Warren, in memory of his father, John C. Warren, being the income of $2,000 for three years, will be awarded, after Feb. 1871, to the author of the best original dissertation, considered worthy of a prize, on some subject in physiology, surgery, or pathological anatomy. The arbitrators to be the medical board of the Hospital.

"Dissertations, accompanied with a sealed envelope containing the name and address of the writer, must be sent on or before the 1st Feb. 1871, to the Superintendent of the Massachusetts General Hospital."

On Jan. 21, a Committee, to whom had been referred a circular addressed to the Trustees asking a contribution to a fund to be raised for the benefit of the family of the late Dr. Morton, and to pay for a monument to be erected over his remains, reported a form of reply to be sent by the Secretary, which was adopted, as follows: —

"The Trustees beg to say, that, while they are deeply sensible of the great blessing Dr. Morton conferred on mankind by proving that sulphuric ether can safely be used to produce insensibility to pain, even under the most serious surgical operations, they nevertheless feel that the appropriation of any portion of the funds of the Hospital for the purposes named in the circular would not be consistent with the uses for which they have been bestowed."

The annual meeting of the Corporation was held at the Hospital on Feb. 2, 1870. The only change among its officers of last year was in the election of Messrs. George S. Hale and Samuel W. Swett, as Trustees in place of Messrs. Lowell and Storrow, who resigned after they had been chosen. The report for 1869 shows that there had been nothing of special or marked importance in the recent experience of the institution, its appropriate work having gone successfully forward under able and faithful officers, Drs. Shaw and Tyler, with their valued assistants. The large number of nurses, whose assiduous and patient duties are so essential, so trying and exhausting too, are not forgotten, though their names are of silent fame. The expenditure at the Hospital has been $62,238.60; at the Asylum, $138,132.02. The weekly cost of a patient has been, at the Hospital, $10.14; at the Asylum, $14.20. The receipts have exceeded the expenditures by $3,445.21. Besides the donation from John C. Gray, the further sums of $49,500 had accrued under the will of the late John Redman, and of $18,690.10, under the will of the late M. P. Sawyer. There had been admitted to the Hospital 1,390 patients, of whom 834 were free; of the greatest total at any one time, of 139, there were 98 free. The out-patients treated had numbered 6,953. The new surgical instruments and electrical apparatus, selected abroad by Drs. Bigelow and Ellis, had been received with much satisfaction. The death of Dr. S. D. Townsend on Sept. 17, and his long and devoted services, are appropriately noticed. The Resident Physician writes: " What cannot always be said may be said of him — that, as Consulting Surgeon, he always punctually and conscientiously attended the consultations, and gave his advice and assistance in the most important operations."

Dr. Tyler reports that there had been under treatment during the year, at the Asylum, 284 patients, of whom 184 remained. He regards the cases of insanity most proper for his Institution to be the violent and dangerous, and also the recent and curable. The soundness of the general principles of treatment adopted there is year by year verified. The study of French has been introduced with marked success into the Asylum, Madame Harney attending weekly upon separate classes of either sex. Mrs. Bunker, on another day, has classes in drawing. Mr. Moorhouse presides over an orchestra of twelve or fifteen male patients, one of the Trustees having generously given instruments for the purpose. A "singing-school" under Mr. Hadley has united both sexes. These exercises have varied the inevitable monotony and cheered the weariness of life within the walls. Flower-beds, garden grounds, chickens and ducks, embroidery, needle-work for the poor, the carpenter's shop, concerts, readings, dancing parties, excursions in the harbor, festivals, waxworks, and observance of holidays, have furnished their resources. More rooms like those in the Appleton wards are very much needed, as also an amusement hall, and a chapel. The religious services, under Rev. D. G. Haskins, are greatly prized; their omission for a single Sunday having been much mourned.

Mr. Rogers was chosen Chairman of the Board of Trustees for 1870. The Board of Consultation was changed only by the loss of the name of Dr. Townsend. The Medical and Surgical Staff and the officers of the Hospital and Asylum were the same as last year. The Standing and Visiting Committees were designated and arranged. The resignation of Messrs. Lowell and Storrow was received with regret, and thanks were voted to them for their long and efficient services. On March 18, the resignation of Mr. James L. Little, as Trustee, was announced to the Board, with the appointment by the Governor of Dr. George E. Ellis, to fill the vacancy. Thanks were voted to Mr. Little for his valuable services during the past four years. Six young ladies were appointed as assistant visitors to the female wards of the Hospital; viz., Miss Mary I. Bowditch, Miss Henrietta Townsend, Miss Helen A. Perkins, Mrs. Otto Cüntz, Miss Annie Putnam, and Miss Caroline Young. A communication was received, on April 1, from Dr. J. C. White, resigning the office of Visiting Physician of the Hospital, and asking to be appointed Physician to a department for skin diseases, which he recommends to be established at the Hospital. The communication was referred to Messrs. Rogers and Bullard for consideration and report. The sum of two hundred dollars was, on April 15, placed at the disposal of the lady visitors of the Hospital for procuring pictures to be hung upon the walls of the wards. On May 6, a conference was asked for with the Visiting Physicians and Surgeons, by the Trustees, or a communication in any other form, on the subject of the proposed department for skin diseases. The illness of Dr. Tyler made it necessary to procure assistance for Dr. Whittemore at the Asylum. On June 3, the lady visitors of the Hospital were authorized to visit the male wards also, at their discretion. A case of interest, which had occurred at the Hospital in connection with an autopsy, led to the appointment of a Committee, whose report was accepted by the Board on July 15, with a vote, by which the attention of the officers of the Hospital was called to the rules relating to autopsies, and another that a "Post-mortem Register" be kept to meet the requirements of those rules, — each entry in which shall be examined and signed by the Visiting Committee, — the book to be laid before the Trustees at their regular meetings. The Resident Physician was requested to keep a press copy of his official correspondence, including notices to relatives and friends of deceased patients.

Mr. Dalton made a communication from Dr. Henry J. Bigelow, presenting to the Hospital " a collection of instruments lately procured by him abroad, which are now placed in new cases in the operating theatre, at an aggregate cost of about three thousand two hundred and fifty dollars ; " also giving " the further sums of one thousand dollars, and of five hundred dollars, the income of the former to be used exclusively for the purchase of surgical instruments required by the attending surgeons, not including ' apparatus,' splints, nor general appliances, — and the latter sum to be devoted to the maintenance of a free bed for five years." It was voted that these very valuable gifts be accepted with gratitude, and that Mr. Dalton, with the Chairman, be requested to communicate the fact of their grateful acceptance to Dr. Bigelow. On July 22, the resignation by Miss G. W. Mills of the office of female Supervisor of the Asylum was accepted; and the nomination of Miss Lucia Woodward, as her successor, was confirmed. An expression of high appreciation of her services, and a testimonial of approbation, were voted to Miss Mills. The Committees on Free Beds and on Repairs were requested to consider and report, respectively, " on the advisability of preparing a general review of the financial wants of the Hospital, with a view of appealing to the public for contributions to the Free-bed Fund," and "what new buildings and improvements, if any, are desirable at the Asylum." The Vice-president, Mr. Thayer, was added to the latter Committee.

On Aug. 5, Dr. Robert Willard resigned his office of Physician to out-patients; and his resignation was accepted. On Sept. 2, the Treasurer announced that he had received from Dr. Henry J. Bigelow an additional sum of seventeen hundred and fifty dollars, making the whole amount of his donation six thousand dollars. It was thereupon voted, —

"That the Treasurer be directed to establish the Henry J. Bigelow Fund in the sum of $1,750, of the principal of which one hundred dollars *per annum*, for five years, shall be appropriated for Dr. Bigelow's free bed, and the income of which shall be applied annually to the purchase of surgical instruments, as may be agreed upon by the Surgeons and Trustees."

Dr. Bigelow having suggested the appointment of a Committee of the Surgeons to have the care of the surgical instruments, &c., it was —

"*Voted*, That a Committee of two Surgeons be appointed to take charge of the surgical instruments recently presented by Dr. Bigelow, to make future purchases of instruments from the income of funds provided for such purpose by Dr. Bigelow, and to make such rules for the use and keeping of the instruments as may seem to said Committee to be best."

Drs. Bigelow and Hodges were made such a Committee. The instruments here referred to make a collection in itself of a curious and strangely fascinating interest. They are of an amazing ingenuity, variety, and adaptation; keen of temper, brilliant in polish, mysterious in their uses to any but experts, and exhibiting with great impressiveness the triumphs of scientific and mechanical skill. Of course this impression, with the accompanying associations and feelings, are very unlike for those who gaze upon them in safe security and those on whom their use is to be tested.

A legacy from the late Rev. Dr. S. M. Worcester was announced to the Board on Oct. 14, making, with the amount given by him during his life, the sum of nineteen hundred dollars. There was a special significance in the gift of Dr. Worcester from his slender means, as a token of his gratitude for the kind care which his wife had received at the Asylum. Thanks were voted to Mr. Walter K. Bigelow for the manner in which he had carried out the wishes of Dr. Worcester. Dr. Daniel Hyslop Hayden was elected a Physician to out-patients, in place of Dr. Willard, resigned.

After the Board had given a full and deliberate consideration to the subject, with the help of a Committee and a knowledge of the views of Dr. Shaw and of the Medical and Surgical officers, it was voted, on Oct. 21, to establish a separate ward for the treatment of patients with skin diseases, and to appoint Dr. White as Physician to that department; it being understood that the measure was but an experiment, and the appointment but temporary. Rules were adopted for carrying out the provisions of the vote, in the arrangements of the room designated, and the disposal of patients of either sex. The resignation of Dr. White as a Visiting Physician was accepted, and Dr. Edward B. Dalton was chosen in his place.

On Dec. 16, Messrs. Ellis and Swett were appointed a Committee to prepare the annual report. Dr. Calvin Ellis sent in his resignation of the office of "Microscopist and Curator of the Pathological Cabinet," and the Board accepted it. On Jan. 13, 1871, the Treasurer announced the gift of $20,000 to the Hospital Free-bed Fund from Mr. John L. Gardner, whereupon it was —

"*Voted*, That the Secretary be directed to communicate to Mr. Gardner the thanks of the Board for his very liberal and timely gift; and that the Treasurer be directed to invest and hold the same as the 'John L. Gardner Free-bed Fund.'"

The annual meeting of the Corporation was held at the Hospital Feb. 1, 1871; and the first subsequent meeting of the Trustees for organization was held on Feb. 17. It appeared that the only change in the officers of the Corporation from the previous year was that already noticed in the resignation of Mr. Little, and the appointment of G. E. Ellis as a Trustee. The Trustees re-elected the same Boards of Consultation, and of Visiting Surgeons and Physicians, save that, on the last Board, Dr. E. B. Dalton took the place of Dr. J. C. White, resigned. Dr. D. H. Hayden takes the place of Dr. R. Willard, as a Physician to out-patients; Dr. Reginald H. Fitz takes the place of Dr. Calvin Ellis, as Microscopist and Curator of the Pathological Cabinet; the other officers of the Hospital being re-elected.

The report for 1870, being the fifty-seventh, notices the changes in the Board of Trustees already specified. The Treasurer congratulates himself and the Corporation that he is able this year to make the most favorable statement of the financial affairs of the institution which it has been in his power to present since he had filled the office, — he was elected Feb. 18, 1859. The income of the property had exceeded the expenses of the two departments by $9,126.19. The average number of patients at the Hospital had been $120\frac{1}{4}$; weekly cost of each patient, $10.04. Average number at the Asylum, 187; weekly cost of each, $13.81. The dividends, interest, and rent amounted to $38,334.18, being 7.70 *per cent* on the investments.

The donations and legacies received during the year amounted to $49,074.85; and, after the Treasurer had closed his accounts and before he had made his report, accrued the gift already mentioned of $20,000 from Mr. J. L. Gardner, and another of $1,000 from Mr. B. T. Reed. The lady visitors at the Hospital had added much to the comfort and enjoyment of the patients. The Young Men's Christian Union had also provided for them dramatic representations and other entertainments. The Committee charged with the subject had reported an appeal to the community for increased subscriptions to the free-bed fund, which was adopted. The Trustees had acted upon the subject of a communication, dated Nov. 17, from the Surgeons, expressing their views on the management of the Hospital, warming, ventilation, diet, &c., and asking for more beds for the Surgical Department. The temporary and experimental measure for the treatment of skin diseases in a separate ward is referred to. Dr. White had visited during the year patients by such diseases 2,045 times; the new patients had been 638; the specifications of the diseases treated were 656. There had been treated during the year 7,370 medical, and 2,192 surgical out-patients. There had been 1,427 patients in the Hospital, of whom 958 were free. There had been under treatment at the Asylum 263 patients; 178

remained at the close of the year. Since April, Dr. Tyler had been taken from his duties by illness; and Dr. Whittemore, with his assistants, had borne the pressure of responsibility. Some improvements in the treatment of mental disorder had been verified during the year, and the well-established principles and methods of moral treatment had received new confirmation. A fund had been contributed by some friends of the Asylum for the supply of amusements by music and concerts. Mrs. S. Cabot, of Brookline, had sent weekly gifts of rare flowers during the winter. Other ladies had participated in extending these favors. Rev. Mr. Worcester had officiated most acceptably as chaplain. Dr. A. A. Porter, appointed Assistant Physician in June, had acceptably performed his duties till ill-health had compelled him to resign in November, when Dr. F. A. Stillings succeeded him.

It was with profound sympathy and deep regret that the Trustees learned that Dr. Tyler's health and strength were not fully restored by the leave of absence that had been granted him. They received a note from him on Feb. 17, resigning his office as Superintendent of the Asylum. The subject was referred to Messrs. Rogers, Eliot, and Bullard, for consideration and report. The election of officers for the Asylum was postponed. Mr. Rogers was re-elected Chairman of the Board, and, with the approbation of the Trustees, designated the usual Committees. The "Benjamin T. Reed Free-bed Fund" was established. Three dissertations were presented for competition for the Warren Prize, and they were referred to the Medical Board for examination and adjudication. At the meeting of the Board on March 3, the first business being the election of officers for the Asylum, the ballots were all cast for Dr. Tyler as Superintendent; Mr. and Mrs. Whittle being re-chosen Steward and Matron. But the hope of continuing Dr. Tyler in their service was at once precluded by the following report of resolutions proposed by Mr. Rogers for the Committee: —

"*Resolved*, That this Board, after due consideration of all the facts and circumstances in the case, accept, with great reluctance, the resignation tendered them by Dr. John E. Tyler.

"*Resolved*, That Dr. Tyler, during the thirteen years of his administration of the Asylum, has, by his professional skill, sound judgment, self-sacrificing spirit, and conscientious discharge of the duties of his arduous and responsible office, not only maintained the very high standard of excellence which this Institution had previously attained among similar institutions of the country; but, by his courteous manners, well-balanced temperament, and loving heart, has, to a singular degree, won the esteem and affection of the large number of patients who, from time to time, have been under his charge; the confidence of their relatives and friends, and the respect of the public at large. And therefore this Board deem it their duty to tender to him, in behalf of the Institution, their warmest thanks for the services he has rendered; their deep regret at the circumstances which make him unable, at present, to perform the duties they would have so gladly continued to him; and their sincere wishes and prayers for his speedy and complete restoration to health and usefulness."

. . . .

"*Resolved*, That the Board is unwilling to conclude its action in this regard without noticing the valuable voluntary services rendered to the Institution by Mrs. Tyler. In their belief, by her good judgment, her quick sympathy and constant kind attentions and care, she has done a great deal to soothe and mitigate the sorrows of the patients, and promote the happiness and welfare of the household; and they beg leave respectfully to tender to her, with their hearty acknowledgments, their personal esteem and their best wishes."

The report was accepted, the resolutions were adopted, and the Secretary was directed to send a copy of them to Dr. Tyler. Nor was this the only loss the Asylum was to meet with in this emergency in its history. Dr. Whittemore had found his responsibilities so arduous as to impair his health, and he desired also to go abroad for professional study. A note was received from him at the same meeting resigning his office of Assistant Physician. The same Committee was asked to consider and report upon this subject. Mr. Beebe was added to the Committee to consider and report upon filling the office of Superintendent at the Asylum. Mr. Dalton was requested to consider and report upon the subject of a yearly publication of important medical and surgical cases at the Hospital.

A letter was received from Dr. Tyler, on March 17, in grateful response to the action of the Board at its last meeting.

Mr. Rogers, for the Committee on the resignation of Dr. Whittemore, presented a report, recommending the adoption of votes, the first of which follows. The report was accepted, the votes were adopted, and the Secretary was directed to send a copy to Dr. Whittemore.

"*Voted*, That in accepting the resignation tendered to them by Dr. J. H. Whittemore, Assistant Physician and Apothecary at the Asylum, in order that he may be at liberty to pursue the general practice of medicine, and to take place on the first of July next, the Board desire to express their entire satisfaction with the manner in which he has performed the duties of his office; and especially would they recognize and commend the ease and readiness with which he assumed, in addition to his own, the duties and responsibilities thrown upon him by the illness of the Superintendent, and his very able, wise, and faithful conduct of them since the first of April last. With a deep sense of obligation to Dr. Whittemore for these voluntarily rendered services, and a high appreciation of his capacity and character, the Board beg him to accept their best wishes for his future happiness and success."

On March 31, Dr. Whittemore gratefully acknowledged the action of the Board.

An effort was made by the Trustees on April 14, by the appointment of a Committee, to secure the removal of at least ten incurable female patients at the Asylum, who could be removed without injury to them. It was known and well understood by the Trustees, in their constant visits, that there were such patients within the walls whose condition was hopeless, who would be as well provided for in some other institutions, who would not suffer from a change of place and surroundings, while, as coming perhaps from outside the State, or from other circumstances, they had not as strong a claim to be retained here as some other applicants had for admission who were necessarily excluded from lack of room. The Committee engaged the most earnest attention and effort in the matter, and put themselves in correspondence with the friends of the patients under consideration. But very slender results followed of the nature desired. It was found very difficult in any case, and impossible in most cases, to induce the friends of such patients to consent to their removal. In one point of view the incidental measures brought into action called out gratifying evidence of the high consideration in which the Asylum was held by the parties concerned, and of their full confidence in and grateful appreciation of the kind and faithful care bestowed upon the afflicted objects of their solicitude. The fact is a striking comment on one of the inconsiderate imputations upon institutions like this, as forcibly or unnecessarily detaining patients who might as well be discharged. The Asylum would best reward the hopes and labors of its friends by receiving almost exclusively curable patients, and by discharging them on the earliest day on which their restoration is assured. But it must meet the wishes and needs of the community as a merciful refuge for many incurables.

A communication was received by the Trustees, on April 21, from Dr. Hodges, announcing the award of the Warren Prize, by the medical board of the Hospital, to the dissertation on "The Physiological Effects of the Nitrate of Amyl," by Dr. Horatio C. Wood, jun., of Philadelphia. The Treasurer was instructed to pay the writer of the dissertation the amount of the prize, $388. Dr. Wood was permitted to take a copy for publication, on condition of returning the original manuscript to the Hospital, and indicating any additions he might make as not having passed under the eye of the Prize Committee.

The continued encroachments by railroads upon the grounds of the Asylum had now resulted in completely encircling them with the iron tracks, and dividing them so as to make them unavailable and dangerous for the uses for which large portions of them had been purchased. The Trustees were compelled to admit the almost proximate necessity of a removal of the institution to another site. The prospect of this necessity also prevented the Trustees from making any plans or large outlays for improvements, for new buildings, or even for repairs. On April 21, the Trustees voted that Messrs. Eliot, Dalton, and Ellis be a Committee to make such inquiries as they deem expedient for a new site for the Asylum, and report to the Board. A Committee "on Improvements at the Asylum," which had been appointed nearly a year before, was discharged. It was voted, on May 5, "That the Secretary request the Medical Board to select 'some subject in physiology, surgery, or pathological anatomy,' which may be advertised as the subject for the next Warren Prize, if approved by this Board." At this meeting a note was received from Mr. Farnsworth, announcing his resignation of the office of Trustee; and it was voted that the Chairman communicate to Mr. Farnsworth the appreciation of his services by this Board. The Secretary was directed to communicate this resignation to the governor, with the request that an appointment be made to fill the vacancy. The thanks of the Board were voted to Edward Jackson, Esq.,

Treasurer, for a donation of $450 from the Amateur Dramatic Association, of Boston; and to Miss Homer and others, trustees, for the manner in which they have conveyed to this institution the sum of $1,000, being a bequest from the late Sydney Homer, Esq.; also to George Gardner, Esq., executor, for the manner in which he has conveyed to this institution the sum of $2,000, being a bequest from the late James Read, Esq. The Treasurer was directed to establish the James Read Fund, in the amount of $2,000, the income of which shall be annually appropriated, one half to the support of free beds, and one half to the Asylum. On May 29, temporary arrangements were made for the superintendence of the Asylum till the existing vacancy should be filled. Dr. Hall Curtis, on June 2, resigned his office of Physician to out-patients. His resignation was accepted, and Dr. William L. Richardson was elected to fill the vacancy. A communication was received from Dr. Hodges, for the Medical Board, informing the Trustees that that Board had passed the following votes: —

"1st. To recommend the following as a subject for the Warren Prize for 1874; viz., 'Experimental Researches on the Elimination of Drugs by the Mammary Gland.'

"2d. That the Trustees, in advertising the above, or any other subject, be requested to announce that no person connected with the Medical Board of the Hospital is to be regarded as a competitor for the Warren Prize.

"3d. That, in the advertisement of a subject for the year 1874, the Trustees be requested to give notice of the award of this year's prize, for the information of unsuccessful competitors, as well as of the public in general.

"4th. That the Trustees be asked to confer with the Prize Committee, Drs. Minot, Hodges, Ellis, Cabot, and Warren, in regard to the choice of medical journals, in which the subject for 1874 should be advertised."

This communication was referred to the Visiting Committee with full powers. On June 10, the Board were informed that Dr. Ray, of Philadelphia, had consented to act as temporary Superintendent of the Asylum, until that office could be permanently filled. On June 30, Mr. Sweet, for the Committee, reported the following form for an advertisement, which was approved: —

"WARREN TRIENNIAL PRIZE.

"The Trustees of the Massachusetts General Hospital give notice that the first Triennial Prize (amounting to $388), from the fund bequeathed to the Hospital by the late Dr. J. Mason Warren, has been awarded to Horatio C. Wood, jun., M.D., of Philadelphia, for an essay on 'The Physiological Action of Nitrate of Amyl.' The next Warren Prize will be awarded to the author of the best essay considered worthy of a prize on the subject of 'Experimental Researches on the Elimination of Drugs by the Mammary Glands.' Each essay should be accompanied with a sealed envelope containing the author's name and address, and be transmitted to the Resident Physician of the Hospital on or before Feb. 1, 1874."

The Treasurer was requested to have the advertisement inserted in the " Boston Medical and Surgical Journal," the " New York Medical Record," and the " Philadelphia American Journal for Medical Sciences."

On the recommendation of Dr. Shaw, it was voted, —

"That the article and tables of statistics of surgical operations at the Hospital, recently prepared by Dr. Chadwick, be published in the ' Boston Medical and Surgical Journal,' with an edition of five hundred copies for distribution, at an expense not exceeding one hundred dollars."

On Oct. 13, Mr. Rogers, for the Committee, recommended Dr. George F. Jelly as a candidate for the office of Superintendent of the Asylum. The ballot being taken, Dr. Jelly was elected. The Chairman was requested to inform him of his appointment, and his salary was fixed at $3,000 per annum. The thanks of the Board were tendered to Dr. Isaac Ray " for his very acceptable services during the last three months, as temporary Superintendent of the Asylum;" and the Treasurer was directed to send to him the sum of fifteen hundred dollars. On Oct. 20, Dr. Henry P. Quincy was elected Artist of the Hospital. The Chairman was requested to confer with the Superintendent relative to the nomination of two Assistant Physicians of the Asylum, and to consider the appointment of a medical student to act as Assistant Apothecary without salary. Mr. Samuel D. Warren took his place at the Board on Dec. 1, as a Trustee, by appointment of the governor, in place of Mr. Farnsworth, resigned. Dr. John E. Tyler was elected a member of the Board of Consultation.

The date has now been reached at which it was proposed that this summary sketch of the more important incidents in the history of the Hospital for the last score of years should close. As, however, between the writing of these pages and their passage through the press several incidents of interest have transpired, a brief record of them may properly follow here.

The experiment of a separate ward for the treatment of patients afflicted with skin diseases, though by no means unsuccessful in its especial results, was regarded by the Trustees as open to some general objections, and was discontinued at the close of the year. Dr. James C. White had on his own part made a most faithful trial of the experiment, and had devoted to it his skill and experience in his specialty. He continues to serve the institution as Chemist and Physician to patients with diseases of the skin.

Munificent additions were made to the funds of

the institution near the close of the year. Mr. James McGregor, of Boston, sent to the Treasurer the sum of $10,000, which now constitutes the "McGregor Fund," half of its annual proceeds to be devoted to the Hospital and half to the Asylum, according to the wishes of the donor. The executors of the will of Miss Nabby Joy, of Boston, in the exercise of the discretion according to which she had directed that they should appropriate and distribute a very large sum of money from her estate among various objects of benevolence, put themselves in communication with the Trustees of the Hospital in reference to a proposed donation to them. At the meeting of the Board on Dec. 15, 1871, the following proposition was read: —

"The executors of the will of Nabby Joy propose to make to the Massachusetts General Hospital a donation of $20,000, to be appropriated to the maintenance of free beds, subject to the payment of an annuity of $500 for the benefit of —— during his life, and of a further annuity of $200 to —— during her life: the right of appointment (subject to the rules of the Hospital) to two free beds to be in the executors during their joint lives, and the life of the survivor."

The communication was, by vote, referred to the Chairman, with Mr. Hale and the Treasurer, with authority to accept the offer and to execute the necessary papers.

Soon after the organization of the staff of the Hospital for 1872, the Trustees were compelled with much regret to contemplate a change in its leading office caused by the resignation of its incumbent. Dr. Benjamin Shurtleff Shaw had been elected Resident Physician at the Hospital on May 23, 1858. For most of the time since that date he had been also Acting Steward, the Trustees finding practical advantages in the union of the two offices under one head. A severe domestic affliction, with the natural weariness incident to the continuous discharge for so many years of such confining duties, led Dr. Shaw, in the beginning of April, 1872, to tender his resignation to the Trustees. He asked to be relieved as early as convenient in the coming autumn, and that a successor might be appointed ready to take his place. The Trustees, at their meeting on May 3, accepted his resignation, and instructed the Secretary to express to Dr. Shaw "their grateful appreciation of his long, assiduous, and valuable services; their regret at the loss this institution sustains in his retirement, and their sympathy with him and Mrs. Shaw in their recent domestic affliction."

Dr. Norton Folsom was unanimously elected by the Trustees as successor of Dr. Shaw as Resident Physician of the Hospital, and will enter upon the responsible office though young in years, yet with much experience hard won in peace and war, and with many favoring auspices.

These pages close at a critical point in the history and future prospects of the Asylum at Somerville. The spacious edifices which have gathered by enlargements, and the erection of new structures around the original dwelling purchased by the Trustees, even with all the ingenuity and skill, and all the large outlays of money spent upon them, have never been regarded as wholly satisfactory in their arrangements. Successive changes have had to conform their qualified improvements to defects and to previous conditions in the forms and positions and internal structure of the buildings which could not be altered. Mr. Bowditch has well said of some of the labyrinthian passages, above and below, that, if the oldest Trustee were left in them without a guide, he could not well find his way out. Still, the edifice bears, from its foundations to its domes, a sort of history of the course of the wiser science and the tenderer humanity which have gradually been brought to the treatment of insanity. Some of the old strong-rooms, now disused except for the autumn stowage of fruits and farm vegetables, present us one page in that history which we are all glad to forget, as we mount from them towards the domes, through the sunny and cheerful apartments lighted by their bay-windows, with their fountains, flower-stands, and aquaria. It is safe to say that, rating money at its

A NEW SITE FOR THE ASYLUM.

valuation a half-century ago, structures of the same capacity, and with far ampler conveniences, might be erected for less than half the outlay that has gone to those edifices. In the mean while, steadily, with the successive purchases by the Trustees of new acres of ground around the Asylum, their intended uses as quiet and secluded spaces for the exercise and refreshment of the inmates have been impaired and well-nigh prevented by the encroachments of traffic, with its noise and its risks. Those spacious and beautiful grounds, with their fertile soil and pleasant undulations of surface, are not only completely encircled by railroads, but their breadth is twice cut through by them. When the first of these railroads was opened, Dr. Bell, then in charge of the Asylum, had the gravest apprehensions that the clatter of the iron wheels and the shrieks of the steam-whistle, combining themselves with the delusions of some of the patients, might have a very deplorable influence upon them. But, contrary to what might have reasonably been feared, very limited, if any, mischief of this sort has been realized. Yet the Trustees, under the present condition of things, have been brought to the conviction that it is highly desirable for them to find a new site for the Asylum. It has been slowly and with reluctance that they have come to this conclusion. They have realized many advantages in the present location. The proximity to the city has made access to the Asylum very convenient to the friends of patients, so large a portion of whom are from the immediate neighborhood. The references made in the preceding pages to the abundant resources of relaxation and amusement furnished to the patients show a large dependence upon the city for making them convenient and varied. But, in deciding upon a change of site, the Trustees have hoped that it may, and will do all in their power to insure that it shall, result in gain, with no loss, to the best interests of the institution. Our architects, mechanics, and builders will find themselves engaged in perhaps the most exacting demand that has ever been made upon their skill, ingenuity, and executive abilities, in meeting the wishes and purposes of the Trustees, in the planning, disposing, and completing such structures as will be desired under conditions that must be combined and harmonized.

As to the questions still kept under discussion, — not always judicious or discreet, — in our community and elsewhere, relating to the internal discipline of an asylum, and the mode of treatment which humanity and science commend as best for the patients and most satisfactory to their friends, all parties to these questions are concerned only to reach the fair, full truth. Putting out of view, as a matter of course, the differences of opinion, — not to say the prejudices, — which are found to influence those whose feelings and fancies serve them in place of reflection, experience, and candid, intelligent inquiry, there may yet be allowed a limited range still left open for theoretical and practical divergence of judgment on some of the subjects involved in this specialty. The preceding pages furnish abundant evidence of the efforts of the successive Boards of Trustees to secure to the Asylum the services of the ablest, the most accomplished, and the most devoted men. And the series of Reports of the Superintendents, from which summaries have been sketched, certify to the qualifications, the fidelity, and the self-consecrating earnestness of zeal and effort which they have given to their work. Men, in whom a self-respecting regard for their own reputation, and a conscientious sense of responsibility, have been traits so evidently prominent in character and in work as in the writers of those Reports, are not likely to need any incentive from the community to quicken them in the search for and in the appreciation of any new methods or appliances for the advancement of their science. Those who, either as partially recovered patients, or as the friends of patients, criticise the management of this Asylum in a querulous or distrustful spirit, will naturally urge the objections, which unprofessional persons encourage each other in repeating, against experts and functionaries who in the exercise of their trusts have common principles for their guidance. Such officials are said to carry their professional rules and methods into a rigid and unyielding application; to become formalists, stiff in their prepossessions, mechanical in their theories, averse to changes, and mischievously restrained by an *esprit du corps*, which makes them stoutly conservative, as they follow routine, and shut their eyes to new light. On the other hand, those who are thus criticised and censured turn towards their questioners with a silent or an avowed remonstrance at the presumption which so positively condemns or distrusts, without due qualifications of knowledge or experience. These outside critics may be idealists or theorists, with visionary fancies which they themselves would have to abandon as impracticable if they should have an opportunity of testing them in trial. These theorists and idealists, however, are found to have a legitimate and sometimes a most effective influence for good in very many of the interests of society, compelling conservatism and professional and official routine to flow with the stream of progress. Only our progressionists sometimes seem to forget that we can, from almost any outlook, see into spaces where there is no foothold.

It is claimed that those who as professional experts have had the oversight of the insane have become, in some few very important practical principles of their science, advocates of different methods, and so are now divided among themselves. Thus we are told of some who are of the highest repute in this specialty who disapprove of the aggregation of patients in an asylum, and prefer the distribution of them over a rural village, and in cottages where more personal freedom is enjoyed, while still the necessary oversight, with more hopeful curative results, may be obtained. Also a few asylums are adduced in which " the moral treatment" is very different in some important respects, and in which likewise no forms or modes of physical restraint whatever are employed; and much less, if any, of the restrictions heretofore considered necessary, are put upon interviews and correspondence of patients with their friends. The alleged differences of opinion and practice on these points, between men of repute and experience in the guardianship of the insane, may be made to appear really serious when stated in unqualified terms and brought into strong contrast. If, however, a searching, discriminating, and candid inquiry is brought to bear upon the facts, we discover that misunderstanding, misrepresentation, and a wrong statement or coloring of the truth greatly perplex the issue. Indeed, considering how largely our age is characterized by individuality, eccentricity, and the love of novelty in theory and practice, and by the spirit of rivalry in adapting and commending institutions to the caprices and whims of patrons, it is somewhat remarkable that there is so general an accord of opinion and method among the guardians of the insane. The local peculiarities of some communities, and the former condition and habits of life of those who require treatment, must be taken into account in deciding between an asylum like our own and the village system, like that of Gheel, for instance. Again, there are two asylums in England, in which it is professed that recourse is in no case had to physical restraint in any form of it which confines the body or the hands or arms of a patient, in the bed or out of it, so as to interfere in the least degree with the free exercise of the limbs within the walls or the grounds of the refuge; and thus it is said all the fretfulness and exasperation which excited patients feel when under such fetterings is saved them. But there is no satisfactory statement of the substitutes for physical restraint which are relied on. Such substitutes there must be; for there are patients who would exhaust themselves by intensely excited muscular activity, and who would never occupy a bed if allowed their perfect bodily freedom. The substitutes which suggest themselves are the use of anæsthetics and drugs, or a recourse to the restraining power of the presence, the voice, and the muscles of an attendant, — perhaps of more than one attendant. It is not for the writer to plead or to arbitrate in this issue. So far as the method and practice of this asylum are concerned, it may be said, that all of its successive superintendents, disapproving the use of drugs for subduing excited patients, and believing that a sole reliance upon the muscular force of an attendant would be either impracticable or otherwise objectionable, especially as being most irritating and offensive to the patients, have reduced the use of physical restraining appliances to the minimum.

A portion of a report made to a Committee of the Trustees by Dr. Jelly, on several subjects relating to the conduct of the Asylum, may fitly be introduced here : —

The " Restraint " used in McLean Asylum during the year ending Dec. 31, 1871.

"The varieties of restraint used are the 'Camisole,' or 'Sleeves,' which restrains the hands, prevents violence, and self-injury, and the destruction and removal of clothing.

"The 'Mittens,' used for the same purpose as the 'Camisole,' which simply cover the hands and are fastened to a belt which passes round the waist.

"The 'Wristers,' which surround the wrists only, allowing free use to the hands, but being also fastened to the waist by a belt, prevent the wearer from striking. This form of restraint is used generally on men who are watching every opportunity to strike those about them.

"The 'Bed Straps,' by which a person is confined to the bed, but can turn on his or her side and move up and down. These are used in the most violent cases of mania, where there is danger of exhaustion, or where a patient will not remain in bed at night; and in desperately suicidal cases, where the presence of an attendant in the room, or the wearing of a camisole, are not sufficient precautions.

"In suicidal patients, our practice differs according to the severity of the paroxysms of suicide. In mild cases, the presence of an attendant in the room, sleeping in the bed, or in a cot, or on a lounge, close by, is considered enough. In more severe cases, the addition of a camisole is necessary; while the very severest forms of suicidal melancholia are not safe without the bed straps.

"Where persons can be made safe without restraint, they are always made so by the presence of attendants in the room, or near by, except in those cases where the patient is too filthy or violent to make it proper for an attendant to sleep in the room.

"In addition to the forms of restraint already mentioned, we sometimes use a chair, for violent patients, who can be allowed to sit up, but who, if unrestrained, throw themselves on the floor, beat their heads against the wall, or otherwise injure themselves.

"The constant effort on the part of the officers is to reduce the use of all restraint to a minimum, to use it only for the good of a patient, and never to use any form of it when the presence and efforts of attendants would do as well.

"No attendant is allowed to put any restraint upon a patient, either day or night, unless by the order of one of the officers, with the exception of the extremely rare cases, where a patient is suddenly seized with a severe paroxysm of violence, rendering him or her dangerous to all around, as well as to himself or herself. In such cases, if an attendant cannot safely leave his or her gallery to find one of the officers, he or she is allowed to put on a camisole, or a pair of mittens, never any thing more, which must be reported to one of the officers, for his approval or disapproval, at the very earliest moment when the gallery can be left. The whole matter of the use of restraint is carefully watched by each one of the officers of the Asylum.

"The Night Watchers are required to make the rounds of the house, and be on every gallery once every hour, that they may be ready to help any one who may need it. They are required to look into the rooms of suicidal patients, and of those who are weak and feeble, or who frequently are up in the night. They are required to move about quietly, and to throw the light of their lanterns into the rooms, but not upon the face of the patient. They look into only about one-fourth of the rooms. They can make use of no restraint, without the order of one of the officers. The house would be very unsafe without Night Watchers.

"During the year ending Dec. 31, 1871, there were in the Asylum 253 persons. The following were the uses made, respectively, of

THE CAMISOLE.

For violence	2
To prevent suicide	7 (at night).
To prevent removing clothing	4
To prevent self-abuse	3 (at night).
	16

MITTENS.

To prevent removing clothing	2
To prevent suicide	3 (at night).
	5

WRISTERS.

To prevent striking 5

THE CHAIR.

To prevent injury to self and exhaustion 3

BED STRAPS.

To keep in bed and prevent exhaustion (at night only)	11
To prevent violence and exhaustion (during day and night)	15
To prevent suicide	6

"Making a total of 61, out of 253 persons, who were under restraint, either twenty-four hours or one night at least, during 1871.

"This includes all the habitual restraint. Occasionally a patient wears the camisole or mittens, for an hour or two only, on account of some special outburst of violence, which is not mentioned in the records.

"GEORGE F. JELLY."

As to the restriction upon interviews with friends of patients from outside the Asylum, who might wish to see their condition and their apartments, popular prejudices have often gone the length of assuming that our gentle and wise Superintendents exercise the functions of those who have prisoners of State or convicts under their charge, with whom they can positively prohibit all intercourse. It is enough to say that no such prerogative is granted or exercised at the Asylum to or by those who have the oversight of it. Recently, of the whole number of patients in the Asylum, — being 167, — the friends of 142 of them could and did visit them at their pleasure. Of course, the friends of the chronic demented very rarely wish to see them. Only 25 of the whole number of the patients were pronounced by the Superintendent as in a condition to render visits from friends, for the time, unadvisable. In no single case, and under no circumstances, is the nearest friend or guardian, having personal rights, precluded from an interview with a patient, or prevented from removing him or her at pleasure. Of course there are cases in which in the exercise of his judgment, and as a prime condition of his qualification for his high trust, the Superintendent will strongly advise, perhaps remonstrate, against allowing an interview between a patient and one who has a right to ask for it. The Superintendent will freely, perhaps earnestly, give reasons for objecting to it. He will speak from his intimate knowledge of each case, and his experience of many cases. He will say that interviews with friends, under this or like circumstances, are purely harmful; renewing and intensifying the force of delusions, reconnecting the chain of morbid associations which it is his object permanently to break, arousing discontent, ensuring a period of excitement with sleepless and wretched nights, and perhaps stirring a suicidal impulse. If the friend, after listening to this kind and wise suggestion, is not convinced by it so as to comply with it, the way is freely opened to an interview with the patient, the friend assuming the responsibility for the consequences. After like advice and remonstrances on the part of the Superintendent, and similar persistency of friends, patients partially recovered, or with a prospect of restoration, may be removed, though to their sure injury. There are always more applicants than can be received; and the gratification of all the officers of the Asylum is the highest only when a new patient can be admitted to fill the place of one discharged perfectly well.

As to the restriction upon the correspondence between patients and friends outside, there is misapprehension here, also, which is made to exaggerate popular prejudice. The figures on this point will be most satisfactory. On the 28th of May, 1872, there were in the McLean Asylum as patients 77 males and 101 females, in all 178; of these, 53 males and 60 females, in all 113, never wish to write; 21 males and 34 females, in all 55, write when they wish, and receive letters, — more than half of these not having their correspondence subject to any prudential oversight whatever. Of those from whom the means of correspondence are withheld, there are but 3 males and 7 females, in all 10. The restriction in these very few cases is imposed for one or both of the two sufficient reasons, either that it would harm the patient for whom there is hope of cure to yield to the excitement of putting delusions and fancies upon paper, or that the morbid communications which they might write would be misleading and harrowing to friends. Reasons there are also, in some of these cases, for leading the friends of patients to enjoin extreme caution on the officers of the Asylum as to the exchange of letters with objectionable correspondents, while they are also earnestly desirous that no letters from the patients be written to themselves.

If, as has been above intimated, there is a limited range for difference of judgment among professional experts still left open, as to principles and methods of general or special application, there are abundant and well-adapted means now in use, through conventions and journals, by which the Superintendents of Asylums can instruct each other.

The preceding pages, devoted to the supplemental

history of the Hospital, have been composed according to the terms of the wish expressed by the Trustees in their vote. The interest of them, limited by the object had in view, will of course be very small, and of no account whatever to a general reader. Far different in tone and contents, in tenor and in impressiveness, would be a work that might be written, concerning either the Hospital or the Asylum, which should be engaged with the aspects and experiences of human life, the incidents of personal history, the secrets and the revelations of character, discipline, sorrow, stern suffering, and the precious resources of patience, fortitude, and submission, — the inner wealth of human spirits, — that have been known within those walls. It has not been a pleasant task to the writer to recognize only as matters of routine business for committees and votes, the oversight of interests which come so tenderly, often so harrowingly, within the sacred privacy of the wards and galleries of these refuges of human suffering and woe. Neither, on the other hand, would it have been an engaging task for the writer to prepare, nor would readers be profited by the perusal of, pages which should furnish details of these inner experiences. Only holy sympathy and a power to minister to and relieve the maladies of humanity in soul or body — sympathy and power like those of the

Great Physician — can wisely or healthfully be brought into contact with, or even into the contemplation of, those varied human woes. As I write these pages, I have before me on the wall a most instructive picture, the groupings of which are suggestive of the partition between the different classes of sufferers engaging my thought as I make my regular visits, as a Trustee, to the Hospital or the Asylum. It is a copy of Ary Scheffer's picture of "Christus Consolator," Christ the Consoler. The Scripture sentence which it illustrates is this: "He hath sent me to heal the broken-hearted, to preach deliverance to the captives." The artist has grouped into two classes the forms of all the varied sufferers by disease and wrong and sorrow, through all the maladies of mind and body; while the Saviour, the central figure to whom they all turn, ministers to them all. The retinue which He drew around him — a following such as no other King or Prince ever coveted or won — is described as composed of " all sick people that were taken with divers diseases and torments, and those which were possessed with devils, and those which were lunatick." They who can help or comfort, with the hand or the heart, any such sufferers, have the right of access to them. But any details or particular relations drawn out on the printed page would be simply distressing to all to whom they would not be hardening.

It is enough for us to have the assurance that, in both Hospital and Asylum, the highest appliances of science and the gentlest ministrations of a refined humanity are engaged for each human malady as if it were a case by itself. When we read in our daily papers of some accident or shocking disaster on the highways, or the wharves, or in a dwelling, and are informed that the victim " was taken to the Massachusetts General Hospital," we need not send our imagination there to fashion the scene that follows. It is a satisfaction for us to know that, by day and night, there are always ready there the services of physician and surgeon, watchman, nurse, and attendant, with all appliances of science and curious skill to restore or relieve. When we are reminded of the many cases of complicated disease, congenital malformations, disabling or malignant in their character, which, after having baffled for a long time the resources of country practitioners, are at last brought from far distances to the Hospital, that the expert, whose skill is divided between his brain and his almost intelligent instruments, may engage it in their behalf, we need intrude no farther. Yet the reserve which then becomes wise for us cannot but enhance the grateful feeling, ever to be associated with the walls of that Hospital so long as they shall stand, that within them was first tried and verified the harmlessness and the potency of the anæsthetic agent in ensuring the painlessness of the most fearful processes of the surgeon's knife. The shrinkings and the quivers which were almost equally distressing in their stages of apprehension and reality have yielded to perfect obliviousness or to sweet dreams and visions. The mechanical devices, in bed and chair, the regulations of diet, the skilled nursings, the discretion exercised in the employment of drugs and medicines, the perfection reached in the construction and use of surgical instruments, the exacting discipline secured by minute rules and by the requisitions of a record, and above all the absolute immunity from all the risks of quackery and irresponsible practice, — these are but a few of the more obvious privileges in which the patients of the Hospital have their equal and impartial shares. What those privileges are to the poor, to those whose only home is the garret or the tenement house, whose only attendants there would be those as poor and almost as inefficient as themselves, it needs no display of contrasts for making the estimate. But the cases are numerous — indeed the list of them begins with the opening of the Hospital and continues to this day — in which the rich and well-befriended have been brought from luxurious homes, to have their full share in the privileges of the institution,— its quiet, its internal discipline, its appliances and resources, its ever-present ministrations of skill and experience. Among those informed on the subject it is very well understood that, if a stranger in the city from any part of this country, or from abroad, however wealthy, refined, or delicate, should be disabled by accident or serious disease, he would do well to exchange his apartments in one of our best appointed hotels for a private room in the Hospital. There have been instances enough, so satisfactory too in their results, in which this exchange has been made, to warrant the above assertion, without a qualification. Indeed, the records of the Trustees and of the Treasurer bear witness to the munificent gifts which have accrued to the Hospital from the grateful returns of such patients.

Among the crude and popular, perhaps natural, expressions of distrust and opposition to the first planning and the supposed subsequent administration of the Hospital, this was prominent, — namely, that poor patients were to be enticed within its walls that they might be made the subjects of experiments in surgical processes or in the trial of drugs, chemicals, and medicines; so that this gratuitous practice might fit a few young doctors and surgeons for safer and well-remunerated professional work for the rich in their luxurious chambers. Now, it may be most emphatically affirmed, that one of the paramount objects had in view, as prompting the establishment of the Hospital, was that by its agency the poor and unfriended might be secured from those very outrages, — to which they were exposed outside of it to an extent and at a cost to them far beyond what any of them realized. It needs only that one should cast his eyes over the newspapers which circulate most among the poor, the ignorant, and unfriended, to learn from their advertisements what appliances are offered them for self-treatment, and what sort of professional aid is commended to them. Indeed, the Hospital, if it had no other claim for regard and consideration, might advance a most substantial one on the score of its quiet and most effective discountenance of quackery and empiricism, and those enormous and villanous outrages which are practised by charlatans on the ignorant and the credulous.

Nor is there a shadow of reason in the allegation that, when it is affirmed that science and humanity preside over the administration of the Hospital, the service of science consists in putting disease and the operations which it requires into subserviency to a Medical School, for the training of classes of young pupils in medicine and surgery. Those who preside over the operating theatre, and make its necessary processes the means of education for their successors, do not need the indorsement of any outside testimony to the spirit and method of their exercises. Delicacy, tenderness, prudential reserve, and all the refinements of professional propriety and courtesy may be taken for granted there. Meanwhile, if it were possible to look at surgical operations abstractly, as performed on insensate materials, — as indeed the anæsthetic agent ensures that they are substantially, — it would be difficult to define a more effective condition for their delicate and perfect performance than is found in the presence of a group of keenly inquisitive pupils. It may be believed that, if a comparison were instituted between the clinical and surgical practices of the best appointed hospitals and those in the chambers of private homes for any class of people, the comparison would at no point be unfavorable to the former as to all the most desirable conditions of skill, tenderness, consideration, and the prospect of benefit in relief or cure.

In closing the work required of him, the writer will indulge himself in expressing, in brief and simple terms, three most pleasing impressions which the study of the records in his hands has wrought in his mind. First comes that grateful sense of the wisely guided and instructed spirit of sympathetic benevolence, considerate generosity, and munificent liberality in our immediate community, by which, from the first proposal of its objects to the present day, persons of all classes among us as regards means, position, and culture, have founded and endowed this institution. Its affluence comes from the transfer to its treasury of the wealth of many kind and Christian hearts. Never has an appeal been made in vain in its behalf. The footings-up of the specific contributions received have always exceeded the amounts asked for. "Father Taylor," the eminent sailor-preacher, — himself for his own sake and for his cause a large sharer in the benevolence which he extolled, — while once thrilling a large audience on a charitable occasion with his fervid, glowing, and unartistic eloquence, not only " lost his nominative case," but became hopelessly involved in his figures of speech and flight of rhetoric. Knowing that he ought to close, and seeing no other way out of his evident embarrassment, he brought his hand down with a heavy blow, and abruptly turning to the chairman, Justice Story, said, " The truth is, Mr. President, the Lord has only one Boston, and we live in it."

A second impression, of an equally grateful character, realized from the review of our records, is that of the free, unpaid daily service, continued on for long years, which the institution has received from the most accomplished, the most eminent, and the most honored and beloved professional men, physicians and surgeons, in this community. Practitioners, whose ability and repute made their labors most engrossing and their time most valuable to them, have put the claims of this institution foremost in their regard. They gave to it themselves while they lived, and left to it their blessing, the memory and influence of their devotion, and their pecuniary aid.

And, last of all, the writer must add, that, as he has read the records before him, with the filed reports and documents to which they refer, he has been profoundly impressed by the dignity, the respectful consideration, and the perfect courtesy of feeling, intercourse, and business which have characterized the relations between the Trustees and the Officers of the Institution. Delicate questions have arisen; some matters of prerogative, precedency, and authority, have required attention. But there never has been a personal issue. Frankness, kindness, and mutual regard, which are themselves forms and qualities of justice, have uniformly prevailed here.

To the residents in this immediate community, the names of those who for so long a series of years have successively served as Trustees of this institution will make it unnecessary to add any thing as to their claims to confidence and respect, for the services they have rendered. It will have been noticed very rarely in the preceding pages that the election as a Trustee has been followed by the declination of one so chosen to serve. Considering what sort of men have been elected, and from what ranges of life they come, the wonder is that the Hospital bears on its records, often for a considerable series of years, the names which are found upon them. Occasionally those names are of professional men of the highest standing. For the most part, however, they are the names of men in the full vigor of life, pursuing actively the higher and most engrossing tasks of business, managing large trusts, and guiding the enterprise of the community. The regular meetings of the Trustees are held at the Hospital on alternate weeks. Quarterly meetings, for the examination of accounts and for receiving the reports of officers, are held at the Asylum. Two of the Trustees, each of them changing his colleague from month to month, so that each serves for two successive months, visit the Asylum every Tuesday, and the Hospital every Friday; seeing every patient and every apartment, examining the entries on the records of each admission, fixing the price of board according to circumstances, disposing temporarily of any question of interest that presents itself, and then making and signing their report upon the ledgers. The Trustees are likewise distributed into Standing Committees on Finance, on Accounts, on Free Beds, on the Book of Donations, on the Warren Fund and Library, and on Repairs. That gentlemen, most of whom might plead the engrossment of their own private affairs or business agencies, have been found from year to year to give their time and the indorsement of their reputation to these exacting tasks, is to be regarded simply as a tribute paid by them to the cause of humanity as represented by the Hospital.

CONTINUATION OF THE LIST

OF THE

OFFICERS OF THE HOSPITAL.

PRESIDENTS.

William Appleton	from 1844	to 1862.
Robert Hooper	from 1862	to 1869.
Edward Wigglesworth	from 1869	to

VICE-PRESIDENTS.

Robert Hooper	from 1850	to 1856.
Nathaniel I. Bowditch	from 1856	to 1862.
Edward Wigglesworth	from 1862	to 1869.
Nathaniel Thayer	from 1869	to

TREASURERS.

Henry Andrews	from 1835	to 1859.
J. Thomas Stevenson	from 1859	to

SECRETARIES.

Marcus Morton, jun.	from 1842	to 1859.
Thomas B. Hall	from 1859	to 1865.
William S. Dexter		for 1865.
Thomas B. Hall	from 1866	to

TRUSTEES.

Nathaniel I. Bowditch	from 1837	to 1856.
Thomas Lamb	from 1839	to 1861.
George M. Dexter	from 1839	to 1853.
Francis C. Lowell	from 1839	to 1853.
Henry B. Rogers	from 1839	to
Edward Wigglesworth	from 1844	to 1862.
J. Thomas Stevenson	from 1846	to 1859
Charles H. Mills	from 1848	to 1859.
Amos A. Lawrence	from 1848	to 1854.
William S. Bullard	from 1849	to 1872.
G. Howland Shaw	from 1850	to 1856.
William J. Dale	from 1851 to 1862, and for 1864.	
John P. Bigelow	from 1852 to 1855, and for 1857.	
Charles H. Warren	from 1853	to 1857.
Robert M. Mason	from 1854	to 1862.
Henry M. Holbrook	from 1855	to 1857.
James B. Bradlee	from 1856	to 1859.
William D. Greenough	from 1856	to 1866
John Lowell	from 1857	to 1870.
Abbott Lawrence	from 1858	to 1859
Nathaniel H. Emmons	from 1859	to 1861.
George Higginson	from 1859	to
Marcus Morton, jun.	from 1859	to 1860.
Martin Brimmer	from 1860	to 1864.
James M. Beebe	from 1860	to
J. Amory Davis	from 1861	to 1866.
Samuel G. Howe	from 1861	to
James C. Wild	from 1862	to 1865.
Harrison Ritchie	from 1863	to 1867.
Henry A. Whitney	from 1863	to 1868.
Charles S. Storrow	from 1865	to 1870.
Charles H. Dalton	from 1866	to
Samuel Eliot	from 1866	to
James L. Little	from 1866	to 1871.

Ezra Farnsworth . . . . . from 1867 . . . . to 1872.
Edmund Dwight . . . . . from 1868 . . . . to
George S. Hale . . . . . . from 1870 . . . . to
Samuel W. Swett . . . . . from 1870 . . . . to
George E. Ellis . . . . . . from 1871 . . . . to
Samuel D. Warren . . . from 1871 . . . . to
Henry P. Kidder . . . . . from 1872 . . . . to

CHAIRMEN OF THE TRUSTEES.

Nathaniel I. Bowditch . . . from 1850 . . . . to 1856.
Henry B. Rogers . . . . . from 1856 . . . . to

SUPERINTENDENTS OF HOSPITAL.

Richard Girdler . . . . . from 1845 . . . . to 1858.
Benjamin S. Shaw . . . . . from 1858 . . . . to 1872.
Norton Folsom elected May 3, 1872.

PHYSICIANS OF ASYLUM.

Luther V. Bell from 1836 to 1856, and temporarily for 1857.
Chauncey Booth from 1856, died January 13, 1858.
John E. Tyler from 1858 to 1871.
George F. Jelly elected October 13, 1871.

Table of Admissions, Discharges, and Results, at the McLean Asylum, from its opening, October 6, 1818, to December 31, 1871, inclusive.

YEARS.	Admitted.	Discharg'd	Whole No. under care.	Died.	Much Improved, &c.	Recovered.	Remaining at end of year.	Average No. of Patients.
1818–19	58	35	58	5	19	11	23	–
1820	44	40	67	1	28	11	27	–
1821	47	46	74	3	33	10	28	–
1822	64	50	92	5	31	14	42	–
1823	73	61	115	2	39	20	54	–
1824	53	56	107	5	28	23	51	–
1825	59	56	110	8	27	21	54	–
1826	47	46	101	5	21	20	55	–
1827	58	56	113	5	17	34	57	–
1828	77	65	134	5	37	23	69	–
1829	73	77	142	9	42	26	65	–
1830	82	78	147	10	34	34	69	–
1831	83	84	152	8	46	30	68	–
1832	94	98	162	10	45	43	64	–
1833	103	100	167	8	50	42	67	–
1834	108	95	174	7	47	41	80	–
1835	83	84	163	11	28	45	77	–
1836	106	112	183	10	38	64	71	–
1837	120	105	191	8	25	72	86	80
1838	138	131	224	12	45	74	93	95
1839	132	117	225	10	38	69	108	112
1840	155	138	263	13	50	75	125	128
1841	157	141	283	11	55	75	142	135
1842	129	138	271	15	43	80	133	143
1843	126	126	260	18	45	63	134	131
1844	158	140	292	20	52	68	152	146
1845	119	120	271	13	33	74	151	149
1846	148	126	299	9	52	65	173	164
1847	170	170	343	33	50	87	173	172
1848	143	155	316	23	50	82	155	171
1849	160	137	321	15	58	64	184	177
1850	173	157	357	28	51	78	200	201
1851	164	173	364	29	69	75	191	195
1852	145	135	336	15	48	72	201	200
1853	114	120	315	17	45	58	195	194
1854	120	120	315	16	45	59	195	195
1855	123	126	318	24	46	56	192	192
1856	149	145	341	19	58	68	196	195
1857	141	159	337	28	60	71	178	191
1858	155	147	333	25	50	72	186	187
1859	131	142	317	28	53	61	175	185
1860	121	109	296	24	46	39	187	185
1861	111	110	298	23	33	54	188	193
1862	82	94	270	18	37	39	176	190
1863	94	69	270	13	20	36	201	191
1864	101	107	302	27	38	42	195	200
1865	82	85	277	17	33	35	192	186
1866	103	98	295	29	23	46	197	197
1867	89	108	286	27	36	45	178	186
1868	92	94	270	23	37	34	176	166
1869	108	100	284	18	31	51	184	187
1870	79	85	263	12	40	33	178	187
1871	75	81	253	13	22	21	172	178
–	5719	5547	–	790	2127	2605	–	–

Table of Admissions, Discharges, and Results at the Massachusetts General Hospital, from Sept. 3, 1821, to Dec. 31, 1871.

Year	Total admitted	Paying board all the time	Free	Paying part of the time	Whole Number treated. Paying board	Whole Number treated. Paying board part of time	Whole Number treated. Free	Discharged well	Percentage on "Total admitted."	Much Relieved, or Relieved in Part	Not Relieved	Not Treated, Unfit, Dismissed, &c.	Deaths	Percentage on "Total admitted."	Greatest number free at one time	Greatest number paying at one time	Greatest total	Least total	Average	Accidents	Percentage	Average time of Paying Weeks	Average time of Free Weeks	Patients remaining under treatment Dec. 31. Paying	Patients remaining under treatment Dec. 31. Free	Out-Patients treated
1821 to 1841	7992	—	354	—	—	—	—	3719	47	2613	815	68	573	6	—	—	61	41	—	—	—	4 5-7	6 6-7	—	—	328
1841	404	168	213	23	—	—	—	151	37	152	53	21	26	7	—	—	62	26	51	—	—	4	6 1-7	—	—	378
1842	347	159	177	11	—	—	—	121	34	137	45	16	25	11	—	—	56	13	43	—	—	4	6	—	—	272
1843	365	170	183	15	—	—	—	136	37	115	55	17	41	11	—	—	71	40	47²	—	—	3 6-7	7 1-7	—	—	294
1844	435	174	265	11	—	—	—	183	43	137	41	23	47	12	44	30	72	37	53	55	12²	5 1-4	6 6-7	—	—	237
1845	453	176	250	12	—	—	—	205	45	130	37	28	54	8	44	34	72	27	56	62	14	3 3-1	6	—	—	248
1846	459	182	250	27	—	—	—	211	46	137	30	23	36	8	82	28	72	37	55	59	13	3 1-2	6	—	—	358
1847	674	279	460	41	—	—	—	340	50	145	54	30	57	13	86	41	123	54	81	74	13	3 1-7	5	—	—	477
1848	804	283	543	61	—	—	—	400	50	219	52	59	103	10	89	38	124	94	108	103	12²	2 4-7	4 1-2	—	—	645
1849	870	273	527	54	—	—	—	436	48	218	75	33	84	9	103	38	127	90	112	97	11	2 4-7	5	—	—	887
1850	746	242	477	77	—	—	—	363	46	200	56	49	76	10	93	33	136	83	108	98	12²	2 6-7	5 5-7	—	—	1574
1851	839	298	487	64	—	—	—	387	50	235	47	63	98	11	105	48	141	77	112	98	11	3 1-4	6	—	—	2223
1852	836	271	472	83	—	—	—	410	46	234	52	47	82	11	108	41	133	104	119	123	13	3 1-6	6	—	—	3523
1853	925	335	490	85	—	—	—	431	50	287	70	66	82	9	112	39	142	125	133	132	15	3 1-4	5	—	—	4433
1854	922	321	415	111	—	—	—	423	46	257	73	41	115	13	107	45	145	108	134	157	16	3	7	—	—	4676
1855	915	352	414	147	—	—	—	456	49	238	59	51	101	12	114	59	152	120	134	189	17	3 3-7	10	—	—	4800
1856	976	335	454	96	—	—	—	478	50	230	57	71	102	14	119	48	153	103	128	186	23	3	114.7	—	—	4987
1857	920	280	549	91	—	—	—	510	50	195	57	60	117	13	120	40	157	91	123	131	17 3-10	2 2-3	5	—	—	5619
1858	1015	251	718	46	287	49	—	514	53	229	65	50	130	11	145	37	144	80	128	212	19	4	7-2	14	140	5356
1859	1240	201	934	49	215	42	1040	653	56	280	54	94	127	9¾	149	33	165	102	140	157	17 7-10	4	3-4	15	121	5608
1860	1240	253	997	42	268	32	1137	698	59	305	73	58	141	6⁴	135	45	175	116	137	292	17	4	6	16	124	4553
1861	1416	283	1131	32	308	15	1252	831	59	318	79	154	121	7⁴	135	29	162	110	134	271	21	4	3-4	25	120	5264
1862	1611	326	1175	17	441	17	1299	843	52	431	96	70	99	8	139	23	166	88	137	242	16 3-4	2 1-10	4.37	24	126	6953
1863	1648	425	1348	17	308	11	1468	856	49	459	77	60	162	8½	139	33	158	78	138	140	15 2-10	3 4-10	4.85	25	123	4553
1864	1599	283	1262	11	350	17	1388	916	55	390	94	74	101	6¼	137	33	157	80	113	132	15 2-10	3.67	5.10	45	123	5356
1865	1199	567	497	68	592	24	687	702	60	295	68	82	104	8⅓	62	45	164	78	95	132	15 2-10	3.40	4.26	45	59	5608
1866	1120	578	626	45	693	45	556	677	56	82	50	74	96	8¼	77	62	109	72	104	98	11	2.37	4.30	39	50	4553
1867	1206	556	771	31	601	26	676	676	60	282	62	84	94	7.8	95	72	126	69	102	93	11 7-10	3.00	3.50	31	69	5264
1868	1265	463	834	24	302	24	840	757	55½	258	64	82	107	7.7	98	56	132	90	118	140	9.36	3.40	4.82	25	96	6953
1869	1390	532	858	30	563	30	930	771	60	352	78	68	85	6.45	106	45	139	98	120	140	7.74	3.37	4.30	24	100	8767
1870	1302	414	858	25	439	30	958	780	60	303	65	73	109	1.64	126	43	137	98	120	140	6.69	3.12	3.92	24	86	8767
1871	1427	432	970	25	456	25	1056	821	57½	322	58	73	109	1.64	126	43	154	91	122	178				28	126	9792
	38550							19855		10185	2721	1922	3409													82252

Table of Applications, Admissions, &c., for Ten Years,—1862–1871.

Years	Applications Hospital	Admissions Hospital	Admissions Asylum	American Hospital	American Asylum	Foreign Hospital	Foreign Asylum	Not admitted Hospital	Discharged, cured, relieved, or improved Hospital	Discharged, cured, relieved, or improved Asylum	Percentage of same, on Admissions Hospital	Percentage of same, on Admissions Asylum	Died Hospital	Died Asylum	Accidents	Whole number under care in the year Hospital	Whole number under care in the year Asylum	No. of Free patients Hospital	Paying all the time Hospital	Paying part of the time Hospital	Greatest total number at any time Hospital	Greatest total number at any time Asylum	Least total at any one time Hospital	Least total at any one time Asylum	Average Hospital	Average Asylum	Greatest number at any one time of Free or Paying at Hospital — Paying	Greatest number ... Free	Average Paying and Free at Hospital — Paying	Average Paying and Free at Hospital — Free	Out-Patients Hospital
1862	1888	1611	82	81	1	893	—	277	1274	76	79.08	92.6	101	18	271	1751	270	1299	441	11	166	193	102	177	134	190	133	45	2.1	4.3	4800
1863	2051	1648	94	92	2	1000	—	403	1315	56	79.18	59.5	162	13	292	1798	270	1468	308	17	158	206	116	179	137	191	135	29	3.4	4.0	4987
1864	1932	1599	101	99	2	945	—	333	1306	80	81.68	79.1	130	27	242	1749	270	1388	350	11	157	208	110	192	138	200	139	33	3.2	4.4	5619
1865	1430	1199	82	80	2	628	—	231	997	68	83.15	82.9	104	17	140	1347	302	637	592	68	164	195	88	181	113	186	137	72	3.7	4.8	5356
1866	1328	1120	103	100	3	587	—	208	909	69	81.17	66.9	96	29	192	1224	277	556	623	45	109	203	78	192	95	197	62	58	3.4	5.1	5608
1867	1419	1206	89	88	1	849	—	213	956	81	79.43	91.0	94	27	113	1301	295	676	601	24	126	200	72	172	104	186	77	62	3.4	4.3	4553
1868	1474	1265	92	92	0	661	—	209	1015	71	80.03	77.1	85	23	98	1373	286	840	502	31	132	181	69	160	102	166	97	56	3.0	3.5	5264
1869	1633	1390	108	108	0	709	—	243	1123	82	80.03	75.9	107	18	93	1217	218	930	563	24	139	196	90	177	118	187	98	55	3.4	4.3	6953
1870	1706	1302	79	76	3	718	—	404	1083	73	88.20	92.4	85	12	140	1427	284	958	439	30	137	195	98	181	120	187	106	45	3.4	4.8	8767
1871	1781	1427	75	75	0	778	—	354	1143	43	80.09	57.3	109	13	178	1537	253	1056	456	25	154	187	91	167	122	178	126	43	3.1	3.9	9792

Table of the Income and Expenses of the Hospital

INCOME.

Year.	Board of Patients at		Free-bed Funds and Subscriptions.	Funds for other Charities at		Total Income of	
	Hospital.	Asylum.	Hospital.	Hospital.	Asylum.	Hospital.	Asylum.
1862	$5,853.89	$65,182.65	$17,175.62	$414.15	$4,106.69	$23,443.66	$69,289.34
1863	6,312.25	67,130.07	17,311.70	695.30	4,514.46	24,319.25	71,644.53
1864	7,714.54	96,960.53	18,832.22	648.21	4,118.29	27,194.97	101,078.82
1865	14,847.27	111,377.98	32,329.06	717.35	4,883.90	47,893.68	116,261.88
1866	14,977.44	125,457.64	23,843.74	1,082.64	7,035.18	39,903.82	132,492.82
1867	16,717.68	134,416.01	27,480.37	1,146.20	5,579.02	45,344.25	139,995.03
1868	14,671.45	127,893.29	27,913.05	1,320.00	5,144.00	43,904.50	133,037.29
1869	13,426.70	140,292.63	30,420.08	1,165.00	4,992.07	45,011.78	145,284.70
1870	12,003.83	141,793.86	31,944.08	807.00	4,659.27	44,754.91	146,453.13
1871	11,078.69	136,194.35	40,311.06	1,042.32	5,031.17	52,432.07	141,225.52
10 yrs.	$117,603.74	$1,146,699.01	$267,560.98	$9,038.17	$50,064.05	$394,202.89	$1,196,763.06

EXCESS OF EXPENSES

Year.	Excess of Expenses over Total Receipts.	Average cost per week per Patient.		Cost of Pay Patients over Board.	Free Patients over Funds and Subscriptions.	Cost of all Patients over Board.
	Hospital.	Hospital.	Asylum.	Hospital.	Hospital.	Hospital.
1862	$18,671.15	6.04	7.27	$774.76	$17,896.39	$36,260.92
1863	23,102.46	6.66	6.98	−160.98*	23,263.44	41,108.46
1864	32,964.58	8.38	9.76	2,510.27	30,454.31	52,445.01
1865	10,075.12	9.86	12.49	8,272.35	1,802.77	43,121.53
1866	28,882.98	13.88	12.30	15,108.64	13,694.38	53,809.36
1867	15,664.97	11.28	13.84	9,368.99	6,277.65	44,291.54
1868	23,659.97	12.74	16.51	8,992.05	14,568.66	52,893.02
1869	17,226.82	10.14	14.21	6,702.16	10,316.36	48,812.90
1870	18,059.91	10.05	13.83	3,840.52	14,143.34	50,810.99
1871	11,094.30	9.96	15.80	4,187.82	6,815.06	52,447.68
10 yrs.	$199,402.26			$59,596.58	$139,232.36	$476,001.41

* Excess this year of Receipts for Board over cost of Paying Patients.

and Asylum, for ten years, — 1862 *to* 1871.

Ordinary Expenses.

Year.	Cost of Paying Patients.	Cost of Free Patients.	Other Charities.	Total Expenses of	
	Hospital.	Hospital.	Hospital.	Hospital.	Asylum.
1862	$6,628.65	$35,072.01	$414.15	$42,114.81	$71,823.46
1863	6,151.27	40,575.14	695.30	47,421.71	69,300.63
1864	10,224.81	49,286.53	648.21	60,159.55	101,484.38
1865	23,119.62	34,131.83	717.35	57,968.80	120,885.84
1866	30,086.08	37,538.12	1,162.60	68,786.80	126,015.83
1867	26,086.67	33,758.02	1,164.53	61,009.22	133,844.14
1868	23,663.50	42,481.71	1,419.26	67,564.47	142,535.36
1869	20,128.86	40,736.44	1,373.30	62,238.60	138,132.02
1870	15,844.35	46,087.42	883.05	62,814.82	134,339.63
1871	15,266.51	47,126.12	1,133.74	63,526.37	146,191.23
10 yrs.	$177,200.32	$406,793.34	$9,611.49	$593,605.15	$1,184,552.52

over Board, etc.

Outlay for Lands and Buildings.		Charges upon the General Funds.	
Hospital.	Asylum.	Hospital.	Asylum.
		$23,451.42	$18,869.36
		27,882.72	13,991.34
		37,744.85	16,740.79
For Nine Years. $43,022.39	For Nine Years. $147,017.13	14,855.38	20,959.20
		33,663.25	9,858.25
		20,445.23	10,184.34
Average per annum. $4,780.26.	Average per annum. $16,335.24.	28,440.24	25,833.31
		22,007.08	9,182.56
28,740.85	....	22,840.18	4,221.73
		39,835.15	4,965.71
$71,763.24	$147,017.13	$271,165.50	$134,806.59

Table showing the Cost of Principal Stores at the M'Lean Asylum.

Articles.		1862.			1863.			1864.			1865.			1866.		
		Quantity.	Cost.	Average.	Quantity.	Cost.	Average.	Quantity.	Cost.	Average.	Quantity.	Cost.	Average.	Quantity.	Cost.	Average.
Beef	lbs.	11,565	$1,231.02	.1064	9,127	$1,196.86	.1311	8,680	$1,513.39	.1743	11,074	$2,508.95	.2265	15,869	$3,343.60	.217
,, Steak	,,	5,725	792.68	.1384	8,540	1,391.62	.1629	7,874	1,717.12	.2180	8,778	2,500.21	.2848	8,204	2,405.10	.29316
,, Corned	,,	11,329	920.24	.0812	11,066	1,083.58	.0979	16,636	2,639.79	.1586	15,090	2,726.49	.186	13,770	2,456.77	.17841
Bread	,,	48,276	1,875.82	.0388	48,637	2,167.26	.0445	53,987	2,936.55	.0543	49,344	3,125.17	.0633	64,995	4,467.76	.06874
Butter	,,	15,965	3,252.58	.2037	16,356	3,988.50	.2438	14,777	5,778.28	.39103	15,557	6,607.67	.42474	17,427	8,016.42	.46
Coffee	,,	3,167	713.30	.2252	2,773½	827.42	.2983	2,570½	1,016.29	.39537	3,153	1,402.27	.44474	3,350	1,301.78	.38859
Eggs	doz.	5,582	905.70	.16223	3,812	777.55	.2039	2,016	618.51	.3068	3,489	1,200.59	.344	5,391	1,719.42	.31894
Flour	bbls.	104	748.62	7.198	113	998.39	8.835	71	776.87	10.94	129	1,665.13	12.908	136	2,182.80	16.05
Hams	lbs	6,052	445.40	.07359	3,602	351.90	.09769	3,043	572.46	.18812	2,115	456.97	.216	1,004	196.15	.19536
Ice	tons	53¾	161.25	3.00	55½	277.50	5.00	57.65	230.60	4.00	78½	314.00	4.00	94	550.46	5.856
Lard	lbs.	55	5.77	.105	410	46.21	.1127	1,573	280.48	.1783	1,173	306.99	.261	960	184.46	.1921
Mutton and Lamb	,,	8,215	715.22	.087	4,791	509.32	.1063	8,454	1,169.26	.1382	9,110	1,542.55	.1693	9,638	1,394.88	.14472
Poultry	,,	10,723	1,320.58	.1231	4,417	551.05	.1247	8,749	1,878.93	.2147	7,323	2,214.59	.3024	13,493	4,072.20	.3018
Sugar	,,	21,869	2,523.06	.11537	21,994	3,214.59	.14615	20,030	4,272.17	.21328	22,000	5,003.46	.22743	24,788	4,098.21	.16533
Tea	,,	1,801	954.62	.5300	1,353	919.48	.68	1,226	966.03	.7879	1,500	1,695.00	1.13	1,240	1,215.20	.98
Veal	,,	5,632	462.72	.0821	5,718	569.35	.0995	5,204	770.30	.1481	4,421	695.17	.1572	4,718	792.06	.1678
Lights		—	1,827.45	—	—	1,786.64	—	—	2,172.95	—	—	3,217.63	—	—	3,738.93	—
Coal	tons	509¾	2,816.45	5.22	126,39	1,167.14	9.25	659.951	8,204.58	12.43	739.75	7,350.83	9.94	809.825	7,848.87	9.69
Wood	cords	134⅗	635.06	4.71	—	—	—	43¼	491.75	11.37	—	—	—	96¼	1,160.56	12.06

Table showing the Cost of Principal Stores at the M'Lean Asylum,— continued.

Articles.	1867.			1868.			1869.			1870.			1871.		
	Quantity.	Cost.	Average	Quantity.	Cost.	Average	Quantity.	Cost.	Average.	Quantity.	Cost.	Average.	Quantity.	Cost.	Average.
Beef . . . . lbs.	13,703	$3,238.85	.2363	13,686	$3,275.73	.2393	10,920	$2,369.34	.2169	11,563	$2,585.68	.22361	11,110	$2,174.02	.19568
,, Steak . . . . ,,	10,879	3,208.50	.2949	10,633	3,235.50	.3043	12,825	3,847.50	.30	13,448	4,391.37	.32654	15,340	4,168.36	.27173
,, Corned . . . . ,,	18,205½	3,129.21	.17188	17,675	3,128.28	.177	15,821	2,579.49	.163	15,731	2,464.90	.15668	16,638	2,250.59	.13526
Bread . . . . . . ,,	52,290	4,293.15	.0823	46,325	3,706.00	.08	53,375	3,951.82	.074	59,423	3,773 69	.06345	58,754	3,474.21	.05913
Butter . . . . . . ,,	16,203	5,624.20	.3471	17,065	7,532.56	.4414	19,168	8,420.53	.4393	18,821	7,214.62	.38332	22,843	8,219.68	.35983
Coffee . . . . . . ,,	3,917½	1,514.29	.3865	4,239	1,541.27	.3621	4,976	1,780.94	.3577	5,152	1,560.33	.30285	4,886	1,302.77	.26663
Eggs . . . . . . doz.	7,332	2,207.56	.30108	6,237	2,001.36	.3208	8,288	2,633.08	.3176	8,299	2,415.59	.29107	9,211	2,537.35	.27546
Flour . . . . . bbls.	149	2,434.75	16.34	139	2,124.75	15.28	154	1,876.88	12.1875	150	1,409.50	9.39	154	1,560.00	10.1298
Hams . . . . . lbs.	1,094½	184.77	.1688	831	143.52	.1727	187⅓	32.35	.168	—	—	—	1,142	169.26	.14821
Ice . . . . tons	102	516.70	5.06	106.65	432.55	4.05	113¼	453 00	4.00	1 623	1,199.15	7.3884	230¾	923.00	4.00
Lard . . . . . . lbs.	1,239	176.56	.1425	1,453	267.25	.1839	1,045	215.36	.206	1,228	227.04	.1847	1,953	231.18	.11837
Mutton and Lamb . ,,	10,515	2,328.12	.2214	9,658	1,519.52	.1573	9,686½	1,534.46	.1584	9,961	1,580.75	.15869	10,405	1,436.53	.13866
Poultry . . . . . ,,	13,143	3,790.55	.2884	17,262	5,048.19	.2924	20,082	6,445.72	.329	21,026	6,117.40	.29094	20,885	5,760.72	.27582
Sugar . . . . . . ,,	26,528	4,173.23	.1573	24,928	3,985.04	.1598	29,324	4,666.54	.1592	28,652	3,924.38	.13696	26,351	3,507.66	.13311
Tea . . . . ,,	1,397	1,467.49	1.055	1,542	1,634.90	1.06	1,616	1,588.15	.9827	1,899	1,648 80	.86824	1,864	1,526.04	.81869
Veal . . . . ,,	5,518	887.26	.1679	3,017	529.43	.1754	4,482½	773.91	.1726	5,247	886.24	.1689	6,811	1,083.01	.15910
Lights	—	3,801.19	—	—	5,600.73	—	—	4,649.13	—	—	4,276.25	—	—	3,938.04	—
Coal . . . . . tons	647.82	5,497.66	8.48	899 121/140	6,956.75	7.73	848 1508/2100	9,692.11	11.4197	688	5,283.98	7.68	713.190	5,899.93	8.27
Wood . . . . . cords	63⅞	559,22	8 75	43¾	409.71	9.36	97¼	984.17	10.12	85¼	869 25	10.19	195⅞	1,837.42	9.38

Table showing the Cost of Principal Stores at the Massachusetts General Hospital.

Articles.		1865.			1866.			1867.			1868.		
		Quantity.	Cost.	Average.	Quantity.	Cost.	Average.	Quantity.	Cost.	Average.	Quantity.	Cost.	Average.
Beef, Sirloin	lbs.	1,789	$396.45	.2216	2,097	$497.14	.2323	2,150	$533.43	.2481	2,347	$645.19	.275
" for Soup	"	7,697	525.73	.0683	5,046	353.22	.07	5,392	377.44	.07	5,525	386.75	.07
" Corned	"	4,436	555.82	.1253	3,228	403.50	.125	3,828	511.56	.1336	4,137	579.18	.14
" Steak	"	2,797	625.12	.2235	3,030	647.39	.2136	4,045	924.37	.2285	3,890	915.37	.2353
" Ribs	"	5,684	947.01	.1666	5,681	908.96	.16	5,648	899.33	.1592	5,968	1,002.62	.168
Mutton	"	4,686	673.47	.1457	6,512	803.78	.1234	6,928	996.91	.1439	6,506	958.66	.1473
Poultry	"	4,213	1,296.72	.3077	3,902	1,202.01	.308	3,944	1,137.84	.2885	3,978	1,189.64	.299
Butter	"	7,606	3,178.38	.4178	7,134	3,132.55	.4391	8,223	3,597.56	.4375	7,517	3,451.31	.459
Eggs	doz.	1,599	535.35	.3348	1,448	496.78	.343	1,490	483.35	.3244	1,459	491.11	.3366
Flour	bbls.	32	398.50	12.45	23	339.71	14.77	34	544.00	16.00	34	496.75	14.61
Bread	lbs.	37,339	2,300.56	.0616	32,521	2,317.91	.0712	33,558	2,616.80	.0779	30,223	2,247.52	.0743
Ice	tons	73¼	293.00	4.00	82.9	475.00	5.73	50½	252.50	5.00	37¾	151.00	4.00
Sugar	lbs.	7,842	1,240.47	.1581	7,867	1,084.29	.1378	8,700	1,200.60	.1380	7,931	1,110.20	.14
Tea	"	848	893.18	1.0532	929	881.18	.9485	497	468.42	.9425	923	833.25	.9027
Milk	qts.	24,103	1,830.31	.0759	25,357	1,845.66	.0728	31,545	2,208.15	.07	34,076	2,385.32	.07
Potatoes	bush.	742	668.22	.90	374	426.36	1.14	560	616.00	1.10	480	639.08	1.33

Table showing the Cost of Principal Stores at the Massachusetts General Hospital, — continued.

Articles.		1869.			1870.			1871.		
		Quantity.	Cost.	Average.	Quantity.	Cost.	Average.	Quantity.	Cost.	Average.
Beef, Sirloin	lbs.	2,922	$800.46	.2739	3,932	$1,061.64	.27	5,582	$1,465.28	.26¼
,, for Soup	,,	6,140	429.80	.07	5,592	391.44	.07	5,852	366.92	.0627
,, Corned	,,	4,161	582.54	.14	4,196	587.44	.14	5,251	674.22	.1284
,, Steak	,,	4,687	1,113.76	.2376	5,601	1,318.13	.2353	5,960	1,311.20	.22
,, Ribs	,,	5,985	984.02	.1644	6,113	978.08	.16	6,822	1,011.00	.1482
Mutton	,,	7,605	993.07	.136	8,716	1,180.66	.1354	8,700	1,185.81	.1363
Poultry	,,	3,926	1,186.60	.3022	3,835	1,096.90	.286	4,942	1,331.37	.2694
Butter	,,	7,690	3,343.31	.4347	8,287	3,300.10	.3982	8,695	3,141.50	.3613
Eggs	doz.	1,924	640.19	.33⅓	1,749	531.33	.3038	2,454	689.08	.2808
Flour	bbls.	24	263.50	10.98	34	315.52	9.28	32	301.44	9.42
Bread	lbs.	35,195	2,367.36	.0672	33,793	2,196.54	.06½	37,110	2,189.50	.059
Ice	tons	43¾	175.00	4.00	58	475.60	8.20	57¾	236.78	4.10
Sugar	lbs.	8,770	1,228.19	.14	9,393	1,122.46	.1195	9,043	1,058.00	.117
Tea	,,	1,161	933.55	.8041	443	328.80	.7422	967	705.91	.73
Milk	qts.	39,216	2,725.20	.0695	42,028	2,912.68	.0693	42,826	2,925.00	.0683
Potatoes	bush.	627	522.85	.8338	685	641.84	.937	590	666.70	1.13

SUBSCRIPTIONS, DONATIONS, AND BEQUESTS TO THE MASSACHUSETTS GENERAL HOSPITAL.

It was the wish and purpose of the writer of these supplementary pages of the Hospital History to close them with a statement, as complete as possible, of all the gifts and bequests which have increased its funds subsequently to the date at which the similar statement by Mr. Bowditch terminates. Had the writer been compelled to prepare such a financial report, it would have required of him a very laborious study of the account-books of the Hospital, which would probably have caused him, as one not an expert, all the more perplexity because of the thoroughness of the system and the minuteness of the details by which they are kept.

He desires, therefore, to express his great obligations to the kindness of the Treasurer, Mr. Stevenson, who has so faithfully done this exacting work for him. And even to the Treasurer himself, who has instituted and carried out the method by which the books in his charge are kept, this was a task by no means light. The funds of the Institution are disposed under the different specifications indicating the uses to which they have been appropriated by the donors.

The whole sum of the donations made to the Hospital from the date of its foundation makes in its aggregate a most striking exhibition of the benevolent feelings which have sway in this community. Is there any other benevolent institution in this city, State, or country, whose treasury has been more enriched?

SUBSCRIPTIONS IN 1856 FOR A BRICK FENCE AT THE HOSPITAL.

Appleton, Nathan	$500.00
Appleton, William	500.00
Bradlee, Josiah	500.00
Brooks, P. C.	250.00
Cushing, John P.	250.00
Phillips, Jonathan	500.00
Sears, David	500.00
Sturgis, William	250.00
	$3,250.00

SUBSCRIPTIONS IN 1863, FOR NEW COTTAGE AT ASYLUM FOR MALES.

Amory, William	$500
Bacon, Francis	500
Bacon, William B.	250
Bates, Benjamin E.	1000
Ballard, John	300
Beebe, James M.	2000
Bowditch, Mrs. Nath. I.	5000
Bradlee, J. Bowdoin	500
Brewer, Gardner	2000
Brimmer, Martin	1000
Brooks, Peter C.	1000
Bullard, William S.	2000
Davis, J. Amory	500
Edgerton, J.	1000
Edmands, J. Wiley	500
Fay, Joseph S.	500
Gray, John C.	1000
Grew, Mrs. Henry	300
Higginson, George	500
Hooper, Robert	250
Howe, George	1000
Howe, Jabez C.	1000
Hubbell, Peter	500
Hunnewell, H. H.	1000
Jones, Miss Anna P.	400
Lawrence, James	1000
Lawrence, Abbott	1000
Lyman, Charles	300

SUBSCRIPTIONS FOR NEW COTTAGE.

Lyman, George W.	$500
Mason, Robert M.	500
Oxnard, Henry P., Ex'rs of	500
Paige, J. W.	500
Reed, Benjamin T.	250
Richardson, George C.	1000
Rogers, Henry B.	1000
Sears, David	1000
Shaw, G. Howland	1000
Skinner, Francis	1000
Sturgis, Henry P.	500
Sturgis, William	1000
Thayer, Nathaniel	3000
Wales, George W.	500
Wales, Miss Mary Ann	500
Weld, William F.	1000
White, B. C.	300
Whitney, Joseph	500
Wigglesworth, Misses	1000
Wigglesworth, Edward	500
Wigglesworth, Thomas	300
Williams, Moses	1000
Wolcott, J. Huntington	300
	$44,450

SUBSCRIPTIONS IN 1866, TO PAY OFF DEBT AND IN AID OF FUNDS.

In 1866, at the suggestion of Nathaniel Thayer, Esq., subscriptions were solicited to pay off the debt and in aid of the funds of the Hospital. Mr. Thayer proposed to contribute twenty-five thousand dollars to those purposes if the sum could be made up to one hundred thousand dollars.

The appeal then made by a committee of the Trustees was promptly responded to, and the following is a list of subscribers for one hundred thousand and eight hundred dollars.

Andrews, William T.	$500
Amory, William	250
Appleton, Charles H.	500
Appleton, Nathan, jun.	250
Appleton, Thomas G.	1000
Appleton, William, jun.	500
Appleton, William S.	500
Anonymous, by W. S. B.	500
Bacon, Francis	500
Beebe, James M.	5000
Blake, George B.	100
Borland, John	300
Boston Stock Exchange Board	1000
Bowditch, Mrs. N. I.	5000
Bradlee, F. H. and J. B.	500
Brimmer, Martin	1000
Brooks, Edward	500
Brooks, Peter C.	1000
Brooks, Peter C., jun.	1000
Brooks, Shepherd	1000
Bullard, William S.	5000
Codman, Edward A.	500
Curtis, Greely S.	500
Curtis, Caleb A.	100
Cushing, Thomas F.	500
Cushing, John G.	500

SUBSCRIPTIONS TO PAY OFF DEBT.

Cushing, Robert M.	$500
Daniels, Otis	500
Dexter, F. Gordon	500
Danforth, Isaac Warren	500
Fearing, Albert	500
Flagg, Augustus	100
Gardner, George	300
Gardner, Henry J.	500
Gardner, John L.	5000
Gardiner, William H.	250
Glover, Joseph B.	300
Goodwin, the Misses Eliza and Lucy	500
Grew, Mrs. Henry	500
Higginson, George	250
Hall, Andrew T.	100
Heard, Augustine	250
Hemenway, Mrs. Augustus	1000
Hooper, Robert	200
Hovey, C. F. & Co.	1000
Howe, George	1000
Howe, Jabez C.	2000
Howe, Thomas	250
Hunnewell, Horatio H.	2000
Iasigi, Goddard, & Co.	500
Inches, Herman B.	250
Lawrence, Abbott	500
Lawrence, Amos A.	500
Lawrence James	1000
Little, James L.	1000
Lodge, Mrs. John E.	300
Lowell, Francis C.	250
Lowell, John Amory	1000
Lyman, George W.	1000
Lyman, Theodore	200
Mason, Robert M.	1000
Mason, William P.	500
Matchett, Theodore	200

SUBSCRIPTIONS TO PAY OFF DEBT. 717

Matthews, Nathan	$200
McGregor, James	250
Minot, Charles H.	100
Minot, George R.	200
Mudge, Enoch R.	1000
Merriam, Charles	250
Parker, E. Francis	100
Parker, John Brooks	500
Payson, Samuel R.	1000
Perkins, William	500
Pierce, Andrew J.	100
Pratt, Miss Sarah P.	1000
Pratt, Miss Mary	1000
Richardson, Jeffrey	1000
Rogers, Henry B.	1000
Shattuck, George C.	500
Skinner, Francis, & Co.	2000
Sturgis, Henry P.	500
Swett, Samuel W.	250
Thayer, Nathaniel	25000
Thomas, William	100
Thomas, Mrs. William	100
Wadsworth, Mrs. William W.	500
Wales, Miss M. A.	300
Weld, William G.	250
Welles, George D.	100
Welles, Miss Susan J.	500
Welles, Miss Jane	500
White, Benjamin C.	200
Whitney, Joseph	500
Wigglesworth, Miss Anne	1000
Wigglesworth, Miss Mary	1000
Wigglesworth, Edward	1000
Wigglesworth, Thomas	1000
Williams, Moses	3000
Winthrop, Robert C.	100
	$100,800

FREE-BED SUBSCRIPTIONS.

	Before 1851.	1851–1872.
Adams, Horatio	$183	
Appleton, Nathan	200	
Appleton, William	800	
Appleton, Samuel	100	
Appleton, William, jun.		$1100
Appleton, Charles H.		600
Appleton, William S.		200
Amory, William	100	700
Amory, Charles	200	200
Amory, James S.	400	
Austin, Edward		100
Baxter, Daniel	13	
Brooks, Peter C. Life	910	
Brooks, P. C., jun.		1700
Brooks, P. C., 3d		200
Brooks, Mrs. Gorham		100
Brooks, Shepherd		200
Belknap, Jeremiah. Life	654	
Bradlee, Thomas D.	100	
Bradlee, Josiah	800	1000
Bradlee, F. H.		300
Bradlee, J. Bowdoin. Life		1000
Bowditch, Nathaniel I.	1000	1200
Bowditch, Henry I.	100	
Bowditch, Mrs. N. I.		1100
Bowditch, J. Ingersoll		200
Bumstead, John	100	
Bryant, John	100	200

FREE-BED SUBSCRIPTIONS. 719

	Before 1851.	1851–1872.
Bryant, Miss Mary C.		$200
Bullard, William S.	$100	1034
Brimmer, Martin	300	
Brimmer, Martin, jun.		900
Babcock, Mrs. Mary		100
Brewer, Gardner		1333.33
Bradford, M. L.		100
Burnham, John A.		300
Boston Gas L. Co.		200
Baker, Richard, jun.		200
Bigelow, George Tyler		200
Bigelow, Erastus B.		100
Cabot, George	40	
Cabot, Mrs. Samuel		400
Cabot, Frederick		300
Coolidge, Joseph	500	
Coolidge, T. Jefferson		200
Cushing, John P.	2900	
Cushing, John G.		200
Codman, Henry	400	
Codman, Edward		100
Cary, Thomas G.		100
Cutler, Pliny	100	
Cutler, William C.	200	
Curtis, D. Sargent		100
Curtis, Greely S.		200
Curtis, Benjamin R.		200
Chase, Mrs. Theodore		200
Dwight, Edmund	1100	
Dixwell, John James	100	
Dowley, Levi A.		100
Davis, James		700
Davis, J. Amory		300
Davis, Miss Annie W.		200
Dalton, Charles H.		100

FREE-BED SUBSCRIPTIONS.

	Before 1851.	1851-1872.
Dale, Theron J.		$100
Dexter, F. Gordon.		200
Ellis, Jabez.	$5	
Everett, Otis.	50	
Eliot, Samuel A.	600	
Eliot, Catherine.	100	
Eastburn, John H.		800
Edmands, J. Wiley.		600
Emmons, Nathaniel H.		200
Endicott, William, jun.		200
Friend, Anonymous.	10	300
Fay, Winsor.	5	
Fay, Mrs. S. S.		100
Francis, Ebenezer.	700	
Fales, Samuel.	100	
Ferriera, L. C.	100	
Fearing, Mrs. Albert.		200
Farnsworth, Ezra.		200
Freeland, Charles W.		200
Gassett, Henry.	50	
Guild, Charles.	5	
Gray, John C.	500	1400
Gray, Francis C.	600	
Gray, William.		600
Glover, Joseph B.		800
Greene, Gardiner.	500	
Greene, J. S. Copley.	600	
Grew, Mrs. Henry.		700
Goodwin, Miss Eliza.		600
Goodwin, Miss Eliza, jun.		200
Goodwin, Miss Lucy.		200
Goodwin, Ozias.		200
Gardner, John L.		1100
Gardner, J. P., G. A., and J. L., jun.		1100
Gardner, George A.		600

FREE-BED SUBSCRIPTIONS. 721

	Before 1851.	1851–1872.
Gardner, John		$100
Gardiner, William H.		200
Greenleaf, R. C.		200
Humane Society of Mass.	$9700	4400
Head, Joseph and Joseph, jun.	1200	
Head, Joseph	200	
Howard Benevolent Society	100	
Hallett, George. Life	600	
Hallett, Mrs. E. Life	608	
Hallett, George W.		100
Hallett, Henry S.		100
Howe, George	200	1300
Hubbard, Samuel	100	
Hemenway, Augustus		900
Hemenway, Mrs. Augustus		400
Hooper, Mrs. Eunice		300
Hooper, Robert William		800
Hooper, Misses Eunice and Mary I.		200
Higginson, George		800
Hovey, George O.		200
Ives, Robert H.	100	
Jackson, Patrick T.	1460	
Jackson, Charles	1800	
Jeffries, John	800	800
Joy, Miss Elizabeth	166.67	
Joy, Miss Hannah	900	
Jackson, James	40	
Johnson, Samuel, jun.		200
Kidder, Henry P.		300
Lambert, William	400	
Lowell, John, jun.	50	
Lowell, Francis C.	500	
Lowell, J. Amory	500	500
Lawrence, Abbott	300	
Lawrence, Amos	800	

FREE-BED SUBSCRIPTIONS.

	Before 1851.	1851–1872.
Lawrence, William	$100	
Lawrence, William R.		$200
Lyman, Theodore	900	
Lyman, Theodore, jun.		1900
Loring, Miss Abby M.	400	1100
Loring, Caleb William		100
Lawrence, James		100
Lee, Mrs. Hannah F. Life		1000
Lee, William P.		100
Lee, Francis L.		100
Lodge, John E.		100
Lodge, Mrs. John E.		200
Little, James L.		500
Longstreth, M.		100
Munson, Israel	1200	
Mass. Charitable Fire Society	2025	3900
Mills, Charles H.		100
Mixter, Charles		1600
Minot, William		200
Minot, George R.		100
Mechanics M. F. Ins. Co.		200
Matthews, Nathan		200
Mason, Robert M.		100
Mackay, Robert C.		100
Monroe, William		100
McGregor, James		100
May, Miss Josephine		100
May, Miss Ernestine		100
Oliver, Miss Betsey		600
Oxnard, Henry	100	
Perkins, Thomas H.	820	
Perkins, James	200	
Perkins, William		300
Pratt, William	400	
Pratt, Miss Elizabeth	200	900

FREE-BED SUBSCRIPTIONS.

	Before 1851.	1851–1872.
Pratt, Miss Sarah P.	$300	$2100
Parker, John	1500	
Parker, Daniel P.	100	
Phillips, William	300	
Phillips, Jonathan	1200	1000
Parsons, William	100	
Prescott, William	100	
Parker, John Brooks	237.50	
Parker, James		1200
Parker, Harvey D., & Co.		100
Page, Edward		200
Pickman, William D.		900
Peabody, Francis H.		300
Payson, Samuel R.		200
Parkman, George F.		200
Richards, Paul	5	
Robbins, Edward H., jun.	270	
Reed, Mrs. William	700	600
Rogers, Henry B.	500	1900
Railroad Co., Boston and Lowell	150	2000
,, ,, Boston and Maine	100	2400
,, ,, Boston and Providence	150	1832.50
,, ,, Eastern		500
,, ,, Metropolitan H.		500
,, ,, Union H.		1000
,, ,, Boston and Lynn H.		100
,, ,, Old Colony		100
,, ,, Boston and Worcester		600
Robeson, William R.		200
Redman, John	300	
Raymond, Edward A.	100	
Read, James		100
Safford, Daniel	20	
Shaw, Lemuel	20	
Shaw, Robert G.	1000	200

FREE-BED SUBSCRIPTIONS.

	Before 1851.	1851–1872.
Shaw, G. Howland		$500
Shattuck, George C.	$100	
Sears, David	200	
Sturgis, William	1300	200
Salisbury, Mrs. Elizabeth	1600	200
Salisbury, Stephen		2000
Stone, William W.	100	
Stanton, Francis	100	
Sargent, Ignatius		100
Sargent, Horace Binney		100
Sargent, Turner		100
Skinner, Francis		100
Schlesinger, Sebastian B.		200
Snelling, Samuel G.		200
Sawyer, Joseph		100
Saltonstall, Henry		200
Thompson, John	5	
Tappan, John	100	
Thorndike, Israel	100	
Ticknor, George	500	
Tuckerman, Edward	500	
Thayer, Nathaniel		6100
Thayer, John E.		300
Thayer, E. Francis		100
Tucker, William W.		200
Upham, Henry		100
Williams, John D.	2300	
Williams, Moses	400	2200
Williams, Mrs. Elijah		200
Wales, Thomas B. Life	825	100
Waldo, E. S. and R.	2300	100
Waldo, Daniel	100	
Wigglesworth, Edward		2100
Wigglesworth, Miss Ann		2400
Wigglesworth, Miss Mary		1600

FREE-BED SUBSCRIPTIONS.

	Before 1851.	1851–1872.
Wyman, Rufus		$500
Whitney, Joseph		100
Wolcott, J. Huntington		200
Webster and Co.		100
Wharton, William C.		100
Welles, Miss Jane		250
Welles, Miss Susan J.		250
Warren, Samuel D.		200
Young, Charles L.		200
	$59969.17	$94399.83

From 1822 to Dec. 31, 1850 . . . $59969.17
From 1851 to June 1, 1872 . . . . 94399.83

Total subscriptions from the foundation
of the Hospital to June 1, 1872 . . . $154369.00

DONATIONS AND BEQUESTS.

	Prior to 1851.	Since 1851.
Appleton, Samuel. Bequest. Income for patients		$10,020.00
Appleton, William. Donation. $20,000 for buildings. $20,000 inc. for patients .	$10,000.00	30,000.00
Austin, Mrs. Agnes. Bequest. Inc. of $5000, patients, Asy.; $7,500 unrestricted . .		12,500.00
Amateur Dramatic Association. Donation .		450.00
Bowditch, William I. Donation, bill for professional service		274.25
Bowditch, Nathaniel I. Bequest. $5000 for Wooden Leg Fund, $2000 for republication of History		7,000.00
Belknap, Jeremiah. Bequest. Income for free beds	10,000.00	
Belknap, Miss Mary. Bequest	89,882.60	
Brimmer, Miss Mary Ann. Bequest. Income for free beds	5000.00	
Brown, John. Donation	100.00	
Bromfield, John. Bequest. Income of $20,000, patients at Asylum; income of $20,000, free beds		40,000.00
Bullard, William S. Donation of land. Asylum		800.00
Commonwealth of Mass. Province House; hammering stone	75,070.27	
Crocker, Allan. Donation	100.00	
Curtis, Ambrose S. Bequest, settled for . .	2,500.00	
Clough, Sarah. Bequest	601.16	
Bradlee, J. Bowdoin. Donation for purchase of books		500.00
Dowse, Thomas. Bequest. Income for free beds		5,000.00
Davis, Miss Elinor. Bequest. Income for free beds	900,00	

DONATIONS AND BEQUESTS.

	Prior to 1851.	Since 1851.
Bigelow, Henry J. Donation in addition to surgical instruments valued at $3,250		1,750.00
Eliot, Samuel. Donation for Asylum	10,000.00	
Everett, Moses. Donation	116.00	
Everett, Miss E. G. Sundry donations	150.00	325.00
Friend desiring to be unknown. Bequest		1,900.00
Greene, Benjamin D. Bequest. Income for free beds		5,000.00
Gray, John C. Donation. Income for free beds		1,000.00
Gardner, John L. Donation. Income for free beds		20,000.00
Hill, George. Bequest		1,000.00
Hill, Elizabeth. Bequest		237.50
Harris, Charles. Bequest. Income $1,000 for free beds, $1,000 unrestricted		2,000.00
Homer, Sidney. Bequest		1,000.00
Ingersoll, James. Bequest		2,000.00
Joy, Miss Nabby. To establish Joy Fund, &c.		20,000 00
Kittredge, Rufus. Bequest		3,857.22
Lee, Joseph. Bequest for use of Asylum	20,000.00	
Lucas, John. Donation	900.00	
Lee, Mrs. Hannah F. Donation		1,000.00
Lassell, Ellison. Bequest		6,888.60
Loring, Mrs. Abigail. $5,000 for Loring Fund, balance unrestricted		43,901.67
McLean, John. Bequest	119,858.20	
Moseley, Jonathan	753,46	
Munson, Israel. Bequest	20,000.00	
Minot, William. Donation		100.00
Mitchell, F. N. Bequest.		67.50
Mason, William P. Bequest. Income for free beds		9,400.00
McGregor, James. Donation. Income for free beds		10,000.00
Nichols, Benjamin R. Bequest. Income for free beds	6,000.00	
Oliver, Thomas. Bequest	22,438.70	
Oliver, William. Bequest		57,760.04
Phillips, William. Donation for free beds	5,000.00	
Pickman, William. Bequest		4,000.00
Pratt, Miss Elizabeth. Bequest. One-half Asylum, one-half Hospital		20,000.00
Pratt, Miss Sarah. Bequest. One-half Asylum, one-half Hospital		18,800.00

728 DONATIONS AND BEQUESTS.

	Prior to 1851.	Since 1851.
Phillips, Jonathan. Bequest. Income for free beds		10,000.00
Poland, J. Donation		15.00
Percival, John. Bequest. Income for free beds		950.00
Pickens, John. Bequest. Income for free beds		1,676,75
Russell, Polly. Donation	400.00	
Russell, William. Donation	100.00	
Richardson, Susan. Donation for free beds	250.00	
Raymond, Edward A. Bequest. Income for free beds		2,820.00
Reed, William. Bequest to accrue to $5000, then income to free beds		2,000.00
Redman, John. Bequest. Income to free beds		137,614.50
Reed, Benjamin T. Donations. Income to free beds		1,000.00
Read, James. Bequest. Income, one-half to patients asylum, one-half to free beds		2,000.00
Savage, James. Donation	100.00	
Salisbury, Mrs. Elizabeth. Donation		4,000.00
Salisbury, Stephen. Donation		5,000.00
Sawyer, Matthias P. Bequest. Income of $7,000 to free beds, balance unrestricted		99,003.63
Sever, Miss. Bequest. Income to free beds		500.00
Spaulding, Rev. Mr. Donation		500.00
St. Stephen's Chapel. For two free beds for ten years		2,000.00
Shaw, Miss M. Louisa. Donation for free beds		500.00
Shaw, Mrs. Q. A., and other ladies. Donation. Income for amusements for asylum		5,000.00
Thomas, Isaiah. Bequest	5,256.83	1,113.50
Tucker, Beza. House in Boylston Place	5,350.00	
Tucker, Margaret. For free beds	2,929.97	
Touro, Abraham. Bequest	10,000.00	
Touro, Judah. Bequest		10,000.00
Todd, Henry. Bequest. Income to free beds	5,000.00	
Treadwell, J. G. Bequest. Income of $5,000 to care of library, and balance to free beds together with library		43,703.91
Thompson, Miss S. B. Bequest. Income to free beds		492.40
Townsend, Miss Mary P. Bequest. Income for free beds		7,500,00
Webber, Seth. Donation	1,000.00	
Westerfield, Peter. For poor patients	165.67	

DONATIONS AND BEQUESTS. 729

	Prior to 1851.	Since 1851.
Warren, John C. Donation. Income to purchase books	1,000.00	
Waldo, Daniel. Bequest	40,000.00	
Williams, John D. Bequest. Income to free beds	13,000.00	
Wilder, Charles W. Bequest		20,000.00
Whitney, Edward. Donation		5,000.00
Wigglesworth, Edward. Donation		1,000.00
Warren, J. Mason. $2,000 for new operating-room, $1,880 for Warren Prizes		3,880.00
Wyman, Morrill. Donation		200.00
	$483,922.89	$706,001.47

Amount from 1811 to Dec. 31, 1850 . . . $483,922.86
Amount from Jan. 1851, to June 1, 1872 . . 706,001.47

Total . . . $1,189,924.33

N.B. Upon the final settlement of the estate of the late John Redman, the corporation will come into possession of real estate in the City of Boston, the present valuation of which is about three hundred thousand dollars, to be added to the "Redman Fund for Free beds," which will make the whole amount of that fund not less than four hundred and forty thousand dollars.

SUMMARY OF DONATIONS, SUBSCRIPTIONS, &c.

Original subscriptions $146,992.55
    As per Bowditch, viz., for Hospital $101,619.21
    „   „   „   „ Asylum .   45,373.34
                                              $146,992.55

Subscriptions for enlargement of the Hospital in 1844, as per Mr. Bowditch's list 62,550.00
Subscriptions for a brick fence at the Hospital in the year 1856 . . . .   3,250.00
Subscriptions for new cottage for males at Asylum, in the year 1863. . . . .   44,450.00
Subscriptions to pay off debt of the Hospital, and in aid of its funds, 1866 . . . . 100,800.00
Annual subscriptions for free beds. 154,369.00
    Before 1851 . . . . $59,969.17
    From Jan. 1851 to June, 1872 .   94,399.83
                                                $154,369.00

Legacies and donations 1,189,924.33
    Before 1851 . . . . $483,922.86
    From Jan. 1851 to June, 1872 . 706,001.47
                                             $1,189,924.33

                                                            $1,702,335.88

    Before 1851 . . . . . . $753,434.58
    Since 1850 . . . .   948,901.30
                                      $1,702,335.88

OFFICERS OF THE INSTITUTION.

1872.

EDWARD WIGGLESWORTH . . . . . *President.*
NATHANIEL THAYER . . . . *Vice-President.*
J. THOMAS STEVENSON . . . . . . *Treasurer.*
THOMAS B. HALL . . . . *Secretary.*

TRUSTEES.

HENRY B. ROGERS	*Chairman,* — 5 *Joy Street.*
JAMES M. BEEBE	30 *Beacon Street.*
CHARLES H. DALTON	*Sears Building.*
EDMUND DWIGHT	60 *State Street.*
*GEORGE E. ELLIS	110 *Marlboro Street.*
SAMUEL ELIOT	44 *Brimmer Street.*
GEORGE S. HALE	39 *Court Street.*
GEORGE HIGGINSON	40 *State Street.*
*SAMUEL G. HOWE	20 *Bromfield Street.*
*HENRY P. KIDDER	40 *State Street.*
SAMUEL W. SWETT	60 *State Street.*
*SAMUEL D. WARREN	67 *Mt. Vernon Street.*

BOARD OF CONSULTATION.

JOHN JEFFRIES, M.D.	H. I. BOWDITCH, M.D.
EDWARD REYNOLDS, M.D.	D. H. STORER, M.D.
JOHN B. S. JACKSON, M.D.	CHARLES E. WARE, M.D.
WINSLOW LEWIS, M.D.	C. E. BROWN-SÉQUARD, M.D.
JOHN E. TYLER, M.D.	

* Appointed by the Governor of the Commonwealth.

OFFICERS OF THE HOSPITAL.

NORTON FOLSOM, M.D.	*Resident Physician.*
GEORGE C. SHATTUCK, M.D.	⎫
FRANCIS MINOT, M.D.	⎪
CALVIN ELLIS, M.D.	⎬ *Visiting Physicians.*
SAMUEL L. ABBOT, M.D.	⎪
H. K. OLIVER, Jun., M.D.	⎪
EDWARD B. DALTON, M.D.	⎭
HENRY J. BIGELOW, M.D.	⎫
HENRY G. CLARK, M.D.	⎪
SAMUEL CABOT, M.D.	⎬ *Visiting Surgeons.*
GEORGE H. GAY, M.D.	⎪
RICHARD M. HODGES, M.D.	⎪
ALGERNON COOLIDGE, M.D.	⎭
GEORGE G. TARBELL, M.D.	⎫
JOHN COLLINS WARREN, M.D.	⎬ *Physicians to Out-patients.*
DAVID H. HAYDEN, M.D.	⎪
WILLIAM L. RICHARDSON, M.D.	⎭
J. THEODORE HEARD, M.D.	⎫ *Surgeons to Out-patients.*
CHARLES B. PORTER, M.D.	⎭
JAMES C. WHITE, M.D.	*Chemist and Physician to Patients with Diseases of the Skin.*
REGINALD H. FITZ, M.D.	*Microscopist and Curator of the Pathological Cabinet.*
HENRY P. QUINCY, M.D.	*Artist.*
CHARLES WILSON, D. M.D.	*Dentist.*
A. L. MASON	⎫ *Medical House-Pupils.*
E. G. CUTLER	⎭
WM. J. MORTON	⎫
F. A. HARRIS	⎬ *Surgical House-Pupils.*
JAMES E. TOBEY	⎪
WALTER CHANNING, Jun.	⎭
MISS G. L. STURTEVANT	*Matron.*
DANIEL G. WILKINS	*Apothecary.*

OFFICERS OF THE M'LEAN ASYLUM.

GEORGE F. JELLY, M.D. . . . . . . *Superintendent.*
CHARLES F. FOLSOM, M.D. . . } *Assistant Physicians*
FERDINAND A. STILLINGS, M.D. } *and Apothecaries.*
WALTER J. NORFOLK . *Medical Student and Apothecary.*
GEORGE W. WHITTLE . . . . *Steward.*
MRS. ABBY M. WHITTLE . . . . *Matron.*
ELBRIDGE S. UPHAM, }
MISS LUCIA E. WOODWARD, } . . . . . *Supervisors.*

COMMITTEES.

Committee on Finance.

MESSRS. BEEBE AND HIGGINSON.

Committee on Accounts.

MESSRS. SWETT AND WARREN.

Free-bed Standing Committee.

MESSRS. HIGGINSON AND KIDDER.

Committee on the Book of Donations.

MR. ROGERS.

Committee on the Warren Fund and Library.

MESSRS. ELIOT AND DWIGHT.

Committee on Repairs.

MESSRS. ROGERS, BEEBE, AND DALTON.

VISITING COMMITTEE.

February	MESSRS. ROGERS AND KIDDER.
March	,, KIDDER AND DWIGHT.
April	,, DWIGHT AND ELIOT.
May	,, ELIOT AND BEEBE.
June	,, BEEBE AND HIGGINSON.
July	,, HIGGINSON AND SWETT.
August	,, SWETT AND HOWE.
September	,, HOWE AND HALE.
October	,, HALE AND WARREN.
November	,, WARREN AND ELLIS.
December	,, ELLIS AND DALTON.
January	,, DALTON AND ROGERS.

LADIES' VISITING COMMITTEE.

January	MRS. ELIOT AND MRS. STEVENSON.
February	MRS. STEVENSON AND MISS GOODWIN.
March	MISS GOODWIN AND MISS LORING.
April	MISS LORING AND MISS TORREY.
May	MISS TORREY AND MISS YOUNG.
June	MISS YOUNG AND MRS. ROGERS.
September	MRS. ROGERS AND MISS REVERE.
October	MISS REVERE AND MRS. BEEBE.
November	MRS. BEEBE AND MISS HEMENWAY.
December	MISS HEMENWAY AND MRS. ELIOT.

Medicine & Society
In America

An Arno Press/New York Times Collection

Alcott, William A. **The Physiology of Marriage.** 1866. New Introduction by Charles E. Rosenberg.

Beard, George M. **American Nervousness: Its Causes and Consequences.** 1881. New Introduction by Charles E. Rosenberg.

Beard, George M. **Sexual Neurasthenia.** 5th edition. 1898.

Beecher, Catharine E. **Letters to the People on Health and Happiness.** 1855.

Blackwell, Elizabeth. **Essays in Medical Sociology.** 1902. Two volumes in one.

Blanton, Wyndham B. **Medicine in Virginia in the Seventeenth Century.** 1930.

Bowditch, Henry I. **Public Hygiene in America.** 1877.

Bowditch, N[athaniel] I. **A History of the Massachusetts General Hospital:** To August 5, 1851. 2nd edition. 1872.

Brill, A. A. **Psychanalysis: Its Theories and Practical Application.** 1913.

Cabot, Richard C. **Social Work:** Essays on the Meeting-Ground of Doctor and Social Worker. 1919.

Cathell, D. W. **The Physician Himself and What He Should Add to His Scientific Acquirements.** 2nd edition. 1882. New Introduction by Charles E. Rosenberg.

The Cholera Bulletin. Conducted by an Association of Physicians. Vol. I: Nos. 1–24. 1832. All published. New Introduction by Charles E. Rosenberg.

Clarke, Edward H. **Sex in Education;** or, A Fair Chance for the Girls. 1873.

Committee on the Costs of Medical Care. **Medical Care for the American People:** The Final Report of The Committee on the Costs of Medical Care, No. 28. [1932].

Currie, William. **An Historical Account of the Climates and Diseases of the United States of America.** 1792.

Davenport, Charles Benedict. **Heredity in Relation to Eugenics.** 1911. New Introduction by Charles E. Rosenberg.

Davis, Michael M. **Paying Your Sickness Bills.** 1931.

Disease and Society in Provincial Massachusetts: Collected Accounts, 1736–1939. 1972.

Earle, Pliny. **The Curability of Insanity:** A Series of Studies. 1887.

Falk, I. S., C. Rufus Rorem, and Martha D. Ring. **The Costs of Medical Care:** A Summary of Investigations on The Economic Aspects of the Prevention and Care of Illness, No. 27. 1933.

Faust, Bernhard C. **Catechism of Health:** For the Use of Schools, and for Domestic Instruction. 1794.

Flexner, Abraham. **Medical Education in the United States and Canada:** A Report to The Carnegie Foundation for the Advancement of Teaching, Bulletin Number Four. 1910.

Gross, Samuel D. **Autobiography of Samuel D. Gross, M.D.**, with Sketches of His Contemporaries. Two volumes. 1887.

Hooker, Worthington. **Physician and Patient;** or, A Practical View of the Mutual Duties, Relations and Interests of the Medical Profession and the Community. 1849.

Howe, S. G. **On the Causes of Idiocy.** 1858.

Jackson, James. **A Memoir of James Jackson, Jr., M.D.** 1835.

Jennings, Samuel K. **The Married Lady's Companion, or Poor Man's Friend.** 2nd edition. 1808.

The Maternal Physician; a Treatise on the Nurture and Management of Infants, from the Birth until Two Years Old. 2nd edition. 1818. New Introduction by Charles E. Rosenberg.

Mathews, Joseph McDowell. **How to Succeed in the Practice of Medicine.** 1905.

McCready, Benjamin W. **On the Influences of Trades, Professions, and Occupations in the United States, in the Production of Disease.** 1943.

Mitchell, S. Weir. **Doctor and Patient.** 1888.

Nichols, T[homas] L. **Esoteric Anthropology: The Mysteries of Man.** [1853].

Origins of Public Health in America: Selected Essays, 1820–1855. 1972.

Osler, Sir William. **The Evolution of Modern Medicine.** 1922.

The Physician and Child-Rearing: Two Guides, 1809–1894. 1972.

Rosen, George. **The Specialization of Medicine:** with Particular Reference to Ophthalmology. 1944.

Royce, Samuel. **Deterioration and Race Education.** 1878.

Rush, Benjamin. **Medical Inquiries and Observations.** Four volumes in two. 4th edition. 1815.

Shattuck, Lemuel, Nathaniel P. Banks, Jr., and Jehiel Abbott. **Report of a General Plan for the Promotion of Public and Personal Health.** Massachusetts Sanitary Commission. 1850.

Smith, Stephen. **Doctor in Medicine** and Other Papers on Professional Subjects. 1872.

Still, Andrew T. **Autobiography of Andrew T. Still,** with a History of the Discovery and Development of the Science of Osteopathy. 1897.

Storer, Horatio Robinson. **The Causation, Course, and Treatment of Reflex Insanity in Women.** 1871.

Sydenstricker, Edgar. **Health and Environment.** 1933.

Thomson, Samuel. **A Narrative, of the Life and Medical Discoveries of Samuel Thomson.** 1822.

Ticknor, Caleb. **The Philosophy of Living;** or, The Way to Enjoy Life and Its Comforts. 1836.

U.S. Sanitary Commission. **The Sanitary Commission of the United States Army:** A Succinct Narrative of Its Works and Purposes. 1864.

White, William A. **The Principles of Mental Hygiene.** 1917.